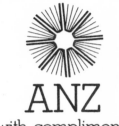

ANZ

with compliments

MISS JOAN E. GODFREY

QUEENSLAND INSTITUTE OF TECHNOLOGY.

AUSTRALIA & NEW ZEALAND BOOK CO PTY LTD
23 CROSS ST BROOKVALE NSW 2100 PHONE 938 2244

NURSING MANAGEMENT

SECOND EDITION

Joan M. Ganong, R.N., M.S.
and
Warren L. Ganong, C.M.C.

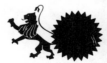

AN ASPEN PUBLICATION®
Aspen Systems Corporation
Rockville, Maryland
London
1980

Library of Congress Cataloging in Publication Data

Ganong, Joan M.
Nursing management.

Includes bibliographies and index.

1. Nursing service administration.   I. Ganong,
Warren L., joint author.   II. Title.
[DNLM: 1. Nursing, Supervisory.   WY105 Gl98n]
RT89.G33   1980   362.1'068   80-10865
ISBN: 0-89443-278-8

Library of Congress Catalog Card Number: 80-10865
ISBN: 0-89443-278-8

Printed in the United States of America

1 2 3 4 5

To
Nurses in the 1980s:
Decade of the Nurse

Table of Contents

v

Preface

Decade of the nurse! The 1980s may well deserve such a designation. Certainly this decade offers nurses unique challenges and wide-ranging opportunities. The stress, struggle, and striving of recent decades is paying off. A new positive thrust is abroad in the land. Nurse managers, educators, and researchers are, more and more, talking the same language. Career refocusing and job interchanges facilitate a cross-fertilization of ideas. Diversity increases; yet strong, positive forces are at work within nursing practice, education, and healthcare administration, and these forces bode well for nurses and healthcare consumers. The public press reflects this situation ("For 'New Nurse': Bigger Role," 1980).

Nurse managers at all organizational levels, in whatever work setting, exert an increasingly vital and healthy influence. As a group, they took giant strides during the 1970s to improve their managerial competence. Examples abound and range from head nurses and directors of nursing to RN hospital administrators. Peter Drucker (1979) predicts that in the 1980s we will see greater numbers of RNs functioning as chief executive officers in hospitals and other healthcare agencies. Attesting to this trend is the fact that at this writing the president of the Board of Trustees of the American Hospital Association is a nurse, Sister Irene Kraus.

We had this in mind as we prepared this second edition. This is a book not only for nurse managers but for all nurses, including students of nursing. All nurses use the management process in their work, though they may not recognize it by that name. Every nurse learns and uses—or is expected to use—the four steps of the nursing process: assessing, planning, implementing, and evaluating. This nursing process model is based upon the same model as the management process of planning, doing, and controlling.

Our purpose is to provide a practical, easy-to-use guide to the understanding and implementation of management concepts, functions, techniques, and skills as they apply in healthcare agencies. Thus, the book will be helpful to nurse managers at all levels of responsibility in hospitals, nursing homes, public health agencies, mental health clinics, schools of nursing, and related facilities that provide all types of acute, short-term, extended, home, in- and outpatient healthcare services, and education. Nurses who have their own independent practices can benefit from this book as fully as can those in the customary agencies.

Our theme is the effective management of patient care as provided by nurses, in whatever setting, to the healthcare consumer (i.e., the patient/client/person seeking assistance as an individual or as a member of a group). We elaborate on this theme through a continuing emphasis on the management process as it is carried out by nurses who understand and use management functions, techniques, and skills. We build upon proven concepts and practices of modern management as they are being applied successfully by nurses in an ever growing number of healthcare agencies. Our focus is always on the management of patient/client care and services—with all of the implications suggested by that phrase.

Throughout the book we use the term *patient* to designate the person who is the recipient of the services, recognizing that other terms may be more appropriate in particular settings. Whenever we use the phrase *management of patient care,* we mean only the patient's direct involvement in the patient care process (or, when necessary, with the involvement of the patient's family and/or significant others). Our use of the term *nurse manager* rather than *administrator* is deliberate. The term manager is all-inclusive, meaning any person whose title is administrator or director. By definition, an administrator is one who performs management functions at the executive level, and a manager is one who manages others, providing leadership for individual and group activity.

Organizational principles and leadership skills are treated throughout the book rather than in separate chapters. In fact, the management functions themselves are not compartmentalized. Hence our emphasis continues to be on managing as a process and on systems concepts. To this end we have attempted to achieve effective cross-referencing between chapters and subject areas.

As in the first edition, whenever we refer to *nurses* or *nursing staff* we mean registered nurses. We use *unit personnel* or *nursing personnel* to include all personnel on the nursing department (or unit) payroll. For dictionary references, consult the *American Heritage Dictionary of the English Language,* Peter Davies, editor; and the *Dictionary of Psychology* by J. P. Chaplin. See the Glossary for definitions of many nursing and management terms used throughout this book.

Our psychological orientation is more humanistic than behavioral, more Maslovian than Skinnerian. We subscribe to the third-force concepts of Abraham Maslow. This is apparent throughout our professional work and throughout this book. We believe that helping others to meet their own needs is the most potent motivational force available to managers and nurses. We strive for an appropriate balance between the technical mode and the human mode in the practice of management. This kind of goal-oriented management seeks to create a working environment in which all employees are encouraged to participate to the maximum extent possible in decisions affecting them and their work. We apply the same concept in the nursing care of patients.

The greatest demand for nurse managers is within institutional settings. Thus, many of our examples are drawn from experiences in hospitals and related types of healthcare agencies. At the same time, all of the materials included herein have direct application in other types of settings, such as community mental health centers, public health departments, and independent nursing practice. The problem-oriented nursing system, the nursing process, performance appraisal, patient teaching, nursing by objectives, budgetary planning and control, staffing and scheduling, career planning, motivation, leadership, and other essentials in the effective delivery of patient care services are treated consistently as interrelated components of a humanistically oriented management process.

In summary, our goals for this book are to:

1. set forth a philosophy of nursing management that embraces enunciated value concepts, the importance of each individual as part of the work group, goal-oriented management practices, the time-tested motivational theory of Abraham Maslow, and the precepts of humanistic psychology that both recognize and transcend individual differences,
2. contribute toward the understanding and use of modern management concepts in nursing practice and education,
3. present process-oriented nursing as a system for managing patient care, and to describe the organizational structure required to support it,
4. explain the management functions, techniques, and skills that are necessary to implement the foregoing,
5. provide specific guidance in the use of the management process for the benefit of patients, staff, employees, and the community at large,
6. emphasize the financial impact of the nurse manager's performance, and how to achieve a necessary balance between patient care goals and the realities of budgetary planning and control,
7. offer an integrated concept of organizational structure and practices as

related to the agency mission, nursing modality, legal considerations, and changing demands, while continuing to be responsive to innovative management, and

8. assist nurse managers at all levels in accepting and fulfilling their necessary roles as effective hospital-wide integrators of patient care services.

This book is organized into four parts: Part I provides an overview of the workworld of the nurse manager. Each individual manager is viewed as the center of his/her working environment. Personal attributes and environmental factors are described that influence each person's performance as nurse, as manager, and as a professional in a helping relationship to others. The three major areas of responsibility of the nurse manager are described as patient care management (the clinical aspects), operational management (the business-related aspects), and human resources management (the personnel and staff development aspects). Part I now includes a new chapter on the framework for nursing management. It provides a pragmatic model to conceptualize and integrate the subject areas of the book. An understanding of this model as related to the workworld model is fundamental to achieving goals and objectives through each of the basic units of organization—the people on your payroll. Also included is new material on the nurse manager's workworld environment (both internal and external), legal aspects in nursing practice, and creative problem solving with the Golightly PRESEARCH model.

The understanding of and ability to use management concepts, functions, techniques, and skills are seen as necessary supportive elements to permit adequate performance of nurse manager responsibilities. Also stressed are the requirements of a suitable organizational structure with adequate policies and practices, not only in nursing but throughout the agency as a whole.

Parts II, III, and IV deal with each of the three major areas of the nurse manager's responsibility. Part II presents the Problem-Oriented Nursing System (PONS) as the process model for patient care management. Five essential components of PONS are described. These are the foundation (the principles of nursing practice), the nursing process, the problem-oriented nursing record (PONR), nursing audit, and education (for patients and staff). The new chapter on primary nursing presents its implications for nursing management, the organization of the nursing department, and the clinical aspects of patient care.

Part III deals with operational management. Specific management techniques are explained, with emphasis on their importance in achieving patient care goals. The selected techniques, presented in sufficient detail to serve as a guide to their implementation, are management by objectives, results-oriented performance evaluation, nursing audit, and annual budgetary planning and control. This section is enriched and updated with innovations in cost containment, staffing and scheduling (as a new Chapter 9), and budgetary control.

Part IV deals with human resources management. Particular attention is given to motivation, employee relations, patient and staff education, and the "wide-track careers" concept in nursing. Recent developments are cited that contribute to getting, training, and retaining the members of a productive, stable workforce.

We have tried to provide in this second edition an even more practical desk reference and major resource for the *nurse* managers and nurse *managers* of the 1980s—both the students and the practitioners. May this book serve you well in this *decade of the nurse*—a decade in which nurse managers become positive forces for change through exemplary leadership and colleagueship in a healthcare system that needs so much of both.

Joan and Warren Ganong
Chapel Hill, North Carolina
June 1980

POSTSCRIPT: FEBRUARY 12, 1980

We have just received a bill from our R.N. friend (a former English teacher) whom we asked to read and correct every page of the galley proofs for this second edition. She works as a staff nurse in a local regional medical center hospital, having graduated from nursing school one year ago at a later age than most of her classmates. We respect both her nursing and writing skills. With her bill she attached the following note.

> *I hope you two will either start your own hospital or call my hospital and help them with their nursing service. I want to work where all these goodies are going on!*

We know what she means. Most staff nurses believe there is a way to improve their lot —and patient care too. When promoted to head nurse and other management positions, staff nurses usually discover that the roadblocks to improvement appear more formidable. The most successful ones learn to practice, in some form, what is contained in this book. In addition, they discover the wisdom in this adage, modified slightly from its usual form:

Yard by yard, it's pretty hard.
Inch by inch, it's no cinch...

—but it's easier, and it works!

NOTES

Drucker, P. How to be a more effective administrator. Presentation at *JONA's 2nd National Conference,* Los Angeles, California, March 9, 1979.
For "new nurse": Bigger role in health care. *U.S. News & World Report,* January 14, 1980, pp. 59-61.

Acknowledgments

We continue to express our indebtedness to the professional educators and managers who were recognized by name in the first edition. They still influence us. They, and numbers of other nurse managers, educators, writers, and other healthcare professionals have helped greatly to enrich this second edition. They are recognized individually throughout the text.

Our warm appreciation to our exceptional nurse consultant associates—Cecelia Golightly, R.N., M.P.H.; Davina Gosnell, R.N., M.S., Ph.D.; and Martyann Penberth, R.N., M.S., M.P.H.—for their individual contributions on PRESEARCH, on education, on legal aspects, and on the work-world environment. And hearty thanks to Barbara Hoecke, Anita Marten, and Judith Wray, whose combined talents helped make this edition possible.

Part I

Workworld of the Nurse Manager

Chapter 1

The Nurse in the Organization

CHALLENGE AND OPPORTUNITY

The tides of change in our healthcare system affect everyone. Nurses especially feel the impact of new demands upon healthcare agencies. Nurses have to *do* something about meeting the more stringent accreditation requirements, standards imposed as a result of federally funded services, quality assurance, cost containment, budgetary planning, PSRO, POMR, HMO, unionization, inflation, national health insurance, community accountability, and all the rest. And nurses have to maintain their professional integrity and personal commitment to patient care while coping with the welter of wonderful work.

One of the reasons for studying nursing is to become a professional helper. Nurses learn how to provide skilled help to other persons with healthcare needs. The student of nursing typically learns to visualize the nursing role as a one-to-one relationship between the individual as nurse and another individual as patient. And so it may be. But more often than not the graduate nurse begins to practice nursing as a member of a complex organization—a healthcare agency made up of groups of individuals with varied competencies who provide necessary services for the patients or clients being served.

You undoubtedly first began to realize the need for finding your place in a healthcare organizational hierarchy as a student. You learned to understand your role within the formal organizational structure of a nursing department, and became familiar with the complexities of the interrelationships among departments, professional disciplines, patients, employee groups, and administration. You may have begun to wonder then, or later, how you could achieve the type of nurse-patient relationship once visualized. As a student you learned that your function was to become well acquainted with the needs and problems of each individual patient and then to use your knowledge and skills to help meet those patient needs in a personal way. Instead, as a staff nurse you were assigned a workload of tasks, procedures, and routines for a group of patients being served en masse by a variety of members of the patient care team. You observed too that those nurses who progressed to higher-level nursing positions spent less and less time in individual patient care, and you learned that to progress in your profession and earn higher monetary rewards you would have to accept responsibility for others as a head nurse or supervisor.

For years this has been true and is still true in many organizations. Yet today in most areas of the healthcare industry, nurses are finding that they can make progress professionally and financially without moving into the ranks of management. Job opportunities and earnings on the clinical, education, and research tracks parallel those on the management track. Job titles such as clinical specialist, nurse clinician, primary nurse, nurse practitioner, and nursing consultant are providing new advancement opportunities. (See Golightly, 1979, for an exhaustive listing.)

This is, in fact, a time of unprecedented opportunity for nurses. It is a time when, as perhaps never before, nurses are being invited to take new initiatives in many areas of service and organizational leadership. It is a time when all nurses in whatever role—clinician, manager, or educator—can more fully utilize their full range of talents, knowledge, and skills. It is also a time to maintain perspective, to take a balanced view of what nurses—yourself, in particular—should do, can do, and want to do.

It may be timely to set aside some quiet time with yourself to take stock of your life situation. Consider where you have come from, where you are, and where you want to go. Ask yourself, "What do I want to do with my career as a nurse?" We believe that most of us can do what we want to do if we want it badly enough—enough to do what is necessary to achieve a goal that is worthwhile to us. The introspection that is necessary for you to explore your life/work goals is likely to lead to identifying and examining your values and motivation, your knowledge and skills. Cecelia Golightly's aforementioned career-planning workbook can be of major help in this task.

While a wide range of opportunities are available to nurses, they exist within the structure of the healthcare delivery system in general and of the patient care process in particular. Becoming an effective nurse manager is, for many nurses, both a conscious career choice and a means toward an end.

Your reactions to the foregoing are very important. You may be feeling now that "this is not for me" or "this is really what I want." Your reactions are dictated largely by your own perception of yourself and your perception of nursing. You may think of yourself as just a nurse who carries out assigned tasks, procedures, and routines for patients. You may see yourself as a patient care manager who works as a primary nurse with your individual patients to assist them in meeting their objectives through carrying out the medical care plan and the nursing care plan. Or you may see yourself as a nurse manager accepting full responsibility for clinical management, operations management, and human resources management. If one of your reactions is, "Oh, I could never do that!" then you may feel restricted by what you believe to be personal liabilities and roadblocks to your own growth. Whether these are imagined or real, it is possible to know thyself while emphasizing the positive. It is a simple fact of self-development and of assisting with the development of others that you cannot build on personal liabilities. You can build only upon personal assets.

Certainly you must face problems that develop out of your own personal life/work situations and recognize their influence on your own goal achievement. But rather than focus on them as problems, you can elect, if you adopt a suitable frame of mind, to see problems as opportunities. When you do this—when you perceive a problem as an opportunity—you adopt a frame of mind (a "willing mind," to use a southern phrase) that helps to marshal your available resources, utilize your assets and skills, and make progress in spite of the problems. Roadblocks are viewed as temporary obstacles to be removed, not as barriers preventing your further progress.

THE NURSE MANAGER: CHANGING CONCEPTS

The rapid expansion of new career opportunities for nurses is a healthy trend. Yet there is a sometimes unrecognized aspect of what has been happening. The entire concept of the nurse manager function has been changing. The role that was once seen as a supervisory link in a traditional authoritarian chain-of-command hierarchy has changed to the concept of a nurse manager who performs as a true facilitator-coordinator-leader. This is a potent change and one which we seek to encourage. It is based upon the weight of experience as well as the findings of the behavioral sciences.

Another change is also having an impact on nursing. This is the trend toward greater accountability by individual nurses in every work setting. While it has always been true that all professional persons have been accountable for their actions, there is now a far greater stress on clearly defined standards of practice and the auditing of results. This is another aspect of the rights movement. One by-product is a clear recognition that the practice of enlightened management is vital. In fact, it is critical to the future of nursing in the world of healthcare. The nurse as clinician and the nurse as manager must understand and practice—thoughtfully and deliberately—the necessary management functions, techniques, and skills to carry out their performance responsibilities. Professional nurses, by virtue of being licensed to practice, have always been expected to assume responsibility for supervising the work of others in lower job categories. From this point of view nurses always have had the responsibility of managerial leadership and its attendant accountability. But in today's workworld, professional nurses have both expanded opportunities and more clearly defined responsibilities to apply management principles and practices, whether they choose the clinical, education, management, or research track as a career plan. In fact, more and more nurses find it beneficial to switch back and forth among these tracks. In doing so they enhance their ability to use their management knowledge and skills. Thus the term "nurse manager" can be used with either of two different emphases—"*nurse* manager" or "nurse *manager*."

This dual role of nurse and manager applies at every job level in nursing. Whether as staff nurse, head nurse, or administrator, the professional nurse necessarily is both nurse and manager with the emphasis shifting according to need. As *nurse* manager, the emphasis is upon the nurse as clinician practicing one's own professional nursing skills. This may be done simply as another RN member of the patient care staff on a unit, with only nominal responsibility for the work performed by nonnurses within the group. (Here the nurse is managing as a professional helper for one's own patients.) Or the nurse-as-clinician may be serving as a primary nurse or team leader with a more apparent leadership role vis-à-vis the other members of the immediate patient care staff. Or the nurse may be acting as a charge nurse or assistant head nurse with temporary shift responsibility for the management of patient care provided by the unit personnel available for that shift—often a highly mobile group of persons in today's hospital environment. In each of these situations the emphasis tends to be on the nurse-as-clinician providing personal patient care, albeit with a group of helpers to assist with the patient care services. Minimal attention is focused on the managerial components of these roles, except as the individual nurse recognizes his/her professional responsibility for patient care management. The personnel management responsibility, even if recognized, often cannot be assumed effectively. The reasons for this are many and include the nature of the nurse's education, the confusion as to who is really in charge of the unit personnel at any given time, and the inability of nursing administration to establish an effective, decentralized organizational structure appropriate for a modern healthcare agency.

The nurse *manager* role, in contrast, places the emphasis upon the nurse as a professional manager. The nursing knowledge, skills, and philosophy are still essential. The clinical skills will be practiced less and less as the nurse progresses to the higher level of management positions, but the other components of being a nurse will continue to be a requirement. One of the reasons for this is the need for credibility and acceptance of persons in the top leadership positions of the key department in any agency devoted to helping patients meet their healthcare needs. Nursing is, and will remain for the foreseeable future, the key department in such agencies. It is the department that provides patient care services twenty-four hours a day, seven days a week throughout the year. It is the department that spends upwards of forty percent of the operating budget of a typical hospital. It has more people on the payroll than any other department. Clearly, the nurses in charge must be competent managers. More than this, they must be effective agency-wide integrators of patient care services (Ganong & Ganong, 1977). This requirement applies to primary nurses, head nurses, and all other nurse managers.

In view of the foregoing and recognizing the dual clinical/managerial roles of any professional nurse, the contents of this book are intended primarily to assist the nurse *manager* in the role of charge nurse, head nurse, supervisor, coordinator, assistant director, associate director, director of nursing service, director of nursing, vice president for patient care services, chief nurse, college dean, director of nursing education, coordinator of healthcare occupations, inservice education director, director of continuing education, staff development director, and so on. Titles abound. Yet they reflect common management components. Our focus is on these components.

YOUR WORKWORLD BEGINS WITH YOU

You are, quite literally, the center of your workworld. You are unique. Thus your job situation is unique. Regardless of your title, job or performance description, and the nature of the supervision you receive, your workworld is more you than anything else. You have more influence on your job situation, more responsibility and more authority to act than you may realize or utilize. This is a fact often overlooked. Nurses in almost every position are known to complain, "If only I had the authority to go with my responsibility!" Or "I could be much more effective if only I didn't have to get an O.K. on everything from my boss." And "Why can't we make more of our own decisions right here on our own unit?"

Yet the managers of these same nurses have complaints of their own. They often say, "If only my people would show some initiative! Why won't they make a decision on their own? They don't have to check with me all the time." Such comments reflect organizational relationships that are all too common. When such ambiguity about role relationships is allowed to continue, the fault lies with both parties—the manager and the staff member. The manager, recognizing a situation in which nursing personnel are not willing to make decisions that are within the scope of their responsibility and authority, should take the necessary steps to clarify whatever misunderstandings exist. Sometimes the problem is simply a matter of one person misunderstanding the expectations of the other. Frank discussion can clear the air. (See "Developing Mutual Expectations" in Appendix J for a highly useful technique.) Other times the problem involves the complications and nuances of decision making that are in gray areas of role responsibility and authority. The manager's dictum of "When in doubt, check with me," is not adequate except in cases of longstanding relationships. It too easily becomes a crutch for the unsure or indecisive subordinate.

A useful tool that the manager can use in discussions with staff members is a Decision Worksheet to outline the degrees of responsibility and authority. On one side list typical situations and problems found in the nursing situation and on the other a range of action possibilities of which one could be checked off as applicable to the situation. Five action possibilities, coded by letters, are: (A) I act on my own initiative. No need to inform others of my action. (B) I take action, and inform my boss (and possibly others) afterward. (C) I consult my boss in advance and say what I expect to do. (D) I recommend action to be carried out by my boss (or others). (E) I turn over the problem to my boss (or others) with no recommendation for action. The use of this form will help to explore and resolve areas of uncertainty in the minds of the manager and the staff members.

The person in the subordinate position has responsibility too for initiating action to clarify questions about decision-making authority. Once familiar with the Decision Worksheet, the subordinate can fill it in for a range of typical situations and problems.

For example, Peggy Ansel (a head nurse) might select the following problems and indicate the level of action responsibility she believes her own nurse manager expects of her.

PROBLEM	A	B	C	D	E
1. Nurse does not update care plans daily	X				
2. Doctor wants a new setup for stocking treatment cart			X		
3. Nurse aide claims discrimination in work assignments		X			
4. Patient says watch was stolen	X				
5. My neighbor reports that our housekeepers are taking steps to join a union					X
6. Night supervisor provides inadequate patient care support on my unit				X	
7. Unit secretary needs to be replaced			X		

Having completed this listing, Peggy then requests an opportunity to sit down with her own manager to see if they are in agreement. Open discussion will resolve any differences. Follow-through discussions will be required to explore fully the variety of questions that may arise regarding each other's responsibility and accountability.

Another recourse for the person in the subordinate position is to "see what you can get away with." This is suggested in the positive, constructive sense of testing how far you can go in making your own decisions—by making them (within the common-sense dictates of policies, practice, and your inclination for taking risks). Decision making involves taking calculated risks. No manager can be sure of making safe decisions all of the time. As a professional, you will learn quickly through this testing approach the degree of appropriate risks you can assume in your decision making within your organization. Most nurse managers can "get away with" more than they realize—by taking on the responsibility and authority expected of them by a competent leader/facilitator.

Remember also another maxim: Never let your boss be surprised. This applies especially to your own actions and relationships. Your manager should not learn from other sources information that you could have provided sooner or more appropriately. Keep your communication lines open. Your use of the Decision Worksheet will assist in developing the empathy that is needed in an effective superior/subordinate relationship.

THE CENTER OF YOUR WORKWORLD

Figure 1-1 is a conceptualization of you at the center of your organizational workworld. It has great significance, since professional nurse managers must think organizationally. They must be able to comprehend the formal organization of departmental relationships as diagrammed on an organizational chart, understand the informal organization made up of the complex interactions of people who make things happen and get the work done, and recognize that they (and each individual employee at every level) are the smallest unit of organization. Note this well. Remind yourself frequently, "I am the smallest and the most important unit of organization in the workworld of which I am the center. I influence my workworld more than I may realize." The impact you make on your workworld is shown by the four out-pointing arrows in the diagram.

Each day when you—with all of your feelings—enter your workworld, you bring with you your values, your motivation, your knowledge, and your skills. These comprise your apperceptive mass, the associational areas of your brain. What you do with these components of yourself each day affects you and others, including your personnel and your patients. These personal at-

Figure 1-1 Me at the Center of My Workworld

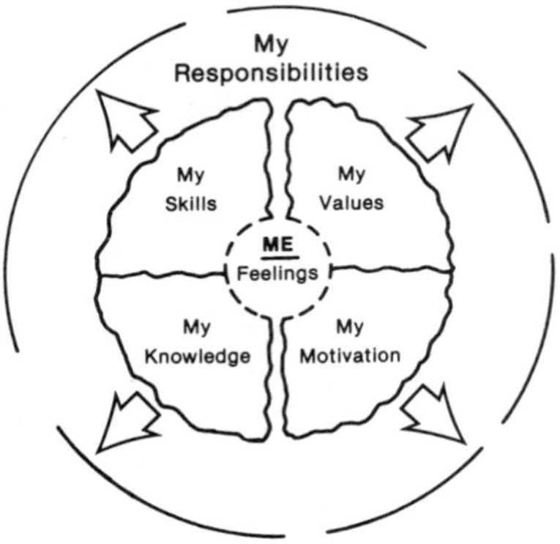

Source: Evolved from Ganong, J. and Ganong, W. *HELP for the head nurse.* Section 3, 1st ed. Chapel Hill, N.C.: W. L. Ganong Co., 1974. (3rd ed. 1978).

tributes comprise the first and central segment of a complete picture of your workworld.

Your values are obviously a highly important part of you and have a sometimes unrecognized influence upon your philosophy and actions as a nurse manager. "A *value* is an enduring belief that a specific mode of conduct or end-state of existence is personally or socially preferable to an opposite or converse mode of conduct or end-state of existence. A *value system* is an enduring organization of beliefs concerning preferable modes of conduct or end-states of existence along a continuum of relative importance" (Rokeach, 1973). Your values affect your life and your work. What do you value? What do you believe in? What is most important to you? What is your attitude toward yourself and others? Is your list of values made up more of things than of people-related items? These are serious questions and deserve your best thought and response, for your values inevitably influence all that you do as a nurse and as a manager. They influence your use of your clinical skills and your managerial skills. They influence the way you react to change. Your values are influencing your response to this material at the present moment. Admittedly, most of your values are acquired subconsciously during your early years and remain relatively unchanged all of your life. Other values may grow or be shaped out of your later life and work experiences.

Your motivation is what causes you to do what you do, to select one course of action instead of another. Your human needs have a great influence on your motivation. One of the most useful and durable theories of human motivation is that of Abraham Maslow. Appendix I provides a personalized adaptation of this theory of motivation. It will serve you well in understanding yourself and others.

A third component of your apperceptive mass is your knowledge. It has been said that chance favors the prepared mind. This is a way of saying that you make your own luck and that there are certain requisites for experiencing personal satisfaction from your work. Adequate job knowledge, the kind of technical and managerial knowledge that gives you confidence in your own ability, is one such requisite. There can be no substitute for necessary job knowledge acquired through study and experience.

Your skills comprise the fourth component. Competence involves not only knowing what to do but being able to do it well. You can perform satisfactorily as a nurse manager only when you have sufficient skills in both the technical and human modes of the nurse manager's role. These include both clinical and managerial skills. You acquire some of these skills prior to becoming a nurse manager. Other skills you develop as you work and learn.

An example of the *human mode* skills is pertinent here. The degree of success with which you exercise your interpersonal skills is related to your understanding of yourself and others. Writing about individuals with neurotic defenses, Yalom explains how such persons with low levels of self-esteem and self-awareness have difficulty in striving toward increased interpersonal competence. They perceive such a goal as incompatible with their need for relief from suffering—from the sense of inadequacy they feel so keenly.

> Their initial response to others is often based on distrust rather than trust, and, most important of all, their ability to question their belief system and to risk new forms of behavior is severely impaired. In fact, the inability to learn from new experience is central to the basic problem of the neurotic. ... The important point is that the individual with neurotic defenses is frozen into a closed position; he is not open for learning, and he is generally searching not for growth but for safety. Argyris (1968) puts it nicely when he differentiates a "survival orientation" from a "competence orientation." The more an individual is competence-oriented, the more receptive and flexible he is. He becomes an "open system" and in the interpersonal area is able to use his experience to develop greater interpersonal competence. On the other hand, an individual may be more concerned with protecting himself in order to survive. Through the use of defence [sic] mechanisms he withdraws, distorts, or attacks the environment (Yalom, 1975, p. 497).

This distinction between survival orientation and competence orientation can be most useful to a nurse manager. It can help in coping with diverse manifestations of closed versus open behavior. You can best help yourself and others when you recognize that unexpected changes in your own customary behavior (or the behavior of others) may stem from a personal need that has not been recognized or acknowledged.

The four personal components comprising your apperceptive mass are the sum total of all your education, training, life experience, parental influence, religion, jobs, prejudices, beliefs, and so on. It is what you have to react with, the associational areas of your brain, your own privately-programmed built-in computer.

Perhaps you feel that you are locked into your apperceptive mass, into being the person you are. This seems to be true for most of us. And that is just fine. What you are today is O.K. But you are not a finished product and neither is anyone else. All of us are in the process of becoming, of continuing to find out how to use most effectively our own personal assets and abilities. With this in mind, let's continue to develop the picture of your workworld.

Your workworld may be an 850-bed acute care hospital, a 10-bed cardiac care unit, a 75-bed nursing home, or a 25,000-population community being served by your home healthcare agency. Regardless of the size or nature of your particular setting, you have three major areas of responsibility. These are patient care management, operational management, and human resources management. Components of each of these responsibilities are summarized briefly as follows:

Patient Care Management	Operational Management	Human Resources Management
Assess problems and needs, Problem identification, Planning of care, Providing care, Teaching, Treatments, Medications, Clinical conferences, and Evaluating results;	Budgeting, Controlling expenses, Staffing, Providing supplies, Scheduling, Communicating, Coordinating, Planning, Evaluating performance, Meetings, Auditing, and Committees;	Teaching, Counseling, Facilitating, Rounds, Conferences, Inservice programs, Continuing education, Bulletin boards, Journals, Career mobility, Peer review, and Research.

Clearly, every nurse manager by whatever title at each level within the nursing department has responsibilities in these three areas. The extent to which these responsibilities are recognized and discharged by individual nurse managers in a given healthcare agency is affected by three major factors. These factors are philosophy, delegation, and competency.

The first factor is the philosophy and organizational concepts of the top administrator in the agency. This has to do with basic beliefs about people and the ways of securing effective performance. It involves ideas about teamwork, risk taking, and support. It includes comprehending the messages of writers like Appley, Argyris, Drucker, Goble, Maslow, McGregor, and Myers. Some administrators prefer to hold the reins tightly themselves and permit little or no initiative and assumption of responsibility by department heads and other supervisory management personnel. Other administrators believe that the best way for the agency to achieve its objectives is to delegate the maximum amount of authority, responsibility, and accountability for results through a decentralized organization structure with adequate centralized control mechanisms. Such administrators tend to believe with Lawrence Appley that "management is guiding human and physical resources into dynamic organizational units that attain their objectives to the satisfaction of those served with a high degree of morale and sense of attainment on the part of those rendering the service" (Appley, 1969, p. 59).

The second factor is the degree of delegation exercised by the top-level nurse manager. Even when the agency administrator believes in and achieves meaningful delegation of responsibility and authority, those at the next level of administration (such as the director of nursing) may not be able or willing to follow the example set for them. When this happens, those persons in the lower levels of management are likely to be restricted in exercising their full potential as managers.

The third factor is the personal competency and accountability of the nurse manager in the subordinate position (patient care coordinator or head nurse, for example). A vital component of competency has been identified as motive force, which is that element in the working relationship between two or more persons which determines whose plan of action is dominant. It is characterized by an ability to see the broad picture, a desire to change things, and a willingness to be measured by results (Ganong, Ganong, & Huenefeld, 1974).

While the nature of managerial performance responsibilities is similar at varying levels of an organization, the degree of responsibility varies depending upon the scope of the individual position. For example, a head nurse assumes only a small share of total managerial responsibility within nursing and does so for an individual patient care unit of limited size with an annual operating budget of perhaps $200,000 or less. A patient care coordinator responsible for a group of units has a broader managerial work load and may be responsible for a budget that is in the $500,000 to $900,000 range. The director of nursing, with the full scope of nursing management responsibility in a hospital of 300 to 400 beds, may have a budget responsibility of somewhere between $6 million and $9 million, representing as much as 40 percent of the operating expense budget for the entire hospital. Obviously, other characteristics also distinguish the job of nursing director from that of head nurse. In developing the concept of the workworld of a nurse manager, the general components apply at all levels of managerial responsibility.

Now, a word about terminology. The professions—such as nursing, medicine, law, and psychology—have their own terminology and a need to use words that convey precise meanings. So does the field of management. As a professional nurse you have learned the necessity for the accurate use of technical terms. Similarly, as a professional manager, you need to be familiar with and make careful use of accurate management terms. Your accurate use of correct management terminology will help reduce misunderstanding and facilitate clear communications. And since "meanings are not in words—meanings are in people," successful communication requires more than your use of precise management terms. Clear communication requires the extra effort of an explanation in words appropriate to the comprehension level of the listener. The Glossary at the end of this book, together with our attempt to use correct terminology consistently, is intended to contribute to your management communication efforts.

MANAGEMENT FUNCTIONS, TECHNIQUES, AND SKILLS

As shown in Figure 1-2, a conceptualization of your workworld as a nurse manager, set within your internal and external environment, can be seen as a supportive structure for you and your responsibilities. This supportive structure is made up of management functions, techniques, and skills. These components of managing are carried out not only by you, but also by your own manager and by your own subordinates in their respective roles. All members of the management team require a clear understanding of management functions, techniques, and skills and how they are applied at various organizational levels to achieve objectives and goals. The primary focus of objectives and goals is to provide the types of care and services that best meet the needs and problems of individual patients and clients. The performance of nurse managers has a critical influence on the caliber of results. We need to examine the ways in which optimum results can be obtained.

Management Functions

Management functions are the basic processes that comprise the work of the manager. These processes are identified as planning, doing, and controlling; their practical application is the main thrust of this book.

Figure 1-2 My Workworld

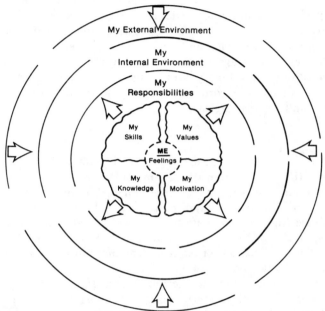

Source: Evolved from Ganong, J. and Ganong, W. *Help for the head nurse.* Section 3, 1st ed. Chapel Hill, N.C.: W. L. Ganong Co., 1974. (3rd ed. 1978).

Planning

Planning is thinking ahead, determining what shall be done. Planning is the process of establishing goals, defining problems and opportunities, setting objectives, and developing strategy and tactics for action. Thus planning involves making decisions regarding such actions as establishing and clarifying organizational relationships; developing broad goals; establishing policies and considering how to implement them; mapping long-range programs and projects; setting specific objectives with target dates for completion; determining specific methods and procedures; fixing day-to-day work assignments and schedules; and estimating budgetary requirements.

Doing

Doing is the implementation phase of the manager's job. It involves carrying out the plans, working on the short-term objectives to achieve the broader purposes and goals. Included in this function are providing leadership and direction for the nursing staff; making use of the necessary leadership tools, techniques, skills, and controls; assuring adequate materials, supplies, and nursing staff; developing objectives and performance responsibilities with the personnel involved; defining standards of performance with personnel; arranging self-development opportunities for personnel; coordinating work activities; integrating viewpoints; building the kind of climate that encourages self-development, motivation, and self-control by personnel; performing direct patient care as required; maintaining strong nurse manager/nursing staff relationships; controlling payroll costs and other expense items; and assuring that adequate records are kept to meet all patient care, administrative, and legal requirements.

Controlling

Controlling is the evaluating, measuring, and feedback function. Controlling provides the link between doing and replanning. Controlling assesses how well the doing achieved the objectives and goals of planning. Controlling encompasses cost containment and sound financial management. Thus controlling provides the objective data for looking back at what has happened, and for looking ahead to what else you want to have happen. In this manner, the recycling of the functions of management continues—the ongoing process of planning, doing, and controlling.

The controlling function involves setting standards for evaluation purposes at carefully selected strategic control points; checking and reporting on performance compared with standards; taking corrective action as indicated; measuring performance results periodically against plans, by (1) appraising departmental and unit results against objectives, and (2) performance reviews, comparing individual results with the criteria for satisfactory performance and specific objectives. Controlling also includes interpreting results, then modifying or expanding existing plans to achieve revised objectives. The feedback aspect of controlling necessitates the use of a suitable performance evaluation procedure such as ROPEP (the results-oriented performance evaluation program described in Part III) so that people know how they are doing and what changes, if any, are desirable for the future.

You will readily recognize that the management functions are not individually discrete parts of the managing process. They do not exist independently of each other. On the contrary, they are interdependent, overlapping, and supportive segments of a continually recycling process. For example, the controlling function has to be planned or it will not be effective. And the measuring and evaluative aspects of controlling, to be most timely and useful, often need to occur during the doing function. A dramatic patient care illustration is the use of the cardiopulmonary resuscitation (CPR) team as an emergency patient care technique on a medical-surgical unit. Consider how the management functions are interrelated.

Controlling: The first indications (objective feedback from the patient) of a cardiac arrest by a medical-surgical patient on such a unit are usually identified by some member of the nursing staff. The staff member takes immediate action: "code blue" (or similar stat call) to secure the CPR team, and immediate emergency measures within the skills and responsibility of the staff member. This is doing in accordance with plan.

Doing: The feedback and evaluative signs which triggered the CPR procedure (observed as part of the controlling function) occurred during the doing function of managing the nursing care of a particular group of patients. (How soon after the patient first showed cardiac arrest symptoms were those symptoms recognized by the nursing staff? Could they have been recognized sooner? How well did the response occur? Was it effective for the patient?) The CPR procedure itself is a doing function, and must be well managed. It obviously requires meticulous planning (the advance selection and training of the CPR team members, the purchase and maintenance of equipment), prompt response and fast teamwork under skilled leadership when a call occurs, instantaneous feedback and response (controlling while doing) during the crisis, and a sense of organized, well-managed effort throughout.

Planning: Several references to planning have been identified in the controlling and doing as described above. The entire CPR procedure, of course, is a masterpiece of management—from conceptualization and planning through implementation and evaluation. The procedure brings into action the coordinated efforts of an interdisciplinary team of members who understand and are skilled in their roles, and who are led by a prepared leader—a model of management in the full sense of purposeful human activity to carry out the necessary functions, techniques, and procedures with appropriate skill and dispatch.

Giving a separate identity (the functions of planning, doing, and controlling) to the major segments of the managing process helps in conceptualizing what management is all about, and assists in differentiating the functions of management from the skills and techniques used by managers.

Management Techniques and Skills

As part of your personal supporting structure for carrying out your performance responsibilities, the management functions are of central importance. The other two parts of your supporting structure are identified as management techniques and management skills. Management techniques are those programs, procedures, and strategies that assist you in performing one or more of the management functions. Specific techniques are presented in

Parts II, III, and IV. A skill is proficiency in a way of doing something using your hands, body, and brain. Thus the management skills are those personal abilities the manager uses to achieve results through the technical mode and the human mode. Such skills include communicating (via one's behavior, body language, eye contact, facial expression, listening, reading, silence, speaking, touching, writing), conceptualizing, decision making, discussion leading, instructing, improving methods, managing time, motivating, perceiving, and problem solving. In summary, managerial performance skills are the ways in which a nurse manager utilizes management techniques to effectively carry out the management functions of planning, doing, and controlling.

Environmental Influences

Refer again to Figure 1-2. Note the arrows that point in to depict the environmental forces that have an impact on you and your workworld. A variety of internal environmental factors influence you in your job. These factors range from the patients and their families to members of the medical staff, members of the nursing department, other employees throughout the hospital, visitors, and so on. External environmental factors also affect you in your job. These include such groups as business, community, educational, governmental, labor, political, international, professional, religious, social, and volunteer organizations. These groups also exert a variety of economic, cultural, and behavioral pressures on your healthcare agency. These groups and the people who represent them—both internally and externally—influence you directly and indirectly whether or not you have regular personal contact with them. They have an impact on your apperceptive mass. They influence your decision making, consciously or unconsciously. As a nurse manager you need to be aware of the environmental factors so that you can give them the attention they deserve, appropriate to decision making at your organizational level. Such factors become increasingly significant as you progress to higher levels of responsibility in any organizational setting. (See Chapter 2 for a more detailed discussion of the environmental factors; see also the section of Chapter 10 on the stages of change and the change agent. These will give added meaning to the in- and out-pointing arrows in Figure 1-2.)

The admonition to consider the environmental factors implies the necessity for a balanced interpretation of what they mean and how they should influence decisions and actions. This is complicated by the fact that we human beings are unable to be purely objective in interpreting what we see. John Ross, an Australian researcher, reports that the human perceptual system draws on unconscious interpretation of visual data and decides what to see.

One research finding indicates that we apparently idealize what we see. Psychologist Ross believes that the visual system may have a program, an arrangement for perceiving shapes in time and space. "What we see is an interpretation. We adopt a perceptual attitude in order to comprehend the world" (Ross, 1976).

Most of us recognize from our own experience the selective receptivity of our senses. When we listen, somehow we often hear what we want to hear and screen out the rest. When we try to identify our feelings, we may be shocked to learn of our seeming inability (or unwillingness) to recognize and express our feelings—as contrasted to our thoughts. We may have difficulty even in recognizing the existence and influence of the affective and cognitive components in learning, teaching, decision making, interpersonal relations, and patient care. When we do discover the productive balanced interrelationship of feeling and thinking, of heart and mind (through transactional analysis, a learning laboratory, an ACT-U-AR,* or similar experience), then our lives and work may become more satisfying.

Much of this chapter is an exercise in conceptualizing your workworld. Conceptual ability is a vital mental skill in your work as a nurse and a manager. A concept is an idea. It exists within your own apperceptive mass, the associational areas of your brain. A concept may be considered a general understanding, thought, or notion that grows out of specific instances or occurrences. We recognize that your workworld can never be as carefully structured, uniformly balanced, or as static a concept as described. On the contrary, it is more like a changing, dynamic, freewheeling, psychedelic, multidimensional kind of a world. Every manager has to conceptualize this big picture, be familiar with its details and how they fit together, and perceive how the meaning of that picture affects day-to-day problem solving and decision making.

We developed the workworld model empirically, based upon our own varied life/work experiences. It has evolved over many years. No doubt some readers will perceive in Figure 1–2 some concepts that parallel Kurt Lewin's Field Theory (Lewin, 1935, 1951; Argyris, 1952), sometimes referred to as the force field theory. As Meissner (1978) indicates, Lewin's field approach has influenced greatly the study of group and social processes.

> The fundamental concept in Lewin's system is the 'life space,' the sum of all facts that determine the person's behavior at a given point in time. The life space includes two primary dimensions: the psychological environment and the person himself. The psychologi-

---

*ACT-U-AR refers to a self-actualizing seminar, to "Act As You Are," your best self.

cal environment is the external or physical environment, insofar as it determines the person's behavior. The second dimension of the life space in Lewin's analysis is the person. The person's motivation comes from need states. The need system is in a state of tension or 'hunger.'

Thus a common-sense approach to understanding how the impact of internal and external forces upon an individual affects that person's behavior as goal-directed action is provided. It is this gestalt which we have tried to delineate in our workworld model.

Your response to the foregoing is likely to be influenced by your own conceptual ability and your position in the management hierarchy. In this regard, Guglielmino (1979) provides the pertinent results of his study of the mix of management skills needed at different organizational levels (Figure 1-3). More than this, he identifies in his article the specific skills included in

Figure 1-3 Hierarchy of Management Skills

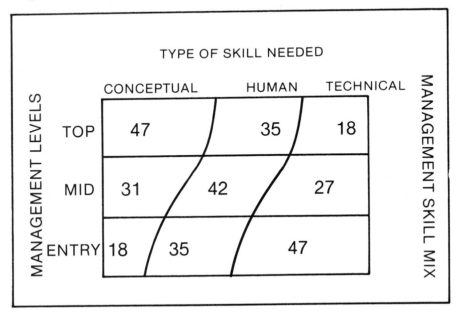

each of the three categories, and the need for an integrated sequence for the effective development of the necessary skills. His findings are consistent with our emphasis on using a suitable mix of technical mode/human mode skills, and on developing your conceptual ability.

THE PERFORMANCE DESCRIPTION

The use of job descriptions has been the traditional way of describing the duties of the person holding a particular job. We much prefer "performance descriptions" (or job performance descriptions) and encourage their use at every opportunity. A performance description has some similarities to a job description, but the two are basically different because they are developed for two different purposes. The job description, by its very title, describes a job. It is prepared by a process of job analysis and its purpose is primarily to provide the necessary descriptive job information for job evaluation purposes. Supplemental uses include orienting a new person to a job and, to some extent, assisting in recruitment.

A performance description, by contrast, describes performance responsibilities and the agreed-upon standards of performance. It is prepared by a process of performance analysis carried out initially by employees with their own managers. Its purpose is to reach agreement and understanding, between superior and subordinate, regarding the subordinate's performance responsibilities so that meaningful ongoing self-evaluation of performance can take place. The emphasis in the preparation and use of a performance description is in reaching a mutual understanding between superior and subordinate regarding who is to do what for whom, when, and how well—so that there can be later understanding and agreement regarding what was done for whom, when, and how well. A further examination of these purposes is included in Part III dealing with results-oriented performance evaluation.

The head nurse example (Appendix G) is used because it is representative of a performance description for any nurse-manager. The descriptions for other nursing personnel, either at the staff nurse level or at higher levels of management responsibility, are similar in form and partially similar in content. First of all, the description provides a simple statement of the purpose of the person in the head nurse position. The major performance responsibilities are listed on the left side of the sheet. These responsibilities are grouped according to the persons for whom they are carried out. Performance responsibilities are always activities that are done for someone else. On the right side of the sheet are statements for each item of responsibility that indicate the measurable conditions which will exist when performance is satisfactory. Thus the head nurse has a responsibility to his or her own nurse manager to "help with budgetary planning and operate the unit within the budget." Performance is satisfactory when "the budget is realistically related to patient care programs and expenses are within the budget." A full examination of these performance descriptions will help to complete the picture of the workworld of the nurse manager. (See Appendix G for an example of a Head Nurse performance description and see Appendix A for a lengthier example of a performance description entitled "General Performance Responsibilities of Administrative and Management Personnel.")

GOALS AND RESPONSIBILITIES

The organizational chart of a department of nursing presents the structure of the department in terms of lines of authority and responsibilities among the members of the department. If you have not seen the organization chart for your department, you should obtain one and review it. Such a chart of organization is another important dimension in your understanding of your workworld.

Every organization exists for a purpose. This purpose is stated in the articles of incorporation, and is often referred to as the statement of mission (Ainsworth, 1976). The purpose or mission is elaborated in the form of a number of specific goals. The broad organizational goals must be translated into departmental and unit goals and objectives. The section on "Management by Objectives" in Part III presents the technique for carrying out such a program. All employees need to understand the goals and objectives of their department and their roles in carrying out the objectives. This concept is diagrammed in the MBO Schematic Organizational Plan (see Figure 5-2 in Chapter 5). The Financial Organization Chart (Figure 8-1 in Chapter 8) emphasizes another important aspect of organization. Everyone knows that everything that happens in an organization costs money. Too few members of the typical nursing department, however, know just how much money is being spent. Usually this is through no fault of the staff members themselves, but it does reflect upon agency administration.

As patients, we have had occasion to ask a variety of members of the patient care staff such questions as, "How much is my daily room charge? How much does it cost to provide me with the daily change of bed linen? Why does the bed linen have to be changed daily when I am ambulatory? Would my bill be less if my bed linen were not changed daily?" Response to such questions is usually a shrug of the shoulders, a guess, or an "I don't know." Such lack of knowledgeable response (and the absence of any apparent interest in the questions) is a sad commentary upon those hospitals' management and nursing leadership in today's healthcare world.

Nurse managers in a modern healthcare setting must be cost conscious themselves and help every staff person be aware that everything he or she does has direct impact upon the expenses of running the department. Such an attitude is important to patient care. In our experience, appropriate emphasis on the financial aspects of nursing contributes to, rather than detracts from, patient care goals.

There is no need to overdramatize here the great significance of this subject of healthcare costs. Professional publications, the daily newspaper, and other media regularly draw attention to the staggering increases in the cost of healthcare.

As much as 40 percent of the annual increase in the cost of a hospital day has been attributed to the use of new health technologies. In the *New York Times Magazine* (August 5, 1979), Laurence Cherry wrote, "But few believe that a Government policy of strict across-the-board cost containment can really work without affecting health care." He went on to describe how the Congress-created National Center for Health-Care Technology within HEW is assessing the value and cost of the pervasive new medical technology—CAT scanners, ultrasound units, microsurgery equipment, and so on. The Center aims "to make sure that medical technology is our servant and never becomes our master," and hopes to influence attitudes toward such technology vis-à-vis limited resources as a basis for deciding which of the new devices should be allowed to survive and spread (Cherry, 1979, p. 22).

The day-to-day operating expenses can be controlled best by those who provide the care. Nurse managers have a vital role in this. As a group, the nurse managers in healthcare agencies have responsibility for spending more of the agency budget than the managers in any other department. This responsibility has had too little emphasis in the past in terms of sound management practices. The chapter on annual budgetary planning provides specific help in this area.

THE NURSING PROCESS AND THE MANAGEMENT PROCESS

During recent decades a great amount of attention has been devoted to defining the practice of nursing. These efforts have been complicated by the variety of changes that have kept nursing in a state of flux. Within a single generation, nurses have seen their responsibilities analyzed, subdivided, broadened, delimited, reorganized, unionized, and role-expanded so often that they can be forgiven if their view of nursing at times seems cloudy and uncertain.

During this period, however, a clearly-defined and well-accepted framework for nursing emerged. This framework is the nursing process. Its significance is underscored by the new Standard IV for Nursing Services of the Joint Commission on Accreditation of Hospitals (JCAH), effective January 1, 1980: "Individualized, goal-directed nursing care shall be provided to patients through the use of the nursing process'' (Accreditation Manual for Hospitals, 1979; see Appendix K). The process includes four phases: assessing, planning, implementing, and evaluating. While the nursing process is an excellent and useful conceptualization of what nurses do, too often the process is not understood or practiced successfully by the nurses themselves. Reasons for this vary, but include educational, organizational, and philosophical deficiencies. Our purpose now is to compare the nursing process to the management process and identify the common source of each.

Ruth Mrozek makes a useful comparison by showing how the nursing process and the problem-oriented charting system are modelled on the pattern of the scientific method (Mrozek, 1973). This is the problem-finding, problem-solving pattern of (1) gathering and interpreting information so that a problem can be clearly defined; (2) considering alternatives for action, making a decision, and developing an action plan; (3) implementing the plan; and (4) evaluating the results, and continuing the cycle of progress toward meeting the patient's problems and needs.

The accompanying diagram of Figure 1-4 portrays the parallel patterns and cyclical relationship of the nursing process, the problem-oriented chart-

---

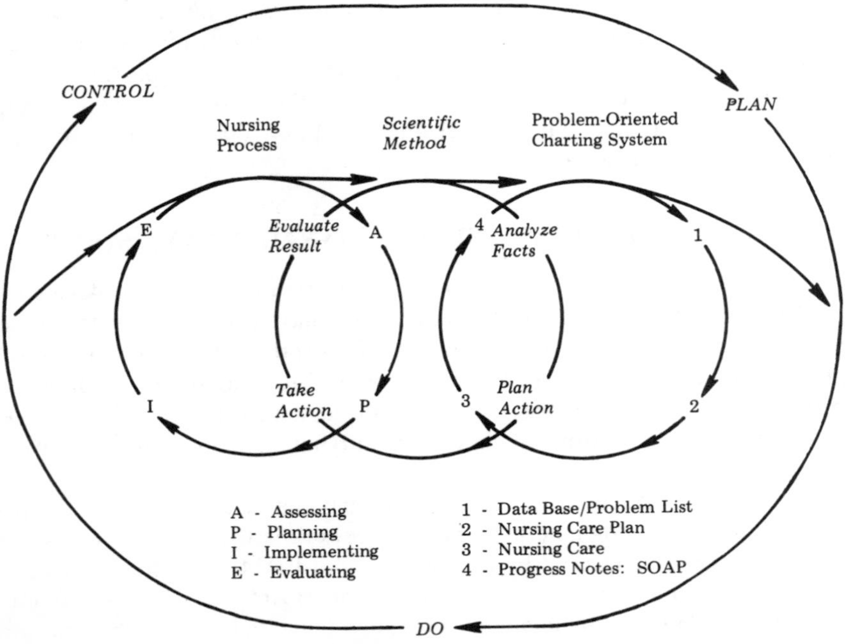

Figure 1-4 An Integrative Functional Comparison of Process, Method, and System

ing system and the scientific method. The three cyclical models are set in the integrative concept of the basic management functions of planning, doing, and controlling. Clearly, the four steps of the scientific method are the core of this diagram. After the term "scientific management" became popular early in this century, it was often described as the four steps of planning, organizing, directing, and controlling. We have used the simpler modern version of three basic functions of the management process shown in the figure as the encompassing cycle that is our theme.

This model is introduced at this point because it is so fundamental to the conceptual structure which we are building with you. Later chapters elaborate upon the various elements of the model. One of the reasons that many good nurses perform so well as good nurse managers is that they have been so well educated in the use of the scientific method. Scientific management is based soundly in the scientific method. And the essence of scientific management is measurement plus control. Clearly the nursing process and the problem-oriented nursing system are specific applications of the management, or scientific, process. The framework for nursing today and tomorrow has evolved beyond the nursing process per se. The nursing process is a component of the problem-oriented nursing system (PONS) which in turn is a necessary part of the patient care process (see Table 3-1 in Chapter 3). The components of PONS, in nurse-management terminology, involve the selective adaptation and use of functions, techniques, and skills directed toward meeting patient/client needs.

THE TRANSITION TO MANAGER

The difference between being a *nurse* manager and a nurse *manager* is more than a matter of semantics. A primary nurse working with a limited number of patients uses the management process is providing and managing the care of those patients. The emphasis is on a personal application of the nursing process while providing guidance and leadership to other members of the patient care team as a secondary responsibility. A head nurse, however, or a patient care coordinator responsible for several units, necessarily has to place major emphasis on the personnel management aspects of the work. Clinical skills are still necessary and important, but the management skills must at the very least be of equal importance.

The career change from being a professional nurse to becoming a professional nurse manager is a big step. For many persons it is the most significant step in a nursing career. The nurse manager is still a member of a patient care team. But now, instead of being one of many persons under the direction of someone else, the manager is the someone else—the person in charge of and responsible for coordinating the work of the other team members (in a unit, section, or department). It is a change from a job status which is primarily one of doing the work oneself to one which involves getting work done through others.

Involved here is a basic change in one's way of thinking. The manager can no longer think only in terms of my work and my job. The manager's concern is about our work and our jobs. No longer are you responsible just for your own work, facilities, and equipment. Now you are responsible for the work, facilities, and equipment of all the nursing personnel on your unit. You may even feel that you have assumed responsibility for the people themselves, your most important asset outside of yourself. And in a way you have. But in another sense you have been given an opportunity to help your people become more responsible for themselves. This opportunity is one of your greatest challenges. It can be met through the ways you shape the working environment and personnel relationships, the ways in which you utilize your human-mode and technical-mode skills. It can mean using the job enrichment concept described by M. Scott Myers in *Every Employee a Manager* (Myers, 1970). Myers explains how the customary ideas about what a manager does (planning, organizing, leading, controlling) compared with the traditional role of the worker (doing manual labor) have contributed to the management/labor gap.

In the traditional organization this view of role relationships has been held by managers and workers alike. Managers are the ones who have been presumed to have the maturity, knowledge, ability, and responsibility to plan, direct, and control what the workers do. And the members of the labor force appear to have been perceived as uninformed, immature, irresponsible, and less intelligent. The result of these commonly held views about the role of managers as compared with the role of the labor group has led to understandable feelings of social distance, of alienation, of differing needs and concerns. While a certain number of such feelings may seem inevitable, many modern managers are finding ways to decrease such feelings and close the management/labor gap.

Myers comments on the role of labor unions in formalizing and widening the gap between the employer and the employees. But he sees two major forces at work to close or eliminate the gap between labor and management. One such force is the rising socioeconomic status of the less privileged members of the employee group, accompanied by rising expectations. The second force is an increasing awareness and acceptance by managers of the democratic pattern in organizational leadership. Myers presents his concept of the enriched job for all employees—not just the manager group—as one that includes the planning and control functions as well as the doing (Figure 1-5).

This is a way to encourage and permit more employees to think for themselves. It encourages more creativity. It permits a wider range of doing. It

Figure 1-5 Meaningful Work Model

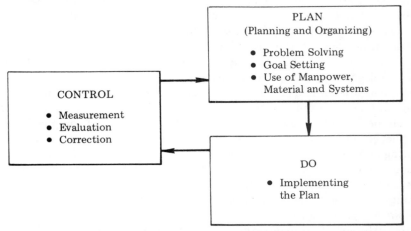

Source: M. S. Myers, *Every Employee a Manager.* New York: McGraw-Hill, 1970, p. 70. Reprinted with permission from McGraw-Hill Book Co.

places more trust in the employee. It builds more interest, self-respect, and pride. In short, job enrichment as envisioned here helps each person to meet his own needs more fully through, and because of, the successful achievement of agency and patient objectives.

As a professional nurse you may never have experienced the feeling of being on the labor side of the management/labor gap. But if you have had that experience at any time during your career, so much the better. It can assist you in having greater empathy for your employees at all job levels. And it may encourage you to learn more of the leadership skills and management techniques that permit all employees to use their maximum capabilities in the kind of enriched job structure that leads to greater self-direction, self-control, and accountability as well as better patient care.

A hospital provides a natural setting for the application of the job enrichment concept. In nursing, many persons already have the experience of managing their own jobs. It is implicit in the earlier discussion of the parallel models of the nursing process and the management process. But nonnurses usually have not been trained in the four steps of the nursing process, and do not have the privilege of using it. And many nurses do not use it either. This may be due to their own lack of initiative or because of the kind of leadership they receive. Some nursing administrators do an injustice to themselves, their patients, and their staff members by placing too little emphasis on the nursing process, the problem-oriented system, and team-building using modern management concepts. Often such administrators understand and agree with the need for these things but fail to implement them successfully because of a blockage in the affective area (emotions and feelings), or because of a leadership style that is too firmly fixed at the authoritarian end of the scale. Such a style is characterized by telling, in contrast to the facilitating behavior of a goal-oriented leader. Between these two styles are varying degrees of selling and involving.

Authoritarian leaders tend to make their own decisions with a minimum of consultation. They tell staff members what to do and how to do it or they try to sell their people on a course of action. They seek prompt compliance and obedience. Goal-oriented leaders usually involve their people in problem solving and decision making whenever possible. They seek self-direction and responsibility from staff members. They are facilitative managers in the sense of making themselves available for help, materials, information—for whatever the staff members need for patient care purposes, for doing satisfactory and satisfying work. The most skillful managers (whether authority-oriented or goal-oriented by inclination) are able to use the basic appropriate combination of telling, selling, involving, and facilitating as suitable to the needs of particular situations.

A nurse manager's leadership style is affected strongly by the kinds of bosses he or she has had in the past who provided early role models. Another influence is the kind of transition the nurse manager achieved in moving from staff nursing into management. For most persons, the necessary change in one's way of thinking referred to earlier does not happen automatically. It has to be learned. Habit patterns are strong. New habits and skills—managerial habits and skills—must be developed and used. Admittedly, professional nurses are likely to make the transition to manager more easily than other healthcare workers. Nurses have carried legal responsibility for their actions and the actions of those coworkers whom they direct. Nurses have learned to understand and accept personal responsibility and liability. Yet when nurses elect to shift from the clinical track to the management track, an adjustment in orientation and performance becomes necessary. Part of the adjustment involves regular reading of management literature. This includes such periodicals as *The Journal of Nursing Administration, Supervisor Nurse, Modern Healthcare, Health Care Management Review, Nursing Administration Quarterly,* and the ever-growing number of clinical journals focused on the clinical specialties.

As a nurse manager you may also wish to expand your membership in professional associations to include such groups as the Society for Advancement of Management, the American Society for Training and Development, or the Association for Humanistic Psychology. Like many other nurse managers you will discover that selective reading of management journals and books and active participation in one or more management groups help with your own self-development as a manager, consciously direct your attention to broad management problems and ways of resolving them, and assist in your change in thinking from professional clinical nurse to professional nurse manager—your big step.

As a manager, your focus is on productive action in achieving desired results through people. This means using their creative talents. These words are just as meaningful for a director of nursing service and a hospital administrator as they are for a new unit nurse manager. Fully understood, this generalized definition of your purpose means that you have to meet patient care goals by guiding the nursing staff into effective action, helping your people attain agency objectives, aiding your people in satisfying their own personal needs, counseling with staff members regarding their performance results, encouraging people to greater self-development and growth, and allowing the staff to use their creative talents.

Surveys and interviews conducted with agency personnel at all levels have told us what their concerns are. These concerns include just about everything from benefits, communications, and job satisfaction to supervisory relations, training, and unions. But there are five which are mentioned most frequently, especially by technical and professional people.

These major concerns are:

1. Relations Between Nurse Manager and Nursing Staff: General rapport; performance reviews; professional guidance.
2. Wage and Salary Administration: Hiring pay vs. pay for performance; understanding agency policy; merit vs. general increases.
3. Mobility: Opportunities for advancement, reassignment, and transfer.
4. Utilization: Good use of education, experience, and abilities; a chance to make a contribution.
5. Recognition: Sense of status; a feeling that my boss knows my worth as a person, and shows it.

These are vital concerns—for the staff, the organization, and patients. Better understanding and improvements can occur only with the help of every individual nurse manager and others with agency leadership responsibility.

THE NEW WORLD OF MANAGER-EMPLOYEE RELATIONS

Let's face it; it's a changing world we live in. For some of us, it changes too fast; for others, not fast enough. Some see the changes as for the better; others, for the worse. Some of us adapt readily to change; others find it more difficult. But saddest of all are those who appear to see no change; or those who, seeing it, recognize no need to adapt to it. One of the significant changes that affects your job as a nurse manager has to do with the nature of those persons you must lead today. Consider today's new generation of employees. Compared with an older generation, your newer staff members tend to be better educated with higher levels of technical knowledge; they have a higher sense of security and high expectations; they question the values of the previous generation; they see interpersonal relations as either open, honest, and trusting—or characterized by suspicion, dishonesty, and distrust; they may view managers as restrictive and exploitative; they resist manipulation, seek involvement, and take pride in individual accomplishment; they desire to use their full range of abilities and are hostile toward a confining job environment; and they are unwilling to adapt to hypocritical standards of behavior and value concepts.

These facts of your employee environment, together with other changes you can identify, mean that your job as a nurse manager is likely to be challenging and exciting. Sometimes your people will be aggravating to work with and difficult to manage, but they will be interesting and exciting to lead. They will respond, create, grow, and help you—given the opportunity. Most will take responsibility, and you can hold them accountable for it. They'll do a good job for you—if you give them a good job to do. If you are newly promoted as a nurse manager, you are likely to be more fully responsive to the opinions, needs, and feelings of your people now than you will be ever again. One reason for this is that you have so recently been one of them. The coming weeks, months, and years will involve you more and more in concerns of nursing management—objectives, costs, budgets, reports, conferences, quality—to mention a few. These may tend to lessen your responsiveness to your people and their needs to feel secure, respected, recognized, worthwhile, and growing. Protect yourself against this usual trend, since your real success as a nurse manager will come from being able to help your people satisfy their goals and needs through the process of contributing to unit and departmental objectives. You have to do it your own way. That's first. Be true to yourself. Don't try to fit someone else's mold. At the same time, don't miss opportunities to learn better ways to manage. Sharpen your leadership skills. Learn from others. Learn by practicing the best methods. For example, here's something to add to your management tool kit right now. Use it the next time you have a problem to resolve. Make it part of the usual steps of getting facts, defining the problem, developing alternative solutions, taking action, and following through.

Problems are caused by persons who...
- Don't Know—and who need—Job Knowledge
- Can't Do—and who need—Job Skills

- Don't Care—and who need—Self-motivation, through need satisfaction.

Problems are resolved by persons who . . .
- Consult with others for facts, feelings, and opinions;
- Explore the problem (ask, listen, and discuss);
- Agree upon what will be done;
- Set objectives (for achievement)
- Set a date (for completion)
- Evaluate (for results).

You learn by doing, especially when you practice the best methods. These simple steps, and their more complete presentation in subsequent pages, can help you to:

- Relate and respond to the persons you lead, to recognize and build upon their value systems, dislike of hypocrisy, desire for a sense of community, contribution, and achievement.
- Contribute to improved handling of major concerns of your people: supervisory-subordinate relations (rapport through rapping, honest goal-oriented performance reviews, self-development guidance); salary administration (pay increases when deserved; explanation of reasons when not possible); utilization (achieving full people-potential by making good use of their education and special abilities); recognition (overt action, regularly, to help others meet their needs for status and sense of self-worth).
- Perform your management functions—planning, doing, controlling—most effectively.

THE TRADEMARKS OF A REAL PROFESSIONAL

What makes a person a real professional? Are you a *real pro* in your field? We decided a few years ago to establish for ourselves a set of criteria having general applicability to any field of human endeavor. Then, at rare intervals, we have awarded a suitably engraved certificate to qualifying persons. An accompanying letter includes an appropriate explanation. While originally inspired by a touch of whimsy, we are entirely serious about the significance of the criteria and the award. We hope that you, the reader, feel that you are ready to qualify as a real professional nurse manager—or that the time will come when you will advise us that you are so qualified to receive the award and the following message:

You are cordially welcomed as a newly elected member of PRO, the Realistic Order of Professionals. Your name has been inscribed in the Great Book of the Order, recording for posterity this well-deserved honor and recognition. Henceforth and forevermore you, as A REAL PRO, are entitled to use after your name the distinctive designation reserved for members of the Order in good standing: PRO. May you always continue to exemplify in your life and work the characteristics that have led to your nomination and acceptance into the fellowship of the Order.

Trademarks of a Real Professional

Knowledge: You know your field of activity thoroughly. You have studied and worked to gain your knowledge and are not likely to be fooled or bluffed about your field.

Experience: You have much meaningful experience. You have been exposed to the tough situations and can react spontaneously with the right response.

Skill: You are an expert. You do a top quality job. You out-perform the amateurs. You have learned the best method, practiced it, and can deliver in the pinches.

Confidence: Your abilities and knowledge have bred a justifiable confidence. It shows. Others respect it. Your confidence is not only in yourself, but in your fellow team workers.

Mobility: You are fully mobile. You are secure in your ability, and have no concern for job security as such. You are welcome on anybody's team.

Performance: You like to win. You use all of your talents to come out on top, to get the results you can be proud of.

Recognition: You get much satisfaction from your work, and you are realistic about your own worth. You know that adequate compensation takes many forms.

Leadership: You are willing to provide leadership in your field, devoting a portion of your time and effort to this end, to be known as a giver rather than a taker. You see the value and need of service *pro bono publico.*

NOTES

Ainsworth, T. J., Jr. The statement of mission: Essential ingredient in planning. *Trustee*, September 1976, 34–36.

Appley, L. *A management concept.* New York: American Management Association, 1969.

Argyris, C. *An introduction to interaction theory and field theory.* New Haven, Conn.: Yale University, Labor and Management Center, 1952.

Argyris, C. Conditions for competence acquisition and therapy. *Journal of Applied Behavior Science*, 1968, *4*, 147-179.

Cherry, L. Medical technology: The new revolution. *New York Times Magazine*, August 5, 1979, 12-22.

Ganong, J., & Ganong, W. The head nurse as hospital integrator. *Supervisor Nurse*, March 1977, *8* (3), 27-39.

Ganong, J., Ganong, W., & Huenefeld, J. Motive force: A key to evaluating nurse managers. *Journal of Nursing Administration*, July-August 1974, 17-19.

Golightly, C. *HELP with career planning: A workbook for nurses*. Chapel Hill, N.C.: W. L. Ganong Co., 1979.

Joint Commission on Accreditation of Hospitals. *Accreditation manual for hospitals* (1980 ed.). Chicago: Author, 1979.

Lewin, K. *A dynamic theory of personality*. New York: McGraw-Hill, 1935.

Lewin, K. *Field theory in social science*. New York: Harper and Row, 1951.

Mrozek, R. Incorporating the nursing process into the problem-oriented record. In H. K. Walker, J. W. Hurst, & M. F. Woody (Eds.), *Applying the problem-oriented system*. New York: Medcom Press, 1973, pp. 355-357.

Myers, M. S. *Every employee a manager*. New York: McGraw-Hill, 1970, pp. 55-95.

Rokeach, M. *The nature of human values*. New York: The Free Press, 1973.

Ross, J. The resources of binocular perception. *Scientific American*, March 1976, *234*(3), 80-86.

Yalom, I. D. *The theory and practice of group psychotherapy* (2nd ed.). New York: Basic Books, 1975.

Reading List

Books

A discursive dictionary of health care. Washington, D.C.: U.S. Government Printing Office, 1976.

Albanese, R. *Management: Toward accountability for performance*. Homewood, Ill.: Richard D. Irwin, 1975.

Anderson, P. *Nurse*. New York: St. Martin's Press, 1978.

Argyris, C. *Personality and organization*. New York: Harper & Row, 1957.

Arndt, C., & Huckabay, L. *Nursing administration: Theory for practice with a systems approach*. St. Louis: C. V. Mosby, 1975.

Bennett, A. C. *Improving management performance in health care institutions: A total systems approach*. Chicago: American Hospital Association, 1978.

Combs, A. W., Avila, D. L., & Purkey, W. W. *Helping relationships: Basic concepts for the helping professions*. Boston: Allyn and Bacon, 1971.

Cunningham, R. N., Jr. *Governing hospitals: Trustees and the new accountabilities*. Chicago: American Hospital Association, 1975.

DiVincenti, M. *Administering nursing service* (2nd ed.). Boston: Little, Brown, 1977.

Dowling, W. (Ed.). *Effective management and the behavioral sciences*. New York: AMACOM, 1978.

Drucker, P. *Management: Tasks, responsibilities, practices*. New York: Harper & Row, 1974.

Frankel, V. *Man's search for meaning*. New York: Simon & Shuster, 1970.

Ganong, J., & Ganong, W. *HELP for the head nurse: A management guide* (2nd ed.). Chapel Hill, N.C.: W. L. Ganong Co., 1975.

Ganong, J., & Ganong, W. *Cases in nursing management*. Germantown, Md.: Aspen Systems Corp., 1979.

Goble, F. *The third force: The psychology of Abraham Maslow*. New York: Grossman, 1970.

Goble, F. *Excellence in leadership*. New York: American Management Association, 1972.

Golightly, C. *HELP with career planning: A workbook for nurses*. Chapel Hill, N.C.: W. L. Ganong Co., 1979.

Haimann, T. *Supervisory management for health care institutions*. St. Louis: The Catholic Hospital Association, 1973.

Hampden-Turner, C. *Radical man*. Cambridge, Mass.: Schankman, 1970.

Hersey, P., & Blanchard, K. *Management of organizational behavior* (2nd ed.). Englewood Cliffs, N.J.: Prentice-Hall, 1972.

Herzberg, F., Mausner, B., Peterson, R. O., & Capwell, D. F. *Job attitudes: Review of research opinion*. Pittsburgh: Psychological Service of Pittsburgh, 1957.

Joint Commission on Accreditation of Hospitals. *Accreditation manual for hospitals* (1980 ed.). Chicago: Author, 1980.

Jourard, S. *Personal adjustment*. New York: Macmillan, 1963.

Jourard, S. *The transparent self*. Princeton, N.J.: Van Nostrand, 1964.

Kirschenbaum, H. *Advanced value clarification*. La Jolla, Ca.: University Associates, 1977.

Kraegel, J., Mousseau, V., Goldsmith, C., & Arora, R. *Patient care systems*. Philadelphia: J. B. Lippincott, 1974.

Lewin, K. *Field theory in social science*. (Dorwin Cartwright, Ed.). New York: Harper and Brothers, 1951.

Likert, R. *The human organization: Its management and value*. New York: McGraw-Hill, 1967.

Marriner, A. *The nursing process*. St. Louis: C. V. Mosby, 1975.

Marriner, A. Leadership and management. In A. Marriner (Ed.), *Current perspectives in nursing management*. St. Louis: C. V. Mosby, 1979.

Maslow, A. *Eupsychian management*. Homewood, Ill.: The Dorsey Press, 1965.

Maslow, A. *Toward a psychology of being*. Princeton: Van Nostrand, 1968.

Maslow, A. *Motivation and personality* (2nd ed.). New York: Harper & Row, 1970.

Maslow, A. *The farther reaches of human nature*. New York: Viking Press, 1971.

Maher, J. (Ed.). *New perspectives in job enrichment*. New York: Van Nostrand Reinhold, 1971.

McConkey, D. D. *No nonsense delegation*. New York: AMACOM, 1979.

McCool, B., & Brown, M. *The management response: Conceptual, technical and human skills of health administration*. Philadelphia: W. B. Saunders, 1977.

McGregor, D. *The human side of enterprise*. New York: McGraw-Hill, 1960.

Meissner, W. "Theories of personality." *The Harvard Guide to Modern Psychiatry*. (A. M. Nicholi, Ed.). Cambridge, Mass.: The Belknap Press of Harvard University, 1978.

Myers, M. S. *Every employee a manager: More meaningful work through job enrichment*. New York: McGraw-Hill, 1970.

Ornstein, R. *The psychology of consciousness*. San Francisco: W. H. Freeman, 1972.

Ornstein, R. *The mind field*. New York: Grossman, 1976.

Powell, J. *Why am I afraid to tell you who I am?* Niles, Ill.: Argus Communications, 1969.

Shanks, M. D., & Kennedy, D. A. *Administration in nursing*. (2nd ed.). New York: McGraw-Hill, 1970.

Simon, S., Howe, L. W., & Kirschenbaum, H. *Values clarification*. New York: Hart Publishing Co., 1972.

Stevens, B. J. *The nurse as executive*. Wakefield, Mass.: Contemporary Publishing, 1975.

Stevens, W. *Management and leadership in nursing*. New York: McGraw-Hill, 1978.

Tarrant, J. *Drucker: The man who invented the corporate society*. New York: Warner, 1976.

Walker, H. K., Hurst, J. W., & Woody, M. F. (Eds.). *Applying the problem-oriented system*. New York: Medcom Press, 1973.

Yura, H., Ozimek, D., & Walsh, M. B. *Nursing leadership: Theory and process*. New York: Appleton-Century-Crofts, 1976.

Articles

Bennett, A. New thinking required for development of management effectiveness. *Hospitals*, 1976, *50*(4), 67–70.

Boccuzzi, N. K. Head nurse growth: A priority for the supervisor. *American Journal of Nursing*, August 1979, *79*(8), 1389–1392.

Brown, B. (Ed.). Organization nurses in action. *Nursing Administration Quarterly, 3*(2), entire issue.

Carper, B. A. The ethics of caring. *Advances in Nursing Science*, 1979, *1*(3), 11–19.

Ferguson, M. (Ed.). *Brain-Mind Bulletin* (Los Angeles: Interface Press), published semimonthly. This bulletin may be obtained from the publisher, P.O. Box 42211, Los Angeles, Ca. 90042.

Ganong, J., & Ganong, W. Good advice: Coping with the changing role of the nurse. *Journal of Nursing Administration*, 1972, *2*(2), 8.

Ganong, J., & Ganong, W. Are head nurses obsolete? *Journal of Nursing Administration*, 1975, *5*(7), 16–18.

Kinsella, C. Nursing. *Hospitals,* April 1, 1975, *49*(7), 101–105.

Nuckolls, K. B. Who decides what the nurse can do? *Nursing Outlook*, October 1974, *22*, 626–631.

Sargent, A. The androgynous manager. *Supervisor Nurse*, March 1979, *10*(3), 23–30.

Uustal, D. Values clarification in nursing: Application to practice. *American Journal of Nursing*, December 1978, *78*, 2057–2063.

Chapter 2

A Framework for Nursing Management

NEW IMPACTS ON YOUR CHANGING WORKWORLD

Chapter 1 examined the role of the nurse in the organization. It presented our reasons for saying that every nurse is a manager—whether serving in a clinical capacity or in an identified managerial role. This chapter continues the same emphasis with a specific focus on the nurse as a member of a division of nursing in a modern hospital setting.

This chapter's focus takes on added significance in view of the publication of the expanded standards for nursing services as published in the Accreditation Manual for Hospitals, 1980 Edition, of the Joint Commission for the Accreditation of Hospitals (JCAH). These standards are reproduced in Appendix K. Included also are the introductory pages of the JCAH Manual. These pages provide a review of the purpose and history of JCAH, and an explanation of the standards development and implementation process. It is highly relevant reading for every nurse manager.

Figure 2-1 expands on the workworld diagram featured in Chapter 1. Still at the center of the workworld is you, the individual. Surrounding you is the framework for nursing management in your healthcare agency, shown in the diagram as a square. We will return to this framework after examining the internal and external environments that directly influence the nursing management framework and each individual within it.

The Internal Environment

The most obvious component of one's internal environment is the department or unit to which one reports for work every day. This department or section, whether large or small, has a particular physical location with its own unique characteristics. The department is comprised of a number of in-

Figure 2-1 My Workworld and the Nursing Management Framework

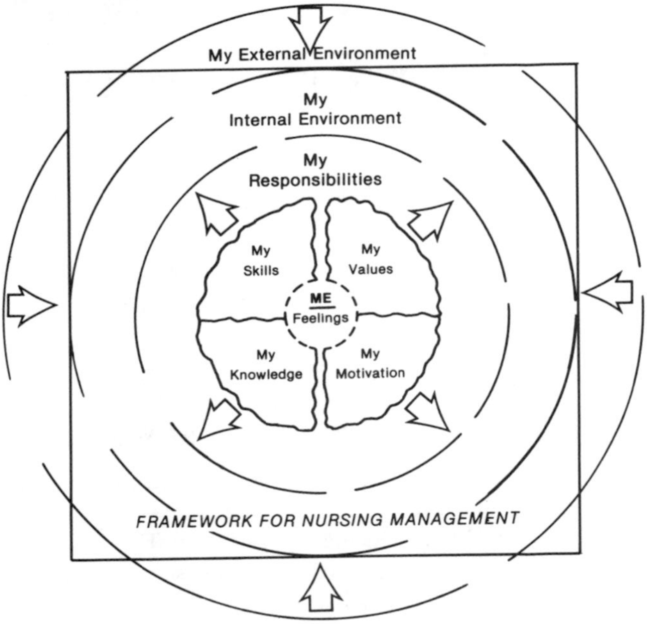

My External Environment

My
Internal Environment

My
Responsibilities

My
Skills

My
Values

ME
Feelings

My
Knowledge

My
Motivation

FRAMEWORK FOR NURSING MANAGEMENT

Source: Adapted from Figure 1–2 by the authors.

dividuals with whom you interact most frequently. This social organization of which you are a part has the most immediate impact on your personal workworld. Similarly, it is within this particular social group that you are most likely to exert your greatest personal influence.

In a hospital, and in many other types of healthcare agencies, the continuing ebb and flow of other persons through your workworld location adds complex dimensions to your internal environment. These other persons may be members of the medical staff, patients, members of other hospital departments, and a wide variety of other visitors. Added to this is the fact that while a great majority of the persons coming and going through your workworld have only a single-shift, or perhaps a two-shift relationship to you and your coworkers, the nursing department itself has the ongoing twenty-four-hours-a-day, seven-days-a-week responsibility for the patients and for patient services.

Someone shared with us a graphic way of summarizing nursing's ongoing responsibility. It was along the following lines:

> Just stop and think for a moment. Ever since this hospital opened
> its doors so many years ago, there has never been a time at any hour

of the day or night when there hasn't been a registered nurse on duty responsible for the continuity of care for each and every patient. Nursing is probably the only department about which this can be said with accuracy.

The medical staff exerts the chief influence within the internal environment. "Physicians hold the key to both costs and quality of care because of their status, power and daily decisions. All other staff provide data for, respond to, or support physicians' decisions" (Weisbord & Stoelwinder, 1979). Every experienced nurse manager can affirm the truth of this statement. Any hospital exists to provide patient care. And it is the physicians whose decisions control admissions, length of stay, and (ultimately) the cost per patient day. The physicians' influence is felt directly by each nurse through the doctors' orders and in a variety of other direct and indirect ways.

Other components of the internal environment are all the other hospital departments that interface with nursing. These include those departments—such as dietary, housekeeping, laboratory, central supply, laundry—whose employees appear regularly on the patient care units. Other departments—admissions, the business office, maintenance, and radiology—may be less in evidence but also have a strong impact as part of the hospital environment. Each department influences every nurse manager's problem solving and decision making.

The External Environment

Recent years have seen many changes in the external environment, including population characteristics, new medical technology, increased government regulation, and healthcare economics, all of which generate new pressures on the healthcare system. The healthcare system is receiving increased attention from both the public and private sectors, heightening the impact of environmental factors on healthcare agencies and nursing management. The nurse manager who has a working knowledge of these factors is in a key position to influence the healthcare delivery system. Consider the following factors in connection with the workworld diagram.

Community

The health status profile of our society is changing. There is a declining birth rate, a growing older population, and increased life expectancy (U.S. DHEW, 1978). The general public is now more urban, better educated, more affluent, and subject to new health hazards. Social problems include increases in drug addiction, alcoholism, environmental pollution, cancer, venereal disease, cardiovascular disease, deaths from suicide and homicide, and accidents (U.S. DHEW, 1978). These factors influence the types of services and programs required in each community, with corresponding effect on nursing management.

Sociocultural

Society's orientation to health is different today from that of earlier years. People view health not just as the absence of disease, but also as the individual's capacity to live most happily and productively. More emphasis is being directed toward primary care and how to stay well than on secondary and tertiary care. The consumer no longer sees the traditional medical system as the only answer. There are a growing number of alternatives to the traditional system. These include more extensive home health care, health maintenance organizations, free clinics, the hospice movement, and a variety of alternatives falling under the rubric of wellness, self-care, self-help, and holistic health. While the traditional system and the alternative modes have been very separate, there is some evidence that shows a slow integration of the two. It seems that our healthcare system could utilize the two philosophies to the betterment of patient care. Some nurses are incorporating alternatives in their patient teaching—i.e., meditation as an adjunct to drug and diet therapy for hypertension.

Economic

No one needs to be reminded of the increasing costs of healthcare. During the past decade the cost of healthcare has been rising at a rate two and one-half times that of the general economy (Cost containment suspended, 1978). Factors influencing rising costs include: present reimbursement mechanisms, physician-dominated decisions as to the nature and extent of services for consumers, lack of rewards in the system for efficiency and cost-reducing innovations, heavy government support of healthcare, increased technology, increased public expectations, and increased malpractice suits. This has forced the federal government to focus on the hospital as the major battleground for cost containment efforts.

While there is much opposition to mandatory cost containment from the hospital industry, there has been a voluntary effort to keep costs down by the American Hospital Association, the Catholic Hospital Association, the American Medical Association, and the Federated Hospital Association. In addition, an increasing number of states have implemented a mandatory rate review system. The long-range strategy of cost containment is to restructure the supply and services through regional planning and the use of alternative delivery systems; to reorient provider practices through incentive reimbursement and utilization review; and to reorient individual demand and behavior through cost sharing and health education. Individual nurses can also contribute to cost containment efforts. To manage a cost-effective patient unit or department, the nurse manager must consider what effect the following items have on the nursing budget: supplies, equipment, personnel policies, hiring practices, type of staffing, and the modality of nursing being practiced.

Business

Technology has invaded the healthcare field from all sides, causing increased costs and increased specialization of providers. As each new or improved piece of equipment comes on the market, every hospital (or its medical staff) wants to have it in the name of better quality patient care. Meanwhile the cost to the patient keeps soaring. The Computer Assisted Tomographic (CAT) Scanner is a prime example. In spite of all of this spending, the Office of Technology Assessment reports that 80 to 90 percent of the medical procedures that cost vast amounts of money have never been proven beneficial (Medical practice called, 1978).

Political

The healthcare industry, once the country's largest unregulated industry, has become one of the country's most regulated industries. Hospitals have to deal with regulations concerning the numbers and kinds of beds and/or services, Professional Standard Review Organizations (PSROs), and utilization review. The Mandatory Certificate of Need (CON) process is an example. The term "Certificate of Need" has become part of the everyday jargon in hospitals. It comes up whenever the hospital wants to add beds or services, buy expensive diagnostic and therapeutic equipment, or undertake a project which will exceed the capital expenditure level stipulated by the state. These decisions are no longer the prerogative of the individual hospital. First the hospital must develop a document that supports the need for the project. Then the local Health Systems Agency (HSA) review board, and later the state planning agency, decide whether the hospital can move ahead with its plan. Many hospitals try to avoid this process by seeking an exemption, or if dissatisfied with the planning agency's decision, by appealing to a higher authority.

Any CON decision contains many factors that will directly affect nursing. If a CON is approved for a new intensive care unit, more nurses will be needed (availability is another question). If an HSA acts to close a unit because there are too many such units in the area, some nurses may lose their jobs. Therefore nursing input is needed during the development of a CON and during the hearings with the HSA and state review boards. Nurses need to participate on the HSA review boards to provide a nursing perspective.

International

The international component of your external environment has become increasingly important. Decisions on the international scene can influence the energy supply for your hospital, the delivery of needed supplies, the construction schedule for an addition or new facility, and even hospital ownership.

Government

Since 1946 when the Hill-Burton Act was passed, the government has been gradually entering the healthcare field. The Hill-Burton Act provided monies to construct hospitals to meet the demand for more beds. In return, hospitals provided certain services for those who could not afford to pay for hospital care. In the mid-1960s, Medicare and Medicaid legislation supplied monies for certain groups of people so they would have better access to care. Another government move was to establish Regional Medical Programs to deal with prominent health problems (cancer, heart disease, etc.). Governmental efforts to establish better health planning were implemented in 1966 when Comprehensive Health Planning Agencies were set up throughout the country. In the 1970s hospitals were dealing with Professional Standard Review Organizations and Health Systems Agencies.

The PSROs were set up in 1972 under an amendment to the Social Security Act. The purpose was to promote effective, efficient, economical delivery of healthcare services of proper quality, and a means to provide public accountability for healthcare. At the institutional level, nurses work toward quality assurance as members of a utilization review team. Their focus is the review of *medical* care, not *nursing* care. Certainly if the intent of the PSRO is to control costs while assuring quality care, nursing services must be reviewed (Bauknecht, 1977). The rationale behind PSROs gives all nurse managers a good reason to question whether patients receive a type of care appropriate for the setting.

With the passage of the National Health Planning and Resources Development Act in 1974, the country was divided into 205 health service areas, each with a Health Systems Agency. The HSA has two broad functions: to develop a Health Systems Plan (Annual Implementation Plan) for the area, and to review the need for new expenditures and the appropriateness of existing services. The HSAs were intended to address the following problems: rising costs, uneven quality of care, and unequal access to healthcare.

Decisions made by HSAs can have tremendous impact on the future of a hospital, and on its nursing department. Nurse managers have an important and worthwhile contribution to make through direct involvement with HSAs.

HSAs are said to be the stepping stone to National Health Insurance (NHI), an idea that has been around since the 1930s. Varied proposals have been introduced in Congress each year, but none of them mentions nursing. Mauksch, a nurse member of the Advisory Committee on National Health Insurance, stresses that registered nurses need to be recognized as providers, and that reimbursement of nursing services is a critical issue in any proposal (Mauksch, 1978). At the institutional and national levels, nurses can serve themselves well by becoming involved in the legislative process and making their voices heard on NHI and other healthcare legislation.

Witness such developments as the following at the state level during 1979. The Maryland General Assembly passed a law that requires insurance companies to provide reimbursement "for any service which is within the lawful scope of practice of a duly licensed healthcare provider." Nurse practitioners were already eligible for such reimbursement through an act passed by the assembly earlier in 1979 (Reimbursement for all, 1979). Effective January 1, 1980, California RNs may own up to 49 percent of professional medical corporations as a result of favorable action by the California legislature. The original state law limited medical corporation ownership to physicians; in 1977 psychologists were included via an amendment. Jean Moorhead, an RN member of the California Assembly, introduced the new amendment that now includes registered nurses (California law lets nurses share, 1979).

Professional

Changes in the nursing profession over the last two decades are a significant feature of the external environment. These changes ultimately affect each nurse practitioner in every type of healthcare setting. Issues of great importance include credentialing, entry into practice, mandatory continuing education, and collective bargaining.

Credentialing (licensing, certification, and accreditation) has become a topic for investigation not only from within the profession but also by groups outside the nursing profession. The main issue here is public accountability and social protection. The public wants to know whether the multiple, elaborate, inconsistent, and expensive mechanisms in credentialing do in fact protect the public or the provider. The credentialing study sponsored by the American Nursing Association (ANA) has been completed and its recommendations may help bring about some order to the credentialing process.

What educational background does a person need to enter the practice of nursing? This question has been debated for years. Once again in 1978, the

ANA House of Delegates endorsed the position that persons need a baccalaureate degree in nursing to enter into practice. Many state associations are following suit and endorsing the same or a similar resolution. However, the details of how to legislate and implement such a resolution have not yet been developed. There is no doubt that this issue carries many emotional overtones that will be heard at all levels of nursing practice. The nurse manager has to cope with this issue while maintaining good working relationships among the nursing staff and carrying out the goals of the nursing department and the healthcare agency.

Mandatory continuing education is one way to assure the public of the continued competence of practicing nurses. This issue was hotly debated in the mid-1970s. Now the notion is more generally accepted and increasing numbers of states are legislating it in their nurse practice acts. The focus now turns to how the nursing department is going to handle decisions on educational leave time, reimbursement for continuing education, and education that can be provided within the institution. A larger question is how nursing will control the quality of continuing education classes being offered.

Collective bargaining is a well-established fact in nursing. As the ANA, through the state professional associations, moved into the bargaining agent position, it diluted its original identity as a professional association and is often referred to as a union. For this very reason, many nurses in administrative positions felt forced to resign their ANA memberships. There is much question as to whether the ANA can be successful at both professional and bargaining functions without a loss in membership. As more nonnursing labor unions are attempting to organize nurses, professional nurses must decide whether to be represented by an industrial or professional model. Can the nonnursing union adequately represent the concerns and needs of nurses who want more than monetary benefits? The ultimate question is whether the union is the only alternative to meeting the needs of nurses. There is much evidence that sound nursing administration in a well-managed healthcare agency can circumvent the need for a union (Ganong & Ganong, 1973; 1979).

Nurse managers do not practice in a vacuum. Their respective healthcare institutions are interacting with the environment constantly. Nurse managers must have a practical working knowledge of these complex environmental factors and understand how to cope with them successfully on a day-to-day basis. This leads us to the framework for nursing management.

FRAMEWORK FOR NURSING MANAGEMENT

Organizations are groups of people working together toward identified goals and objectives. The individual is the smallest unit of every organization. Thus, in looking at organizations and how they function, we need to give as much attention to each individual member as is given to organizational concepts, structures, principles, and design. This is why we presented "The Nurse in the Organization" as Chapter 1; examined the workworld model showing the nurse at the center; and discuss human resources management in Part IV.

Every nurse manager will find it helpful to keep in mind the concept of the individual at the center of, and having a major influence upon, his/her workworld. Every nurse manager also needs to maintain an integrated concept of nursing management within the healthcare agency. A Framework for Nursing Management provides such a model (Figure 2-2). This diagram is not so much a theoretical construct as it is a pragmatic summarization. As you examine the model, feel free to add or change components to fit your idea of a framework in your own setting. Discussing the diagram with other nurse managers in your own agency can be highly productive.

The Glossary provides definitions of specific terms used in Figure 2-2. Regarding the difference between a theory and a model, "Theory is a deeper level of reality representation than a model is, and provides the working insides of a model. Viewed in this way, a model may represent structure while theory connotes function" (Riehl & Roy, 1974, p. 3).

Effective nursing management can make the 1980s the *decade of the nurse*. Nurse managers at all levels are in a key position to implement fully the concept of nurses as the effective integrators of agency-wide patient care.

Segment I of the Framework

At top center in the diagram is the term "Nursing Modality." A variety of nursing modalities are identified to the right. These modalities are defined in the glossary at the back of this book. Someday, perhaps, it will no longer be necessary to use various adjectives to identify different kinds of nursing. Someday, nursing (without a qualifying adjective) will enjoy the same professional status and acceptance accorded medicine. For the immediate future, however, a clear understanding of the various nursing modalities is essential in order to plan for optimal patient care. The entire framework for nursing management can be seen as a plan for progress toward nursing as such. Therefore, the starting point for the model is the nursing modality (or modalities) used in a particular healthcare setting for the individual patient/consumer/client (appearing at the center of the diagram).

Of course there should be more than one nursing modality available in a particular healthcare agency. Different nursing approaches are necessary in caring for different kinds of patients, whether the care is delivered in a hospital or nursing home, at home or in the community. A multiservice

Figure 2-2 Model of a Framework for Nursing Management

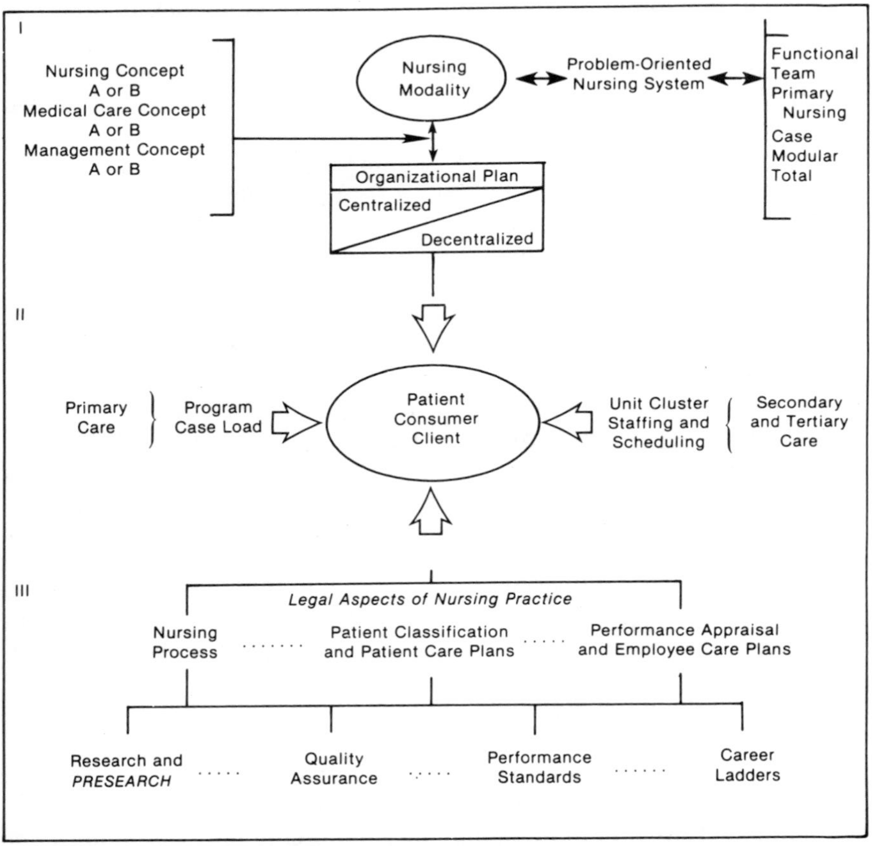

```
I
    Nursing Concept                Nursing        Problem-Oriented       Functional
       A or B                      Modality  ⟷  Nursing System  ⟷    Team
   Medical Care Concept                                                Primary
       A or B                                                            Nursing
   Management Concept                                                  Case
       A or B                                                          Modular
                            Organizational Plan                       Total
                          Centralized
                                        Decentralized


II
                                    Patient
    Primary  }  Program  ⟹        Consumer      ⟸  Unit Cluster  {  Secondary
    Care     }  Case Load           Client            Staffing and    and Tertiary
                                                      Scheduling      Care


III
                          Legal Aspects of Nursing Practice
             Nursing        Patient Classification      Performance Appraisal
             Process  ·····  and Patient Care Plans ···· and Employee Care Plans


        Research and         Quality          Performance          Career
        PRESEARCH   ·····   Assurance  ·····  Standards   ······   Ladders
```

Source: Ganong, J. and Ganong, W. *101 Tremendous Trifles: A Collection of Management Mini-Guides,* 2nd ed. Chapel Hill, N.C.: W. L. Ganong Co., 1979, p. 33.

organization generally offers a variety of nursing modalities because patients may range in age from newborns to geriatric, and the services range from short-term highly acute care, to long-term ambulatory or custodial care, to outpatient and at-home care.

Each modality rests upon a philosophical foundation or concept that reflects the beliefs and goals of nursing leadership. These beliefs may range from Concept A—the nursing workload concept, to Concept B—the patient care management concept. For ease of comparison, concepts A and B of nursing and concepts A and B of management are summarized in Table 2-1.

Table 2-1 Concepts A and B of Nursing and Management

Nursing	Management
Concept A: Functional Nursing	*Concept A: Authoritarian Management*
Workload concept based upon: • Tasks • Procedures • Routines	Managers: • Plan • Lead • Control Employees: • Do
Concept B: Goal-Directed Patient Care Management	*Concept B: Facilitative Management*
Based upon: • The nursing process: —Assess —Plan —Implement —Evaluate • Primary Nursing	Job redesign: • So employees can: —Plan —Do —Control • Managers provide leadership where needed

Source: Ganong, J. and Ganong, W. *101 Tremendous Trifles: A Collection of Management Mini-Guides,* 2nd ed. Chapel Hill, N.C.: W. L. Ganong Co., 1979, p. 13.

We recognize that the performance of nurses and nurse managers is influenced by their perceptions of their roles and of nursing—perceptions that grow out of education and experience. We recognize and lament the seeming wide disparity between the goals of nurse educators and patient care administrators. For the student, there is much merit in a learning focus that emphasizes, "This is how it should be." But for the beginning nurse practitioner, the daily emphasis is necessarily, "This is how it must be." Nurse educators and nurse managers are increasing their efforts to strike an appropriate balance between the two extremes. In the meantime, both groups need to place more emphasis on nursing as such, rather than on the differences between education and service.

The dilemma faced by new staff nurses fresh from nursing education programs was summarized succinctly by Edith P. Lewis, editor of *Nursing Outlook.* She wrote: "To the student we say, 'This is your patient.' To the staff nurse, 'This is your job.' Small wonder that in the transition from the one to the other the nurse ends up by devaluing the patient, herself, and the job" (Lewis, 1974). The role of education must continue not only to emphasize the philosophy, principles, and skills of nursing, but also to provide the student with opportunities to develop the personal skill of conceptualizing ideas and constructs. Part IV of this book deals with these matters more fully. In the meantime, direct your attention again to the two conceptualizations of the nursing role as seen in Table 2-1.

One model is described as the "Nursing Workload Concept" (Concept A), in which the patients are seen as generating a daily volume of routine work handled through the performance of necessary tasks and procedures. This view is symbolized by the question sometimes heard on the nursing units: "Are your patients done yet?" Patients never experience a feeling of being "done" or "finished." Even allowing for the casual quality of day-to-day working terminology, the question is an unfortunate one because it reflects the philosophy of patient-as-workload. Implicit in such a viewpoint is the idea that nurses exist to do things for patients—to carry out procedures, perform tasks, and do all the routine work related to patient care. It is easy to understand how the trend toward measuring workload and work output became common. Over the past two decades, nurse managers have been under strong pressure to contain costs, reduce staffing, and generally keep expenses within the budget.

The other concept, the "Patient Care Management Concept" (Concept B), presents an alternative view of the nursing function. In this view patients are seen as people who seek help for identifiable needs and problems. Patients (insofar as they are able to do so) participate with their doctor, their nurse and their family (or significant others) in developing the goals for their care and the methods by which they can achieve those goals. Where this concept prevails, the relevant day-to-day question is, "How well are the patients meeting their objectives?"

The differences between Concepts A and B are pronounced, not only as two views of nursing but also as they influence the day-to-day operations of patient care units. Procedures and tasks will continue to be necessary in providing patient care. But such procedures should not become mere routines that are carried out for every patient regardless of need. For example:

In a typical general hospital it is four o'clock in the morning. The night nurse discovers that Mr. Jones, a patient, has inadvertently pulled his drainage catheter apart and urine is running out into the bed. He is wet and so are his pajamas and bedding. The nurse reconnects the catheter, washes Mr. Jones, and changes his pajamas and bedding. At seven o'clock there is a shift change; the night nurse goes off duty and another nurse comes on and is assigned to Mr. Jones. Immediately after breakfast Mr. Jones, despite his protests, is helped with a routine bath and a routine change of pajamas and bedding. In all likelihood around ten o'clock the head nurse asks the nurse assigned to Mr. Jones if he is "done yet." The emphasis is on getting the morning routine "done" so that other routines can follow.

Routines may need to be established for particular patients—based upon their needs. But routines are not for everyone regardless of individual needs and desires. Such routines and the time, materials, tasks, and people involved in them are wasteful and costly. In addition the routines may have little to do with the health status of patients like Mr. Jones.

One point must be made here, however. Over the years healthcare consumers have been programmed into expecting these routines when they become patients in general hospitals. More emphasis has been placed on the routines than on involving patients in planning the care designed to meet their needs and resolve their health problems. With the support of administration, nursing can help the consumer toward a better understanding of how nurses can contribute best to health promotion. Fortunately, there are hundreds of hospitals (estimated at close to 10 percent of all U.S. hospitals) now permitting and encouraging patients (who are able) to undertake all the activities—from activities of daily living to making their own beds—formerly done for them by nursing staff members or others. This trend is in the best interests of the patients' health and the economic health of the community at large.

Referring again to Table 2-1, the elements of Management Concepts A and B speak for themselves, contrasting the traditional authoritarian model with the facilitative/consultative model described in Chapter 1. The philosophical orientation of nursing leadership, as capsulized in the contrasting concepts A and B, has a significant impact on the nursing modality of choice. In point of fact, many nursing departments understand and want to implement the concept B models, but for a variety of reasons find themselves caught with functional or team nursing and a continuation of many elements of concept A management. Some organizations see themselves as right in the middle of concepts A and B—moving toward B while going through the change process from concept A. These are the "ABies." From an organizational standpoint, decisions with respect to nursing modality are fundamental to planning and development. Hence, Figure 2-2 shows the nursing modality influencing the organizational plan.

Experience has demonstrated that when doctors themselves examine Table 2-1, they often find it to be an enlightening experience, one that can sometimes lead to worthwhile and productive discussions between nurse managers and medical staff members. Medical care concept A is the traditional diagnose-and-cure approach. Concept B has a more humanistic focus on the spectrum of wellness/illness/prevention. A single medical staff may have physicians and surgeons who practice either concept A or concept B, and some who find themselves somewhere between A and B. This orientation can influence the type of care patients receive and the way personnel are viewed and treated by the doctors. More than this, the A or B orientation of medical staff members can have a significant influence on the way the nursing modality itself can be translated into effective nursing practice.

Figure 2-2 indicates that the use of a problem-oriented nursing system (PONS) has a direct influence on the nursing modality. When concept B of nursing prevails, the problem-oriented nursing system becomes essential. After all, the nursing process itself is based on the model of the scientific method that emphasizes problem identification and resolution. The five components of the problem-oriented nursing system are: (1) the foundation (principles of nursing practice); (2) the nursing process, with a problem-oriented approach; (3) the problem-oriented nursing record (and/or problem-oriented medical record); (4) nursing audit (or a single interdisciplinary quality assurance process); and (5) education for both patients and personnel. As seen in Chapter 3, the problem-oriented record may be introduced within nursing even when the medical staff does not adopt a problem-oriented medical record.

Just as nursing concepts A and B have an influence upon the nursing modality, which in turn affects the plan of organization, so do management concepts A and B influence the organizational plan. Concept A management is an authoritarian model. It goes along very well with concept A nursing. It says, "Look, I'm the boss. I know better than you do. I'll tell you what to do and you just have to do it." Similarly, concept B nursing has a spinoff into concept B management. This type of management is a participative, facilitative model. It recognizes that employees at all levels can participate to a reasonable degree in the planning and controlling functions related to their jobs. Readers familiar with the Theories X and Y of Douglas McGregor, with the writings of Frederick Herzberg, and with the works of M. Scott Myers—all referred to in the reading list following Chapters 1 and 2—will recognize their influence on the foregoing factors that affect the choice of organization design. The alternatives, as shown in Figure 2-2, are either a decentralized or centralized form of organization.

The new breed of employees also has an impact upon the organizational plan. Today's workforce has different characteristics than the one of yesteryear. Examine Table 2-2. How well does your organizational plan and management philosophy accommodate today's new breed of employee?

Table 2-2 The New Breed

The new breed includes individuals (female or male, minority or nonminority, young or old) who share certain attitudes, beliefs, and values—not necessarily radical. What people want is progress toward, and security with respect to, certain goals.

Moving into the '50s and '60s:
Pacifists/Activists *

1. *The respect of their fellows*—The desire to be considered important and respectable by the people with whom you associate.
2. *Creature sufficiency*—The desire to have an amount of food, clothes, shelter, and health that compares favorably with your associates.
3. *Increasing control over their own affairs*—The desire to have your own decisions be effective in shaping your life, and to reduce the amount of control exercised by others over you.
4. *Understanding*—The desire to "know the score," to know the relation between cause and effect.
5. *Capacity performance*—The desire to use the full range of your abilities, to have the chance to do the things you think you can do.
6. *Integrity*—The desire to feel that your actions and principles are consistent; to feel that you are a significant part of the world about you.

Moving into the '70s and Beyond:
The "New Breed" **

1. Recognition as individuals.
2. Treated like adults.
3. Options; choice.
4. Instant gratification (praise now!).
5. Opportunity to use own mind.
6. Continuing education /self-development.
7. Chance to lead whole lives; recreation, social, politics, work—variety.
8. Worthwhile work.
9. Rewards according to accomplishments (anti-seniority).
10. Right to know.
11. Equal opportunity.
12. A voice in decisions.
13. Challenge.

* Adapted from Bakke, W. E. Teamwork in Industry. *The Scientific Monthly*, March 1948, *66*, pp. 213–220. Used with permission.

**Adapted from Peterfreund, S. *Mind-to-Mind Management*. AMACOM, 135 W. 50th St., New York 10020. 1977, pp. 10–12. Used with permission.

Organizational Structure

A decentralized organization permits decision making at the lowest levels of organization consistent with performance responsibilities and accountability. A decentralized plan permits and requires maximum involvement of employees in planning, problem solving, doing, and controlling. Thus it makes possible the application of concepts already discussed under nursing management and administrative management. Other factors that influence organizational planning, and the criteria for an effective organization, are described in another chapter. Experience indicates that decentralization as described here not only provides for more effective patient care but also allows for greater economy in operation.

Functional Models: Figure 2-3 shows six functional models of nursing department organizational structure. Model A is the familiar and traditional hierarchical structure with several layers of administrator/manager positions intervening between the Director of Nursing (DoN) and the nursing staff.

Model B depicts a less familiar decentralized structure with only one manager, the head nurse (HN) between the Director of Nursing and the nursing staff. With this model the head nurse has considerable authority and managerial responsibility for decision making and problem solving.

Model C divides the administrative responsibility between two Associate Directors and decentralizes authority and responsibility for decision making and problem solving to the head nurses. Two levels intervene between the Director of Nursing and the nursing staff. This model is more feasible in a facility with many patient units.

Model D indicates a different title for the director, that of Patient Care Administrator (PCA), which carries with it more administrative power and authority, often at the level of Associate Hospital Administrator. Patient Care Coordinators (PCCs) have decentralized responsibility and authority for clusters of like patient units, and the head nurses have decentralized managerial responsibility and authority at the individual patient unit level. Again, two levels of administrator/manager positions intervene between the PCA and the nursing staff.

Model E is decentralized much like Model B, except that the nursing modality used throughout the patient units is primary nursing. Only the head nurses intervene between the patient care administrator and the primary nurses and unit personnel.

Model F is the ultimate in a decentralized professional clinical structure. Authority, responsibility, and accountability to patients is vested in the primary nurses who have a direct reporting relationship to the nursing administrator. In this model, most appropriate for the all-RN staff, the nursing administrator (as PCA, or Vice President for Patient Care) might report directly to the Board of Trustees.

In most decentralized models there are more functional (*staff*) positions at the administrative level. Most of these are of a special supportive nature to the patient units. They include such titles as director or coordinator of staff development, systems and procedures, staffing and budgeting, and quality assurance. These positions are not shown in the models.

Figure 2-3 Nursing Department Organizational Structure
—Functional Models

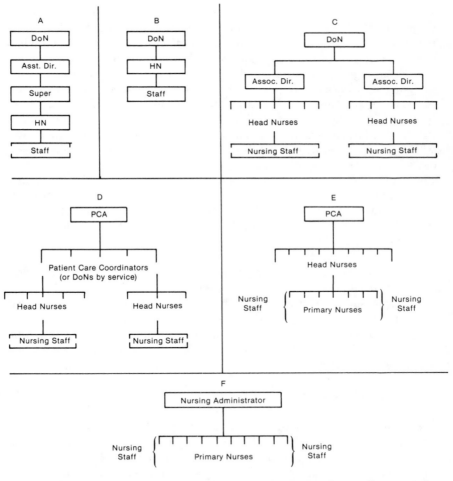

Source: Revised from handout prepared by Joan and Warren Ganong for use at the *Journal of Nursing Administration's* Second National Conference, March 1979, in Los Angeles.

See other chapters, notably Chapter 10, for further guidance in planning nursing organizational structures. Another worthwhile reference is *Primary Nursing: Development and Management* by Karen Zander, 1980.

Segment II of the Framework

The focal point of Figure 2-2 is the patient/consumer/client shown at the center. To the left and right of center, three levels of care are indicated: (1) primary care—entry into the community healthcare system, (2) secondary care—hospital care, and (3) tertiary care—specialized, longer term or intensive care; regional hospital, skilled care facilities.* These three broad categories influence the ways in which nursing staff members are assigned for purposes of patient care. The program caseload is most characteristic of community (public) health agencies. Centralized staffing and/or unit cluster staffing is characteristic in secondary and tertiary care facilities. Unit cluster staffing is most prevalent in medium- to large-size hospitals and other agencies where patient care units can be grouped according to type of service provided. (Such groupings are indicated in some of the organization charts elsewhere in this book.) There are many reasons why unit cluster staffing is so effective from the standpoint of patient care, employee satisfaction, recruiting, and cost containment. These reasons include the following (see also Chapter 9):

1. Recruitment of staff is for specific job openings on a specific service (maternal child care, intensive/critical care, medical/surgical).
2. A condition of employment is that employees will be expected to float only within the individual service.
3. Each unit cluster is responsible for its own staffing. Staff will not be floated off the cluster nor will extra help be provided from outside the cluster—except in the case of true emergencies or disasters.

Segment III of the Framework

The balance of Figure 2-2 includes a variety of factors and management techniques that have a direct bearing on patient care management and human resources management. These factors include the levels of practice among the nursing staff, with the major focus on skill in the use of the nursing process; the levels of patients, with emphasis on patient classification and

---

*For further clarification of terms see the Glossary, and *A Discursive Dictionary of Health Care.* (94th Congress, 2d Session: Committee Print). Washington, D.C.: U.S. Government Printing Office, 1976 (Catalog No. Y 4.IN 8/4:H34/26).

individualized patient care plans; and levels of employees, with suitable performance appraisal and employee care plans. The interrelationship between these factors is shown by the dotted lines on the chart. Legal Aspects is shown as spanning the full spectrum of Segment III and deserves separate consideration later in this chapter. A number of specific management tools and techniques are summarized at the lowest level of the diagram. These are included because of their major impact on the remainder of the framework for nursing management.

The diagram for a framework for nursing management may appear complex. It is. Nursing management itself is complex. Many factors interact to affect both short-term and long-term outcomes. Part of the art of management is to strike the happiest balance among all the factors so that optimal results are achieved. This is not easy since overemphasis on, or neglect of, any single factor will influence the way in which all the factors work together. So *keep the corners off your thinking* while striving for synergy.

For example, the heavy pressures to contain costs may cause a precipitous response, leading to the introduction of management engineering studies that set up patient classification systems and improve personnel utilization. But these actions then have profound impact upon other factors: the plan of organization, quality assurance, employee appraisal, career ladders, and employee morale. Consider the situation if such studies were introduced at a time when nursing is considering a change from functional or team nursing to primary nursing. In this case the investment in the engineering studies is largely wasted, for the well-planned changeover to primary nursing (or similar total care modality) affects all these other factors even more profoundly—but with positive impact and attendant cost containment benefits. Hospital trustees, administrators, and controllers need to fully appreciate these interrelationships. It is to their advantage to consult most carefully with the nursing director or patient care administrator (RN) when deciding whether or not to undertake costly engineering or management studies— whether in nursing or other hospital departments.

LEGAL ASPECTS

The law has a great impact on nursing today. This is especially true in light of rights-conscious consumers of healthcare. Healthcare consumers are more aware of what they "should get," and if wronged or neglected are often prepared to do something about it. Legal Aspects therefore constitutes an important component of the nursing framework. As a nurse manager, one must know the law as related to levels of practice, levels of patients, and performance appraisal (employee evaluation). The following brief summary is from Martyann Penberth (Penberth, 1979).

Levels of Practice

The practice of nursing is governed by the three branches of government and also by the individual institution or agency. The legislative branch of government passes statutes; the executive branch develops and adopts regulations and issues attorney-general options; and the judicial branch hands down court-case decisions. The individual healthcare institution or agency develops policies and procedures governing nursing practice. It is important to realize the hierarchical relationship among these sectors. Regulations can override institutional policies, and statutes can override regulations.

There are two sources of law—statutory and common law. A statute at the federal or state level is the written will of the legislature. Nurses in any setting function under these statutes. Community health nurses are influenced by additional statutes on the municipal level. An important example of a statutory law that directly affects nursing practice is the Nurse Practice Act of each state. A second form of law is common law, or judge-made law, which originated in England. An example of common law is the 1973 Supreme Court decision on abortion. Both statutory and common laws continuously undergo growth and modification. Therefore, it behooves the nurse to stay well informed on laws affecting nursing practice. This knowledge—plus clinical expertise, maturity, self-confidence, and experience—provides an excellent base from which to make decisions.

The Nurse Practice Act is a very important statute in each state, because it regulates the practice of nursing and protects the public. It is imperative that nurses know how the role of the nurse is defined in their state. Although the emphasis is on the registered nurse, the nurse manager must also be aware of the laws and regulations that affect the practice of other levels of employees.

There are several components common to all the nurse practice acts. These include a definition of nursing practice, requirements for licensure and endorsement of persons from other states, specifications for exemption from licensure, grounds for revocation of a license, provision of a board of examiners with specific responsibilities, and penalties for practicing without a license (Kelly, 1975). Since 1971, as a result of internal and external pressures, states have been revising some of these components, specifically, the definition of nursing, requirements for licensure and renewal of licensure, educational standards, and state board composition. The internal pressure stems from overlapping areas in the scope of practice between nursing and medicine. The external pressure comes from an increased interest in health manpower licensing on the part of the state and federal governments.

The key component in any nurse practice act is the definition of nursing. A survey taken in the spring of 1978 showed that nearly all states revised these definitions to deal with the expanded role (Trandel-Korenchuk & Trandel-Korenchuk, 1976). The AHA developed a model Nurse Practice Act in 1955 that was revised in 1976 as follows:

> The practice of nursing as performed by a registered nurse is a process in which substantial specialized knowledge derived from the biological, physical and behavioral sciences is applied to the care, treatment, counsel and health teaching of persons who are experiencing changes in the normal health processes, or who require assistance in the maintenance of health or the management of illness, injury, or infirmity or in the achievement of a dignified death, and such additional acts as are recognized by the nursing profession as proper to be performed by a registered nurse.

The important factor is to have a definition of nursing that is broad and encompassing, to allow for a natural evolution of the practitioners' functions (Kelly, 1975).

An important concept when dealing with levels of practice is malpractice and how it affects each employee. Malpractice is the term applied to professional negligence. Malpractice is defined as bad, wrong, or injudicious treatment resulting in injury, unnecessary suffering, or death to the patient and proceeding from carelessness, ignorance, lack of professional skill, or disregard for established rules or principles (Kelly, 1974). There are three types of negligence: *gross, criminal,* and *contributory.* Gross negligence is defined as failure to exercise even slight care to protect others; criminal negligence occurs when the patient dies; and contributory negligence occurs when the plaintiff has contributed to his/her own negligence (Kelly, 1976).

Nurse as an Employee

The hospital assumes responsibility for the nurse's work and negligence since the nurse is a hospital representative. Under the doctrine of *respondeat superior,* the hospital can be held liable for the employee even though the hospital's actions were without fault. This doctrine can only be applied where a master/servant relationship exists; that is, where the employer has the right to control the physical conduct of an employee's performance of duties (Streiff, 1975). Examples of cases in which the hospital is held liable under this doctrine are situations involving the dispensing of wrong drugs or the use of an overheated water bag.

> *Case Example:* In Parrish v. Clark, [107 Fla. 598, 145 So. 848 (1933)], the hospital was found liable for the nurse's negligence in

continuing to inject a saline solution into an unconscious patient's breast after noticing ill effects. The nurse should have stopped injecting the solution at the first sign of side effects.

A special application of the *respondeat superior* doctrine is the borrowed servant concept where the employer lends an employee to another for particular employment. During this period of special employment, the employer is not liable (Streiff, 1975). An obvious example is the operating room where the physician is considered the "captain of the ship."

Case Example: In Martin v. Perth Amboy Hospital et al., [1969 CCH Neg. 4385 (N.J.)], a surgeon, scrub nurse, and circulating nurse were held liable but not the hospital. The negligence occurred when the nurse reported the sponge count as correct when, in fact, a sponge was left in the patient during abdominal surgery.

Supervisor

The nurse manager or supervisor is responsible for actual supervision and for making assignments that are within the educational scope and experience of staff members. Supervision is incorporated in the definition of nursing in the nurse practice act. Therefore, the supervisor is liable for negligence in carrying out supervisory duties. If a staff person is negligent, and the supervisor made the assignment—with or without the knowledge that the person could do the assignment, then the supervisor is negligent, as is the hospital. The supervisor is not negligent under the doctrine of *respondeat superior* since the hospital is the employer.

Case Example: In Piper v. Epstein, [326 Ill. App. 400, 62 N.E. 2d 139 (1945)], the supervisor and student nurse were held liable when the supervisor reported a correct sponge count when, in fact, a sponge was left in the patient who later died. The student nurse passed out sponges during surgery but never counted them. However, the supervisor was responsible for the count at the end of the surgery.

Private Duty or Special Duty Nurse

Cases involving private duty nurses can be quite complicated in terms of who is responsible. Use of a special nurse does not always exempt the hospital from liability. It depends on who hired the nurse—the patient or the hospital—and what type of negligence was involved.

Case Example: In Emory v. Shadburn, [47 Ga. 643, 171 S.E. 192, aff'd 180 S.E. 137 (Ga. 1933)], the hospital was held liable for the negligence of the private duty nurse. The hospital's liability was due to the fact that the hospital had selected the nurse, received payment for her service, and later settled with her.

Student Nurse

The student nurse is considered an employee of the hospital during clinical experiences. The student should be assigned to procedures and patient care that he/she is prepared to do. If any injury occurs following a procedure the student is prepared to carry out, the student can be found negligent. However, if the student carries out an aspect of patient care for which he/she is unprepared, then the clinical instructor or supervisor can be found responsible. The hospital should have a contract with the affiliated school of nursing which delineates the responsibilities of the instructor, the number of students, and the lines of authority between the student, staff, and instructor (Perry, 1978).

Case Example: In Cadicamo v. Long Island College Hospital, [308 N.Y. 196, 125 N.Y.S. 2d 632, 127 N.Y.S. 2d 855, 124 N.E. 2d 279 (1954)], the parents recovered damages for the death of their newborn daughter. The student nurse had placed a heating lamp with an unguarded bulb within three inches of the bed clothing, causing the blanket to catch fire.

In the everyday workworld there are many opportunities for potential negligence. A preventive approach by both the nurse and the nurse manager is best. Appendix L provides guidelines for such everyday nursing activities as communication, charting, medical records, and medications. General guidelines delineating the legal responsibilities of the staff nurse and the nurse manager follow in Appendix M. In addition to these guidelines, the implementation of nursing concepts expressed in the following documents can enhance the performance of the nursing staff: ANA Code of Ethics, Standards of Care (ANA Standards of Nursing Practice), JCAH Standards for Nursing Services, Nursing Process, and Nursing Audit.

Patient's Rights

When caring for patients directly or indirectly in any setting, both nurse managers and those they supervise must be aware of two major concepts, the Patient's Bill of Rights and informed consent.

In the healthcare field the consumer movement has led to a more humanistic approach to care and the recognition of patients' rights as people. The HEW Secretary's Commission on Medical Malpractice states, "to ignore the rights of patients as human beings is both to betray simple humanity and to invite dissatisfaction that may lead to malpractice suits" (Medical Malpractice Report, 1973).

The National League for Nursing pioneered the patient's rights movement when they issued a document in 1959 called *What People Can Expect From Modern Nursing Service.* It was not until 1972 that the American Hospital Association's Committee on Health Care for the Disadvantaged developed a patient's bill of rights. The AHA document, released early in 1973, formalized rights assumed or taken for granted over many years. See Appendix N for a copy of the AHA's Patient's Bill of Rights.

Such a document reminds people that they have certain rights and encourages them to assert these rights. However, certain problems remain. For one, not all hospitals issue the bill of rights to their patients; second, there is little indication that hospitals have carried out the intent of the bill of rights (Kelly, 1976). Implementation of the bill of rights gives it meaning; otherwise it is no more than a public relations maneuver.

Many of the AHA's statements refer to the concept of informed consent. Consent is an authorization by a patient or his/her authorized representative that changes touching (hands-on care) from nonconsensual to consensual (Streiff, 1975). There are two types of consent—*express* consent, which can be oral or written (either is just as binding in the court), and *implied* consent, where the patient voluntarily submits to treatment. Without consent to touch another, the healthcare provider is guilty of the intentional wrong called battery. Remember that a person can be found liable even if the patient's health improves. Negligence in terms of the consent concept is present in cases where the patient was not given enough information.

The vital concern today is that the consent be an *informed* consent. Informed consent functions in two ways. It promotes both individual autonomy and competent decision making (Besch, 1979). It is not hard to obtain the patient's signature on a piece of paper, and, in so doing, the hospital and physician are protected. However, it is more difficult to be certain that the patient understands the information. The healthcare provider's commitment to human rights is necessary to ensure patient understanding.

The Department of Health, Education and Welfare and the World Medical Assembly have defined the essential elements of an informed consent procedure (Shepard, 1976):

- Explanation of the proposed treatment
- Explanation of inherent risks and benefits

- Alternatives to the proposed treatment
- Adequate time for patient questions
- Option to withdraw at any time.

Performance Appraisal

The role of the nurse manager involves performance appraisal. By law, this process requires scrupulous fairness. Since the Civil Rights Acts of 1964 and 1972, the context within which performance appraisal is conducted has been altered (Odom, 1977). The basis for employment decisions and for performance appraisal must be merit, not race, sex, or national origin. Due to past discrimination, enforcement of these criteria has been directed especially toward females and racial minorities.

Odom, in "Performance Appraisal: Legal Aspects" (1977), summarizes vital legal considerations in performance appraisal. There are two sets of federal guidelines regarding discrimination, one set from the Equal Employment Opportunity Commission and the other from the Equal Employment Opportunity Coordinating Council. These guidelines cover any procedure— formal or informal, scored or unscored—that is used to make a personnel decision (Odom, 1977). Therefore it is imperative to have a formal appraisal system and complete personnel records on all employees and potential employees.

The three government agencies responsible for ensuring compliance with these guidelines are the Equal Employment Opportunity Commission; the Office of Federal Contract Compliance; and the Federal Courts, Department of Labor and the Department of Justice. To prove discrimination, one doesn't need to prove an intention to discriminate. The mere presence of a disproportionate number of employees from either a majority or minority group is sufficient. These differential employment practices are determined relative to the population of potential employees in a given geographical area.

In summary, any performance appraisal system should have at least six characteristics to meet the qualifications of recent court cases (Odom, 1977, p. 12):

- The performance ratings should be job related.
- The variables rated should be developed through job analysis.
- Raters must be able to observe the performance they are to rate.
- Ratings should not be based on raters' evaluations of vague, subjective factors.
- Care should be taken through the choice of measures, through training,

etc., to ensure that ratings are not biased by prejudice regarding race, sex, or religion.

- Ratings should be collected and scored under standardized circumstances.

PROBLEM SOLVING WITH PRESEARCH

No framework for nursing management would be complete without attention to problem solving. This activity consumes a significant portion of every nurse manager's work day. Within any healthcare institution complex problems that cross departmental lines command the attention of department managers. The director of a large department often initiates a solution-seeking process because many people in the department are affected by an interdisciplinary problem. Usually the problem is first viewed symptomatically; each individual symptom of a large, ill-defined problem appears to be an isolated problem. With a complex problem, the most difficult task is problem interpretation and definition. The problems may be numerous, yet so closely interrelated that a solution to only one or two produces no noticeable improvement. Therefore the steps leading up to problem definition are crucial to the success of the problem-solving efforts.

PRESEARCH, developed by Cecelia Golightly, incorporates the method of systematic data collection from a research model into a problem-solving model. PRESEARCH is a process for collecting data from a multidisciplinary sample, analyzing it, and converting subjective material into a usable problem-solving format (Golightly, 1978).

The purists rightfully separate research from problem solving (see Figure 2-4). Mabel Wandelt differentiates the two in their statements of purpose: "The purpose of research is to reveal new knowledge; the purpose of problem solving is to solve an immediate problem in a particular setting" (Wandelt, 1970, p. xvii).

In the research model, information is collected via a standardized, predetermined, carefully designed tool. Uniformity of the data collection tool, and an effort to eliminate researcher bias when obtaining the data, produce the purest information possible within the research design. Likewise, uniformity in the data collection phase of a problem-solving process produces manageable subjective information.

The data collection phase of research can be applied to a problem-solving process and thereby enhances the accuracy of problem definition. Recognizing, refining, and defining a problem are already included in all problem-solving models. In PRESEARCH the data collected support and justify the defined problem(s), whereas in research the data collected speak for themselves (see Figure 2-5). The diagram shows that in the PRESEARCH model

Figure 2-4 A Parallel Comparison of Scientific Research and the Art of Problem Solving

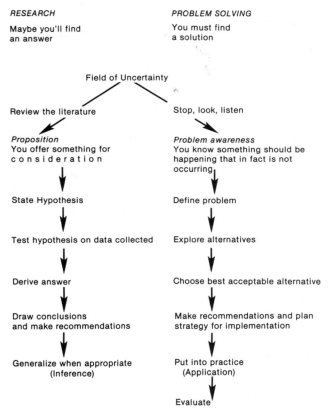

RESEARCH
Maybe you'll find
an answer

PROBLEM SOLVING
You must find
a solution

Field of Uncertainty

Review the literature

Stop, look, listen

Proposition
You offer something for
c o n s i d e r a t i o n

Problem awareness
You know something should be
happening that in fact is not
occurring

State Hypothesis

Define problem

Test hypothesis on data collected

Explore alternatives

Derive answer

Choose best acceptable alternative

Draw conclusions
and make recommendations

Make recommendations and plan
strategy for implementation

Generalize when appropriate
(Inference)

Put into practice
(Application)

Evaluate

Source: PRESEARCH: A new approach to creative problem solving. © Cecelia Golightly, 1978. Privately printed. Used with permission.

data collection occurs *before* information from the "field of uncertainty" is refined into a problem definition, whereas in the research model data collection occurs *after* the hypothesis statement. Regardless of the comparative sequence of events, the significant point is this: In the described process a structured, systematic method is used to collect data prior to problem definition. The data collected then support and justify the problem definition. This process does not change problem solving to research. However, information obtained in the pre-search for the real problem(s) provides the problem solver a base from which to work.

Figure 2-5 A Comparison of Scientific Research and PRESEARCH

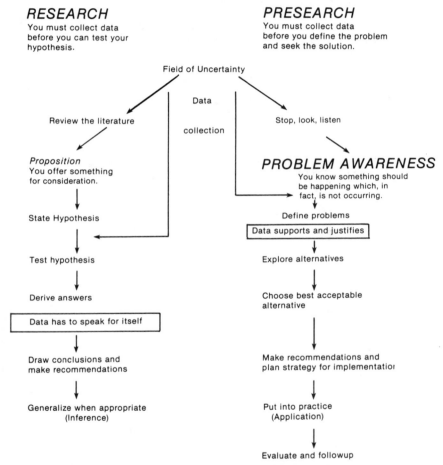

RESEARCH
You must collect data
before you can test your
hypothesis.

PRESEARCH
You must collect data
before you define the problem
and seek the solution.

Field of Uncertainty

Data

Review the literature

collection

Stop, look, listen

Proposition
You offer something
for consideration.

PROBLEM AWARENESS
You know something should
be happening which, in
fact, is not occurring.

State Hypothesis

Define problems

Data supports and justifies

Test hypothesis

Explore alternatives

Derive answers

Choose best acceptable
alternative

Data has to speak for itself

Draw conclusions and
make recommendations

Make recommendations and
plan strategy for implementatioı

Generalize when appropriate
(Inference)

Put into practice
(Application)

Evaluate and followup

Source: PRESEARCH: A new approach to creative problem solving. © Cecelia
Golightly, 1978. Privately printed. Used with permission.

PRESEARCH converts the drudgery of complex problem solving into a
multidisciplinary challenge. The effect of the process on the problem solvers
is fascinating. Since each step means progress toward solution, problem
solvers experience a sense of accomplishment as they progress. Although one
person must function as a coordinator or facilitator, this method lends itself
to group process. There are logical stopping points in the well-defined main
steps and substeps of the PRESEARCH process. These steps can be used as

the framework for a problem-solving workshop. Likewise, many of the individual steps can be used to structure successive problem-solving committee meetings. Because a group or individual can work on a complicated project in blocks of time without backtracking, energy and enthusiasm are sustained. PRESEARCH allows those who will be affected by a solution to participate in various aspects of the problem-solving process. Their involvement makes them more willing to accept a solution and paves the way for solution implementation.

SUMMARY

The Framework for Nursing Management, a plan for progress, is not intended to suggest that there is a specific formula that—when skillfully applied—will automatically lead to improved patient care and employee satisfaction. However, it does provide a conceptual framework that shows the interrelationships between the factors necessary for the effective management of patient care and human resources. Successful patient care administrators are those who can pull together all these factors to provide a new synergy for improved patient and employee satisfaction, coupled with cost containment.

Golightly's PRESEARCH, a new approach to creative problem-solving, provides a suitable ending to this chapter and serves as a transition to Chapter 3. It opens up a way of thinking that can help nurse managers achieve a sense of serendipity with a problem-oriented nursing system.

NOTES

Bauknecht, V. HEW supports participation of more nurses in PSROs. *The American Nurse,* November 15, 1977, *1*(5), 12.

Besch, L. Informed consent: A patient's right. *Nursing Outlook,* January 1979, *27*, 32–35.

California law lets nurses share, *The American Nurse,* Sept. 20, 1979, *11*(8), 1.

Cost containment suspended in house. *American Journal of Nursing,* March 1978, *78*, 348, 478.

Fralic, M. F. The nursing director prepares for labor relations. *Journal of Nursing Administration,* July/August 1977, *7*(6), 4.

Ganong, W., & Ganong, J. Union free health care management. *Journal of Nursing Administration,* January/February 1973, *3*(1), 6.

Ganong, W., & Ganong, J. *Cases in nursing management.* Germantown, Md.: Aspen Systems Corp., 1979.

Golightly, C. *PRESEARCH: A new approach to creative problem solving.* A privately printed introductory booklet (1978) now expanded into a manuscript for a book to be published by Aspen Systems Corp. in 1980.

Kelly, L. Y. Nursing practice acts. *American Journal of Nursing,* July 1974, *74*, 1310–1319.

Kelly, L. Y. *Dimensions of professional nursing.* New York: Macmillan, 1975.

Kelly, L. Y. Keeping up with your legal responsibilities. *Nursing '76,* June 1976, *6*(6), 81-93.

Kerr, A. Nurses notes: "That's where the goodies are!" *Nursing '75,* February 1975, *5*(2) 34-41.

Mauksch, I. On national health insurance. *American Journal of Nursing,* August 1978, *78,* 1323-1327.

Medical practice called unproven. *The Nation's Health,* November 1978, *8,* 12.

Odom, J. V. *Performance appraisal: Legal aspects.* Greensboro, N.C.: Center for Creative Leadership, May 1977.

Penberth, M. *HELP with legal aspects in nursing practice.* Chapel Hill, N.C.: W. L. Ganong Co., 1979.

Perry, S. If you're called on as an expert witness. *American Journal of Nursing,* March 1978, *77,* 458-460.

Reimbursement for all, *RN Magazine,* Sept. 1979, *42*(9), 26.

Riehl, J. & Roy, C. *Conceptual models for nursing practice.* New York: Appleton-Century-Crofts, 1974.

Shepard, D. A. The 1978 declaration of Helsinki and Consent. *Canadian Medical Journal,* December 18, 1976, *115,* 1191-1192.

Streiff, C., & The Health Law Center. *Nursing and the law.* Germantown, Md.: Aspen Systems Corp., 1975.

Trandel-Korenchuk, D., & Trandel-Korenchuk, K. How state laws recognize advanced nursing practice. *Nursing Outlook,* November 1978, *26,* 713-719.

U.S. Department of Health, Education and Welfare. *Medical malpractice report.* Washington, D.C.: U.S. Government Printing Office, January 1973, p. 71.

U.S. Department of Health, Education and Welfare. *Health—United States 1978.* Washington, D.C.: U.S. Government Printing Office, December 1978.

Wandelt, M. *Guide for the beginning researcher.* New York: Appleton-Century-Crofts, 1970.

Reading List

Books

Albanese, R. *Management: Toward accountability for performance.* Homewood, Ill.: Richard D. Irwin, 1975.

Berger, M. M. *Working with people called patients.* New York: Brunner/Mazel, 1977.

Chaska, N. L. (Ed.). *The nursing profession: Views through the mist.* New York: McGraw-Hill, 1978.

Kraegel, J. M., Mousseau, V., Goldsmith, C., & Arora, R. *Patient care systems.* Philadelphia: J. B. Lippincott, 1974.

Lysaught, J. P. (Ed.). *Action in nursing: Progress in professional purpose.* New York: McGraw-Hill, 1974.

Maslow, A. H. *Eupsychian management: A journal.* Homewood, Ill.: Richard D. Irwin, 1965.

Maslow, A. H. *Toward a psychology of being* (2nd ed.). New York: Van Nostrand Reinhold, 1968.

Maslow, A. H. *Motivation and personality* (2nd ed.). New York: Harper & Row, 1970.

Myers, M. S. *Every employee a manager.* New York: McGraw-Hill, 1970.

Roy, C. *Introduction to nursing: An adaptation model.* Englewood Cliffs, N.J.: Prentice-Hall, Inc., 1976.

Warren, D. G. *Problems in hospital law* (3rd ed.). Germantown, Md.: Aspen Systems Corp., 1978.

Zander, K. *Managing primary nursing.* Germantown, Md.: Aspen Systems Corp., 1980.

Articles

Brown, B. (Ed.). Politics and power. *Nursing Administration Quarterly,* Spring 1978, *2*(3), entire issue.

Fritz, S. (Assoc. Ed.). New breed of workers. *U.S. News & World Report,* September 3, 1979, pp. 35-38.

Kinzer, Jeanne. Does nursing administration affect patient care? *Supervisor Nurse,* September 1978, *9*(9), 84-90.

LaViolette, S. Hospital pressures trigger increased democracy in nursing departments. *Modern Healthcare,* May 1979, *9*(5), 62-63.

Lorsch, J. W. Organization designs: A situational perspective. *Organizational Dynamics,* Autumn 1977, pp. 2-14.

Partridge, K. B. Nursing values in a changing society. *Nursing Outlook,* June 1978, *26*(6), 356-360.

Russell, A. Y., Zimmerman, S., & Bruce, R. Organization development at work in a medical center. *Health Care Management Review,* Fall 1978, *3*(4), 59-66.

Stagnitto, M. R. Nursing supervision: Leadership or police work? *Supervisor Nurse,* January 1979, *10*(1), 17-19.

Walton, R., & Schlesinger, L. Do supervisors thrive in participative work systems? *Organizational Dynamics,* Winter 1979, *7*(3), 25-38.

Part II

Patient Care Management

Chapter 3

The Problem-Oriented Nursing System

A CONCEPTUAL MODEL

Nurses need a model for understanding the patient care process in hospitals. A model can help nurses focus their thinking on patient problems and what can be done about them. When nurses are focused on patient problems, they discard the concept A approach of doing things for, at, and to patients, and adopt the goal-oriented concept B approach with its focus on helping patients achieve identified goals for their hospitalization and subsequent health care.

Primary nursing, described in Chapter 4, permits this kind of patient care. But even outside the realm of primary nursing, today's nurses recognize the need for concentrating on patients and their individual identified problems, rather than on the completion of assigned tasks, procedures, and routines. This concentration is most likely to be achieved when nurses have a clear concept of the entire patient care process.

We view the patient care process as being composed of identifiable system elements with which every nurse should be familiar. These system elements provide the basis for both a medical model and a nursing model of patient care. To assist in a consistent use and understanding of terminology, here are definitions of some of the foregoing terms:

Process: A series of actions, changes, or functions that bring about a particular result.
Model: A tentative ideational structure used as a testing device; a means of communicating a concept.
System: A group of interrelated elements forming a collective entity.
Element: A fundamental, essential, or irreducible constituent of a composite entity.

An accompanying diagram, Table 3-1, presents the patient care process and identifies the system elements, the medical model, and the nursing model of patient care. This diagram presents a conceptual framework within which to view the patient care process from the time the person (client) enters the healthcare system as a hospital patient.

The system elements as shown in the center column of the illustration begin with the patient preadmission procedures and follow the patient through the steps of initial assessment, the development of a plan of care and its implementation, followed by the evaluation of the patient's progress and problems. At the next level of the patient's progress is the identification of new problems and the revision of care plans, together with their implementation and evaluation. This sequence, as indicated, is repeated as often as necessary during the patient's hospitalization. The next stages are indicated as the discharge procedure and referral to suitable follow-up care at home or through other agencies. The entire sequence—from initial admission to discharge and referral for home care—may be repeated as required by the patient's condition.

The medical model shown in the left column of the illustration and the nursing model in the right column parallel the system elements as described. The medical model has its focus on the medical care of the patient, while the nursing model has its focus on nursing and other aspects of patient care for which the nursing department is responsible.

An excellent comparison of the key elements of five nursing models is provided by Sister Callista Roy. She writes,

> In recent years nursing has made greater efforts to define its theoretical basis of practice. Each of these efforts has been aimed at defining more clearly the *person* who receives nursing care, the *goal* or purpose of nursing, and nursing *intervention,* that is, what the nurse does. The elements of a nursing model are, thus, the nurse's view of the human being, nursing's goal, and nursing activities (Roy, 1976, p. 5).

Karen Zander, in her book *Primary Nursing: Development and Management,* provides an insightful elaboration on each of these system elements, with a finely balanced emphasis on both clinical and management aspects. After noting that the fundamental tasks for both physicians and nurses are similar, based as they are upon the same system elements, she goes on to say,

> Equal tasks should indicate equal colleagues. The physicians' and primary nurses' roles differ in how the fundamental tasks and priorities are accomplished. Disagreement at any stage of the

Table 3-1 The Patient Care Process: Comparison of Medical and Nursing Models of Patient Care

Medical Model	System Elements	Nursing Model
1. Assess patient, write initial orders	1. Patient preadmission procedures	1. Preadmission procedures
2. Write additional orders	2. Admission	2. Admit
3. History and physical exam	3. Assessment of patient	3. Initial patient interview & observation
4. Problem list	4. Problem identification	4. Problem list
5. Medical plan	5. Plan of care	5. Initial nursing plan & nursing directives
6. Order Rx, medications, record	6. Implementation of care plan	6. Give care, Rx, meds, teach, listen, observe, record, initiate discharge planning
7. Rounds, observe, confer	7. Evaluate problems & progress	7. Give care, rounds, observe, confer, coordinate
8. Write new orders, document on progress notes, Rx, medications, rounds, observe, confer	8. Identify new problems, adjust plan, implement adjusted plan, evaluate problems and progress	8. Revise care plan, write new nursing directives, modify care appropriately & document on patient record, give care, rounds, observe, confer, coordinate
	Repeat Sequence 1 through 7 as Necessary	
9. Order	9. Discharge	9. Finalize discharge plans, write discharge summary, discharge
10. Write order, fill in referral forms	10. Referral	10. Write nursing directives, fill in referral forms
	11. Initial visit and assessment	11. Initial interview, observation, examination
	Repeat Sequence 1 through 7 as Required	

Source: Ganong, J. & Ganong, W. *HELP with a problem-oriented system.* Chapel Hill, N.C.: W. L. Ganong Co., 1975, p. 8.

system elements often causes collaboration breakdown. An analysis of the system elements in relation to primary nursing would benefit the nurse-manager (Zander, 1980).

We recommend careful reading of her line of reasoning.

The model as presented in Table 3–1 is intended to be as simple as possible and yet provide a reasonably comprehensive conceptualization of the patient care process as it exists. As you review it in detail, ask yourself a number of questions about it. Are the system elements as presented consistent with the patient care process in your agency? Is the nursing model compatible with the system elements, based upon your own experience? Are the medical and nursing models correctly interrelated? As you ask these questions and any others that may occur to you, make a note of any exceptions, additions, or corrections that you believe are necessary to make the diagram an acceptable portrayal of the patient care process as you perceive it in your own agency. What other questions are stimulated by your consideration and discussion of the diagram? What additional ideas do you have regarding a more visionary model of what the patient care delivery system should be, as compared with how it is now?

The foregoing provides at least a beginning for, or some elaboration upon, your own conceptual framework for considering patient care, nursing, and yourself in the dynamic healthcare environment of today and the immediate future. As you have considered this conceptual model and attempted to relate it to the workworld of the nurse manager as presented in Part I, you undoubtedly have seen some similarities to the management process and the responsibilities of nurse managers. If such is not the case, we recommend strongly that you review all of this material again to consider its implications not only for yourself as a nurse but also to yourself as a manager. This is important because the whole thrust of this book is to help you develop an integrated view of the patient care process and the management process so that they are seen as inseparable. Admittedly you may not yet have developed the habit of perceiving yourself in the managerial role. We believe that the sooner you do perceive yourself as a manager, the sooner you will—and nursing as a whole—be able to relate most successfully to the other members of the patient care team in meeting the identified needs and goals of patients.

PONS: AN OVERVIEW

The Problem-Oriented Nursing System (PONS) provides an integrated nursing management technique for the implementation of the goal-directed patient care management concept described in Chapter 2. The system is complete and fully effective only when all of the components in the following definition are used as a unified whole.

> PONS is a system based on identified principles of nursing practice; making full use of the nursing process; involving the systematic recording of each patient's data base and identified problems; with

an initial plan of care, progress notes, and discharge planning keyed to the problem list; supported by a nursing audit program; and with inservice and continuing education (for patients and staff) as a relevant component.

Such an approach to patient care that involves identifying the patient's needs and problems is not new. It has a long and highly respected history. A problem-oriented system has a specific connotation and is a fairly recent development. Dr. Lawrence L. Weed, the pioneer who began the development of the Problem-Oriented Medical System (POMS) and the Problem-Oriented Medical Record (POMR) in the 1950s at the University of Vermont College of Medicine, gained renown for his research and developmental work, and for his tireless teaching, speaking, and counseling with all who would listen. His efforts led to gradual acceptance of POMS among his colleagues in medicine and to widespread acclaim by other professional groups—including nurses. For an historical overview and a projection for the future of the computerized POMR, see "Rx for the Maladies of Health Care: A Medical Revolution in the Making" (Cook, 1979).

The problem-oriented system as envisioned and developed by Dr. Weed provides for the use of the problem-oriented record by all members of the healthcare team. The introduction of this system, however, has been delayed or not been attempted at all in many healthcare agencies where the medical staff has had no interest in initiating it. In the meantime, the many workshops, books, and successful applications of the problem-oriented system have been educating more and more healthcare professionals to the benefits it offers for patient care. It is understandable that considerable frustration has existed among some professional groups in situations where they have long awaited leadership from the medical staff in introducing the problem-oriented system. Nurses in particular have wanted to participate in the initiation of the problem-oriented system. Now PONS provides a way for nurses to initiate the system within their own area of responsibility. PONS was developed out of nursing's need for a complete problem-oriented system. The efforts of many nursing departments contributed to PONS as a response to that need.

PONS incorporates a problem-oriented nursing record and the nursing process within a comprehensible system. The system, when introduced unilaterally by the nursing department, can stand on its own, assist in meeting documentation requirements and the standards for the patient's record, contribute to improved patient care, and provide increased support for the members of the medical staff. PONS is so designed that it can be integrated easily with POMS and POMR when the medical staff adopts them. Or, lacking such adoption, PONS may continue indefinitely as the basic model for nursing—using a problem-oriented nursing record and the other components that contribute to optimum patient care.

The benefits are many. Many nurses who have assisted in implementing PONS have found that, for the first time, they have been able to develop a meaningful conceptual framework within which to view all of their efforts, whether as clinical nurses, nurse managers, or nurse educators. One of the reasons for this is the fact that PONS includes a number of components which once received lip service rather than committed application but which now have become, or may soon become, mandatory. These include nursing audit, complete nursing care plans as part of patients' records, greater recognition of patients' rights and legally valid documentation. Another important feature of PONS is its contribution toward the implementation of an effective results-oriented employee performance evaluation program (ROPEP). This is covered in considerable detail in Part III. One of the most gratifying aspects of PONS is the fact that so many nurses who have participated in its implementation in their own agencies have said, "For the very first time, I now feel that I am doing professional nursing!"

PONS: BASIC COMPONENTS OF THE SYSTEM

The accompanying outline presents the five basic components of PONS together with the elements that make up each component. The five components are:

1. The Foundation
2. The Process
3. The Problem-Oriented Nursing Record
4. Nursing Audit
5. Education.

I. FOUNDATION

Principles of Nursing Practice

Goals
Objectives
Definitions
Functions
Education
Research
Philosophy

II. PROCESS

The Nursing Process

Assessing
Planning
Implementing
Evaluating

III. PROBLEM-ORIENTED NURSING RECORD (PONR)

Record

Data Base

Patient Profile
History
Physical

Problem Identification

Asset List

Problem List

1.
2.
3.
etc.

Initial Plans

Numbered and Titled
Activities of Daily Living (ADL)
Therapeutic
Patient Education

Directives/Orders

Progress Notes

Subjective
Objective
Assessment
Plans

Flow Sheets

Discharge Summary

IV. AUDIT

Nursing Audit

Define PONR
What Should Be Included?

Set Standards

Audit PONR

Measure against the Standards
Identify Deficiencies and Strengths

V. EDUCATION

Patient and Personnel

Patient

Teaching and Learning
Correct Discrepancies
Build on Strengths

Personnel

Inservice and Continuing Education

You may find much that is familiar to you in the explanation of these components. This is as it should be. PONS is not something drastically different from what some well-run nursing departments have been doing for many years. Nursing audit, as a management technique (for that's what it really is), is now an accepted part of quality assurance (JCAH, 1980). The problem-oriented nursing record is perhaps the newest component for most nursing departments. But as we have indicated, the basis for this type of nursing record has been available for quite some time. The other components—which include the principles of nursing practice, the nursing process and education for both patients and staff—are much more familiar. A major contribution of PONS is the fact that it brings together all of the components in a meaningful way so that the whole becomes much more than the sum of all its parts. The meaning of the traditional components is enhanced by the addition of the new components. And the newer components, the problem-oriented record and the nursing audit, take on much greater significance when used in the context of the other three. Thus PONS provides the synergy to achieve optimum patient care. In fact, it provides a professional model which sometimes helps to motivate members of a medical staff to take an active interest in the problem-oriented medical record. This is, of course, the ultimate test of success—when something works so well that others see its advantages and decide to adopt it for themselves.

The Foundation for PONS

The problem-oriented nursing system is structured upon a firm foundation of six elements: goals, objectives, definitions, functions, education, and research. Underlying these elements, sometimes referred to as principles of nursing practice, is the basic philosophy (beliefs, values, precepts) that serves as a guide to action and conduct. The foundation for PONS may be seen as a set of firmly interlocked building blocks of these six elements on a base of philosophy.

A statement of one's philosophy is necessarily a personal, individualized expression of the beliefs and values by which one lives. It reflects a person's heritage and early training, education, life experiences, and contemplation of the meaning of what one has learned.

The statement of philosophy for a healthcare agency expresses the beliefs and values by which the organization lives. By definition, a corporation is a body of persons granted a charter legally recognizing them as a separate entity having its own rights, privileges, and liabilities. Thus the philosophy of a hospital, HMO, nursing home, or similar agency is written by a person (or group of people) and reflects that person's (or group's) personal philosophy and views as to the beliefs, values, and precepts that will serve as the guides to action and behavior for all who work for or serve the agency.

Sometimes the organizational philosophy is available in writing as a separate statement. Sometimes it is included in the organizational charter, the legal document issued by a governmental authority creating the corporation and defining its rights and privileges. When not otherwise available in writing, the people in an organization must interpret its philosophy from the pronouncements, actions, and behavior of the recognized leader, the top person. Ultimately, such expressions of philosophy need to be discussed and translated into meaningful departmental and unit philosophies. This can be done as a part of developing unit profiles (Chapter 10) and in conjunction with setting goals and objectives (Chapter 5).

How important is your philosophy, and the philosophy of the leaders in your place of employment? Answers will vary. In Will Durant's introduction to his durable classic, *The Mansions of Philosophy,* he describes graphically the impact of change upon us all and the value of a philosophical outlook:

> All things flow, and we are at a loss to find some mooring and stability in the flux ... we fear the experts in every field, and keep ourselves, for safety's sake, lashed to our narrow specialties. Everyone knows his part, but is ignorant of its meaning in the play.
>
> We shall define philosophy as total perspective, as mind over-spreading life and forging chaos into unity. ... Philosophy is harmonized knowledge making a harmonious life; it is the self-discipline which lifts us to serenity and freedom. Knowledge is power, but only wisdom is liberty (Durant, 1953, pp. viii, ix, x).

For most persons, the philosophy and principles of those who provide agency leadership is of vital importance. These beliefs and values influence the priorities of agency goals and objectives; they influence the performance and work satisfaction of every employee. They influence the caliber of patient care and agency services.

These words may be simply a plethora of pious platitudes unless translated into a program performance plan that includes all elements that comprise the foundation for PONS.

Goals

A goal is a specific statement of purpose, an aim. What is the goal of your unit? Has the goal been communicated to everyone on the unit? Do employees understand the goal and relate it to the purpose of their own jobs?

The goal of a patient care unit must necessarily relate to the goals of the nursing department and the hospital. The primary purpose of the hospital is to meet patient needs. This goal can be achieved most effectively only within a truly integrated hospital system. Such a system is characterized by suitably differentiated activities and functional goals of the specialized departments, but with one primary goal to which all communication and interaction between departments is essential to avoid goal-setting in isolation, and to assure that departmental goals and objectives lead to effective fulfillment of the combined overall purpose of the organization. Indeed, as recognized in *Patient Care Systems* by Kraegel, Mousseau, Goldsmith, and Arora, "A whole new, orderly way of thinking about meeting patient needs has emerged. It presses for a reorganization of resources in the healthcare field which must be recognized. The hospital must be restructured for the patient. This is the growing edge" (Kraegel et al. 1974, p. viii).

Objectives

An objective is a specific task-oriented statement of results to be achieved in order to accomplish a goal. Whereas a goal is a long-term statement of purpose, an objective is a shorter-term statement of a specific target or aim. An objective presents a mutually developed and agreed-upon statement of who is going to do how much of what, how well, and when. The written objective can be clearly stated in a simple declarative sentence: "Somebody does something."

An extensive and detailed presentation of goals and objectives as related to patient care management is included in the chapter on Management by Objectives in Part III. The Objectives Worksheet described therein is helpful in problem solving, planning a mutually-agreed-upon course of action, reminding others of their expected participation, recording progress (one worksheet for each objective), assisting in developing a Program Performance Plan (PPP Schedule) for all objectives, evaluating results, and documenting action (for personnel file, accreditation and auditing purposes, legal evidence, and other reasons related to your management functions of planning-doing-controlling).

The Objectives Worksheet has been helpful to nurses and nurse managers in achieving objectives as diverse as (short term) changing an aide's pattern of arriving late for work, to (long term) implementing a two and a half year program performance plan for a family-centered maternal and child health service.

Definitions

Definitions, as used for this element of the foundation for PONS, refers to the act of making clear and distinct; a determination of outline, extent, or limits. The process of developing meaningful definitions can be exciting, thought-provoking, challenging, and enlightening. Carefully and creatively carried out, it becomes a uniquely educative learning process. A dictionary is helpful—several copies, for expediting work in a group. The dictionary is necessary not for nit-picking, hairsplitting gameplaying, but for reasons of accuracy and precise usage. Professional people, regardless of title, are expected to set a professional example in the use of the simplest accurate words to convey meanings and facilitate understanding.

What needs defining? In the context of the foundation for PONS, the definitions have to do with the answers to such questions as: What's the nature of our business (occupation, concern, interest) on this unit? Whom do we serve? What is our source of patients? What type of care are we expected to provide (acute, long-term, self, out-patient, home, etc.)? Who receives care (children, families, elderly, indigent, etc.)? What do our patients (or clients) expect from us on this unit? To what extent do we expect patients (and/or their families) to participate in their own care? What is our relationship to other agency departments? What does patient care mean to us on this unit? What is the scope of nursing care? What is a patient need? What responsibilities do our unit personnel have to persons other than their nurse manager and patients? How are performance results evaluated?

These questions may suggest others that need answering in addition to or instead of the foregoing for your particular unit, department, or agency. Do not be concerned if such questions seem to overlap with your goals and objectives. They should. They influence one another. Your exploration of such questions with others can lead to a set of definitions and statements that become part of your unit profile, a kind of self-developed charter expressing much that is fundamental to the functioning of your organizational unit and your principles of practice.

Function

A function is the natural or proper action for which a person, office, mechanism, or organ is fitted or employed; assigned duty or activity; specific occupation or role. The functions of the members of the nursing staff comprise another important building block in the foundation for PONS. One of the best ways for clarifying functions is the use of performance descriptions for every person in every job on your unit. Such performance descriptions are described in Chapter 1, and treated more fully in the ROPEP chapter of Part III.

Copies of performance descriptions for all unit personnel need to be available for review and use by every person. More effective team results occur when every person understands not only his own performance responsibilities but also what is expected of all the other team members. We have previously noted that specialization and differentiation of functions, together with a unifying or integrating force, are necessary and desirable for the departments of an entire agency. The same principle applies at the unit level; differentiation of individual performance responsibilities, together with an effective integrating force, are necessary components for goal achievement.

Education

Education is the process of educating; the skills or knowledge so developed. Education has always been, and will continue to be, an essential and respected segment of the principles of nursing practice. Thus education is included as part of the foundation as well as being shown as a separate component. Its several aspects—inservice education, continuing education, and patient education—are discussed in Part IV.

Research

Research is scholarly or scientific investigation or inquiry. Research results are reported regularly in the pages of nursing publications. Increasingly, nurses in agency settings are carrying out research studies and scientific inquiries within their departments of nursing on a specific unit or units. In one notable VA Hospital, the innovative chief nurse stimulated her nurses to initiate a number of mini-research projects on subjects of their own choice. Typical study titles were as follows: How Close Are We to the Patients' Goals?, Evaluation of Patient Bathing, Interdisciplinary Analysis to Meeting Needs of Emphysema Patients, Study of Nursing Assistant Activities on a Single Unit, and Study of Unit Escort Service.

These mini-research projects were carried out by individual nurses, most of whom were previously overawed at the prospect of doing research. Guidance was provided in simple research design. The nurses did an excellent job of presenting oral and written project reports which included: Statement of Purpose, Methodology, Findings, Conclusions, and Recommendations. The process of preparing for, carrying out, and reporting upon these mini-research projects generated much pride, esprit de corps, and useful results. Many recommendations were implemented. This kind of activity at the patient care unit level deserves to be emulated by other nurse managers. It enriches the foundation for PONS.

One form of research is literature research. This is, in effect, researching the research results of others. It involves a systematic inquiry into the investigations of others who have studied one or more facets of the subject in which you are interested. A classic example of this kind of research is the scholarly work by Herzberg, Mausner, Peterson, and Capwell at Psychological Service of Pittsburgh in which they reviewed almost two thousand writings to classify problem areas of job attitudes (Herzberg et al., 1957). As part of their 279-page publication, the authors present results from 15 studies including over 28,000 employees that identify factors contributing to either satisfaction or dissatisfaction. In later writings, the authors concluded that the job factors influencing satisfaction could be grouped in two main classifications—the hygiene factors (affecting job dissatisfaction) and the motivators (affecting job satisfaction). Herzberg's further work led to his familiar and popularized concepts of job enrichment and motivation through the work itself (Herzberg, 1968). Nurses who wish to do so can initiate their own research. It might involve a simple literature review in a specific subject area. Or it might include a limited on-the-job scientific investigation of a specific hypothesis (an assumption subject to verification or proof). For example, after becoming sufficiently familiar with PONS, you may wish to test the following hypothesis (or some limited portion of it): the problem-oriented system leads to better patient care than a nonproblem-oriented system ("better patient care" being defined as a higher level of accomplishment in meeting patient needs).

Then, following some easy-to-understand guidelines, you can observe and evaluate two sets of patients—one group cared for using all of the components of PONS, the other group cared for without using the defined data base, the problem list, the numbered and titled care plans, or the SOAP-oriented progress notes. Your findings and conclusions could become a valuable contribution to your associates and your patients. At the very least, it would be an exciting learning experience for you and your unit associates.

The six building blocks—goals, definitions, objectives, functions, education, research—together with the underlying philosophy, provide a firm, supportive base for a problem-oriented nursing system. Such a solid foundation permits the nursing process to be utilized in ways that provide great satisfaction to the nursing and medical staffs while effectively meeting patient needs.

THE NURSING PROCESS AND PONS

The nursing process was discussed in Chapter 1 in connection with the management process and Figure 1-2. Mention was made of the fact that too often nurses themselves do not comprehend or use the nursing process in any significant way. But when the nursing process is understood as a component of PONS within the framework of the patient care process as depicted in Table 3-1, it acquires renewed meaning and utility. Our purpose now is to review the nursing process as an essential component of a problem-oriented system.

The nursing process includes four phases: assessing, planning, implementing, and evaluating. Yura and Walsh provide this definition: "The nursing process is an orderly, systematic manner of determining the client's problems, making plans to solve them, initiating the plan or assigning others to implement it, and evaluating the extent to which the plan was effective in resolving the problems identified" (Yura & Walsh, 1967). According to Combs, the helping process must be as predictable as the helpers can make it (Combs et al., 1971). When the helper is a nurse, she has a tool at her command—in the very nature of the nursing process—which becomes a facilitator of predictability. This process of improving predictability begins with the assessment of the person who becomes a patient. "Assess" means to appraise; estimate;

form a tentative opinion; form a judgment of worth or significance. It also means to evaluate. In colloquial terms assess means to size up a situation, a person, or a patient's condition. Assessment leads to identification of the patient's problems and needs. This is the basis for a nursing diagnosis.

Assessment in the nursing process begins when the nurse takes a nursing history, by whatever name. This may be recorded on the nursing data base, patient profile, patient history, or initial nursing assessment. It involves communication, observation, and perception. This is a time when needs, problems and some tentative goals are being expressed and identified by both patient and nurse. In some instances the family or significant others may be the only persons able to help with this initial patient assessment.

"Plan" means to formulate a program for the accomplishment or attainment of a goal. Once an assessment of needs and problems has been made, planning begins. Planning, insofar as possible, should be done with the patient and family rather than for them. Goals can be developed, and initial objectives identified, for each need or problem.

Setting patient care objectives is an integral part of the planning phase of the nursing process. The initial objectives are those that are developed upon admission of the patient. As needs change and new problems arise and are assessed, then plans—including objectives—will change too. Since these objectives are intended to be stated as part of the nursing plan, it is not necessary to create yet another nursing form for them. You may want to revise existing forms to assure that the nursing care plans are a part of the patient's permanent medical record.

As you carry out the planning phase of the nursing process, remember that you as a nurse can and must mutually set as many goals and objectives as possible with the patient and family. By so doing, you will be acting consistently within the foundation for PONS and laying the groundwork for a successful discharge plan.

"Implement" is defined as a means employed to achieve a given end; to initiate and complete the actions necessary to accomplish an objective. Implementing implies doing, taking action. The successful achievement of an objective necessitates taking action. The action may involve several steps or just one or two. (The application of the management-by-objectives technique in nursing is presented in Part III.) For example, consider the situation of Mrs. Alexander who is recovering from a cerebral vascular accident which paralyzed her right side. Jane Doe, Mrs. Alexander's primary nurse, identifies the necessary goal as increasing the range of motion of Mrs. Alexander's right arm as much as possible. To achieve this goal, Jane has as one of her objectives to help Mrs. Alexander achieve the following: exercises right arm by herself at least four times a day. Possible steps to achieve this objective might include:

1. Discussing the whole idea of exercising with Mrs. Alexander, including how and why to exercise her arm by herself and her feelings about it (as reinforcement for instruction by the physical therapist).
2. Setting an objective, mutually with Mrs. Alexander, for exercising her right arm.
3. Making suitable entry on the nursing care plan.
4. Beginning the exercises by demonstrating how to do it with the use of her good left arm and hand.
5. Allowing Mrs. Alexander to return the demonstration, assisting her only as necessary.
6. Giving encouragement and praise as appropriate.
7. Having Mrs. Alexander do the exercising on her own schedule and without assistance.
8. Carefully recording Mrs. Alexander's progress in her patient record, using a patient teaching flow sheet.

The implementation phase of the nursing process is the one within which nurses can really make a significant change in the delivery of healthcare. It is at this point—while carrying out the care plan—that nurses can shift their emphasis from performing daily routine chores to a goal-oriented focus on meeting individual patient needs and helping to resolve individual patient problems. In the case of Mrs. Alexander's objective, the purpose is not simply to "get Mrs. Alexander to exercise her arm," but rather to help her understand the need for progressively increasing her range of arm motion so that she continually prevents contractures or muscle atrophy in her paralyzed arm. Having a daily objective in terms of achieving a specified degree range of motion helps Mrs. Alexander's motivation and sense of progress.

The conscious, deliberate, and careful attention to mutual objectives in the implementation phase is the responsibility of nurses, working with their patients.

"Evaluate" means to examine and judge; to ascertain the value of; to appraise. Implicit in the evaluation phase of the nursing process is taking a look at the results of the nursing actions to see how well the nurse, patient, and family have met the objectives (and ultimately the goals) they have established. Thus, at the time of Mrs. Alexander's discharge from the hospital, the nurse's discharge summary will include a notation such as: "Has achieved a 75° range of motion in right arm using lifting exercises which she can do herself unassisted, four times a day. Mrs. Alexander says, 'I know I have to continue these exercises every day in order to achieve my goal of greater range of motion of my right arm.'"

The nurse, as a key member of the helping professions, is in a uniquely advantageous position to lead and coordinate team efforts in meeting patient needs. Skillful use of the nursing process, as an essential component of PONS, will continue to be necessary. The process will be enhanced when the nurse recognizes and effectively utilizes both the technical mode and the human mode in getting results. We will see now how the problem-oriented record simplifies and adds a whole new dimension to the nursing process—and to the opportunities and satisfactions of being a nurse.

THE PROBLEM-ORIENTED RECORD

A problem-oriented record is a written account of events and facts related to identified and numbered problems of a person who has become a patient. The problem-oriented record is a particular kind of documentation for the patient's chart, the medical record kept for each patient. When only nursing personnel are involved in using the charting method unique to the problem-oriented system, then that portion of the patient's record is defined as a problem-oriented nursing record. Components of the problem-oriented nursing record are (1) a nursing data base, (2) a problem list, (3) a nursing plan, and (4) the nursing progress notes, flow sheets, and discharge summary.

Each component needs to be understood and used appropriately if the problem-oriented nursing record is to have real meaning for the patient. And this is what the record is all about; namely, a better means to help meet the needs of the patient. The events and facts alluded to in the definition of a problem-oriented record are very real happenings for the person involved. They are truly vital statistics, events, and facts. As such, they must be recorded accurately and legibly in all details: dates and times of events and facts; signatures (initials alone are not acceptable) and titles of nursing personnel; quotation marks around statements made by patient, family, and significant others; concise statements of observations made by nursing personnel; notation of quantities; and other relevant statistics. We present now each component of the problem-oriented nursing record.

Nursing Data Base

The nursing record begins when a person enters a healthcare agency for care. The agency may be a public health clinic, a mental health center, a general hospital, a state mental hospital, or any one of a number of kinds of specialized hospitals, clinics, or centers. Whatever the setting, basic information about the patient is required to help nursing personnel identify patient needs and problems. A variety of titles are used to identify the patient's data base. Some of these are nursing data base, nursing patient profile, nursing admission history, nursing assessment sheet, nursing history, and nursing interview. Regardless of title, these records provide data that serve as a base line, the basic starting point for measurement and comparison purposes.

The information contained in a nursing data base is obtained by the nurse in the initial assessment phase of the nursing process. Assessment requires proficiency in interviewing and observing. A nurse learns proficiency in these techniques by using the necessary skills, by practicing the right method and using it repeatedly. A skill, remember, is proficiency in a way of doing something using one's hands, body, and brain. During the process of interviewing, the nurse is also observing the patient for behaviors, mannerisms, physical signs and symptoms, and physical expression of feelings. Practice of the necessary skills will help to sharpen observing ability. When skillful interviewing is combined with skillful observing, the assessment process is most likely to yield a meaningful patient data base. Accurate observation depends on the skill of the nurse and the nature of the observation criteria.

Problem List

A problem is anything that causes concern to the patient and his family or to the nursing staff and others concerned with the patient's care. Walker defines a problem as "anything that requires diagnosis or management or that interferes with the quality of life as perceived by the patient" (Walker, 1973, p. 14).

The problem list derives from the data base. It is advisable and desirable to have a complete list of all the patient's problems, such as would be available when a problem-oriented medical record is in use. In any event it is necessary to identify pertinent problems as the patient presents them. The problem list, however, is not fixed and unchanging. The number of problems will increase as new problems are identified and will change as some problems are resolved.

When a problem-oriented medical record is in use, the problem list is usually located at the front of the patient's record for ready reference. When only a problem-oriented nursing record is being used, the problem list may be located at the front of the nursing section of the patient's record as a single sheet. Or the problem list may be combined with the nursing orders, actions, or directives—which constitute the nursing care plan.

The use of the subscript "n" with the problem number is a means of coping with the following question: "If the medical staff adopts a problem-oriented medical record at some later time, will confusion occur in use of problem numbers in prior patient records where only nurses assigned numbers?" One way to avoid any possibility of such confusion is for nursing personnel to use the subscript "n" with each problem number. This identifies it for all time as a problem number assigned by nursing. Later when the

Identifying and Classifying Problems

Categories	Examples
Medical problems	
A diagnosis (if already determined)	Myocardial infarction
Signs or symptoms	Shortness of breath
Abnormal laboratory findings	Abnormal EKG
Surgical problems	
An operation	Myocardial revascularization
Psychological problems	
Psychiatric	Anxiety
Behavioral	Depression
Sociological problems	Loss of income
	Marital friction
Demographic problems	Farmer for 20 years; now unable to farm
Previous problems	
An allergy	Morphine
An operation	Left total hip replacement
A risk factor	Overweight
*Descriptive problems**	Patient must have six personnel and lift to transfer to stretcher
*Anticipated events**	Platelet count: watch for signs of hemorrhage

*We thank Marsha McFall, RN (of St. John's Hospital, Springfield, Illinois) for suggesting these, and for permission to use them here.

medical staff adopts POMR, the "n" subscript no longer is needed since both nurses and doctors will then use the same problem list and numbers.

When many problems have been identified, it is useful and time-saving to refer to the problem by both its number and name rather than using just the number alone (i.e., Problem $\#2_n$—Nausea and Vomiting). Remember that the nurse does not determine medical diagnosis. Once the doctor has made a diagnosis, however, the nurse should include it on the nursing problem list. The above list, Identifying and Classifying Problems, provides some problem categories and examples of specific evidence of such problems.

Each problem is numbered consecutively beginning with one. Once a problem has been given a number, the two become inseparable; the number is not assigned to any other problem, even when the prior problem is resolved. One good reason for this is that the problem may recur. If it does, the same number is there ready to be used, thereby avoiding confusion. Another reason is that the same number is always used to identify the same problem on the nursing care plan, the progress notes, and wherever else that problem is referred to in nursing documentation. So each plan of action, each nursing directive, and each progress note are done in terms of a specific problem rather than at random.

An Asset List

Dr. W. P. Mazur describes a most useful innovation in his adaptation of the problem-oriented system (Mazur, 1974). He and his staff at Osawatomie State Hospital in Kansas have developed a separate form for a listing of each patient's assets, which are whatever may be identified as special attributes and strengths of a patient and his life situation that may be marshalled to assist in his care planning and facilitate his return to normal health and daily functioning. These may include attitudes, habits, beliefs; special skills, talents, hobbies; resources, facilities, and support available from family members and/or the community.

Dr. Mazur suggests listing patient assets in order of availability (how rapidly can they be used?), magnitude or intensity (most outstanding, strongest), and location (intrapersonal, interpersonal, community). A letter-coding of assets (A, B, C, in contrast to the number-coded problem list) makes possible ready cross-reference in the nursing data base, care plans, progress notes, discharge plans, or other records. An asset list has special applicability in psychiatric hospitals and other long-term care facilities. Partly because of our firm belief in the necessity for building on assets, we see significant benefits in the use of the asset list as part of PONS in other agencies, too.

The Nursing Care Plan

No-Nonsense Nursing Orders

The nursing care plan is the document which clearly states the patient's problems, together with the goals, objectives, methods, and strategies for resolving the patient's problems and needs. The medical plan of care is written as the doctor's orders with each order dated, signed, and carried out in strict adherence to the instructions. The nursing plan of care needs to be handled in a similar fashion, with each nurse's order (instruction or directive) dated, signed, and carried out by the nursing staff with the same degree of thoroughness as with the doctors' orders. Doctors' orders are not written in pencil, unsigned, on a Kardex which is erased and discarded upon discharge of the patient. Nurses' orders must no longer be so treated. They, as well as the doctors' orders, must become a permanent part of the patient's chart. Unless and until the nursing care plan is accorded the importance it deserves, there is little likelihood of its being taken seriously by members of the nursing staff. Written policies, procedures, and consistent management follow-through are required to lend meaning and support to the nursing plan of care.

Orders, like objectives, rely on the components implied in the questions, what? who? why? when? where? and how? Here is an elaboration of these components of a nursing order.

WHAT . . . . action is required? (usually an action verb is involved, e.g., check, give, assist, lift)

WHO . . . . . is expected to do it? (RN, LPN/LVN, Aide, Tech, Clerk)

WHY . . . . . is the action being done? (e.g., to reduce swelling, to promote circulation, to encourage coughing, allow verbal ventilation)

WHERE . . . which part or parts of the body are involved? (e.g., left elbow, ankles, right lung)

WHEN . . . . time frame to be used. (e.g., BID, q4h, ac)

HOW . . . . . technique or procedure to be used. (name or description)

Simple, uncluttered forms need to be used for documenting nursing orders. Use experimental forms until nurses become proficient at writing orders that can be taken seriously. The following is an example of complementary medical and nursing care plans that focus on one patient's identified problem.

PATIENT'S NAME: Alexander Watson
CHIEF COMPLAINT: emphysema, heart failure
ONE PROBLEM: fluid retention

MEDICAL PLAN OF CARE	NURSING PLAN OF CARE
(Doctor's Orders)	*(Nurse's Orders)*
Date: 4-17-78	Date: 4-17-78
Time: 7:30 a.m.	Time: 9:10 a.m.
1. Salt-free diet	1. Check lower extremities
2. Lasix 40 mg. po BID after breakfast and evening meal.	at least BID for swelling/ edema by using observation and palpation.
3. Weigh qd before breakfast and record. Report any	2. Elevate both lower extremities periodically

Medical and Nursing Plans of Care continued

weight gain of more than
2 lbs. (signed) Mary Doe
MD

throughout the day and
evening.

3. Teach patient to check
   lower extremities for swelling and to report results
   to nurse. (signed) John
   Jones, RN

The results of using nursing care plans (nursing orders) should be reflected in the condition of the patient and in the documentation on the patient's record. If a problem-oriented nursing record is used, the process and progress should show up in the nurse's progress notes and on the flow sheets. A nursing audit should then be able to pick up in patient outcomes evidence of the planning and follow-through.

Medical orders and nursing orders comprise the plan of care that is used to assure 24-hour continuity of patient care. The use of the medical and nursing orders at change of shift provides an essential adjunct to the oral reporting traditionally used to communicate vital patient care information. When the orders (plans of care) are well executed, the need for oral reporting is minimized.

Planning will be practical and be taken seriously only when the nursing care plan is made simple enough for the nurse to use easily. A complicated care plan may be a good teaching/learning tool, but simplicity is essential in a patient care setting where short-term stays and frequent admissions and discharges are a reality. The patient, regardless of length of stay, has a right to expect both a medical plan of care and a nursing plan of care.

The nursing care plan is intended to be flexible, to change as the patient's needs and problems change. It is important that planning, as evidenced by the nursing care plan, become an integral part of the patient's record. It must not be erased, written over, or discarded. Some interesting ways to achieve this are being utilized in a variety of healthcare settings. It is not essential to use a separate card (such as Kardex) for the care plan. What is essential is that the plan meet the criteria set forth in the following list:

Criteria for the Nursing Care Plan

The nursing care plan:

1. Is initiated on the date of admission.
2. Is in writing as a part of the patient's permanent record.

3. Is based on identification of specific problems and needs of the patient.
4. Is coordinated with the medical care plan.
5. Is based upon scientific principles and is therapeutically effective.
6. Ensures maximum physical and emotional safety and security for the patient.
7. Reflects immediate and long-range planning for regaining or maintaining maximum degree of health attainable for the patient.
8. Identifies and meets the psychosocial and physiological needs of the patient.
9. Provides for patient and family participation as much as possible.
10. Includes patient and family teaching/learning programs and discharge planning.
11. Indicates specific nursing care measures to be taken.
12. Specifies objectives, methods and approaches to assure best results for patient.

Many readers will find the following exercise useful. First select the nursing records for five of your present patients. From these records, identify how well the specific nursing care plans meet the criteria as listed. This simple exercise can be most revealing. You may find more evidence of complete, documented planning than you expected. Or you may find very little such evidence. In effect, you have been performing a nursing mini-audit.

Secondly, review the forms you are now using for their adequacy in filling your needs. Can you create new forms that you think would be more useful than the ones you are using? Remember that the forms you design and use are a means to the end of meeting the criteria for nursing care plans—and thus optimizing patient care. Thirdly, suggest some ways you might meet some of the other criteria as listed.

The total process of planning requires the cooperation of both medical and nursing staffs with the administration of the hospital. The nurse can prove to be of invaluable service to the patient if he/she looks upon the patient first as a person, then as a patient, and then as a part of a planning process. The patient must become a part of the planning process whenever able to do so. It is, after all, the patient's illness. No one is more concerned with it than the patient, even when family and significant others show concern.

The written nursing care plan is intended to be a practical plan of action that individualizes the care of a patient and makes possible meaningful continuity of care. The planning process begins with assessment via the nursing history, interview of the patient, and the medical history. The plan should be based on specific goals of the patient, as well as those of the nurse and physician, and should be flexible. It will change, perhaps daily or hourly, as the patient changes. It becomes a permanent part of the patient's record and is used in any referrals that are made for the patient upon discharge.

Nursing Progress Notes

Once an initial plan of action has been determined for the patient, the implementation of that plan begins. The Joint Commission on Accreditation of Hospitals (JCAH) indicates in its Standard IV for nursing services that, "Individualized, goal-directed nursing care shall be provided to patients through the use of the nursing process" (JCAH, 1979, p. 118). Regarding documentation, the JCAH manual reads as follows: "Documentation of nursing care shall be pertinent and concise, and shall reflect the patient's status. Nursing documentation should address the patient's needs, problem, capabilities, and limitations. Nursing intervention and patient response must be noted" (JCAH, 1979, p. 119). See Appendix K for the complete set of standards and an accompanying interpretation.

There is ample evidence that the JCAH standards must be met for accreditation to be granted (or continued). Here is an example (early 1980) of a specific set of pertinent recommendations by JCAH to one nursing department following a survey visit.

1. The nursing care plan should include "goals" that are based on the nursing assessment and that shall be realistic, measurable, and consistent with the therapy prescribed by the medical practitioner.
2. Documentation should be made in the medical record of nursing intervention and the patient's response to that intervention.
3. The nurse should write a transfer/discharge summary when a patient is transferred from one unit to another or is discharged. This will reflect the patient's status upon leaving that unit.
4. The nursing manual should include a policy relating to the maintenance of required records, reports, and statistical information.

The problem-oriented nursing record provides for the concise, accurate recording of significant information about the patient and his care through the use of (1) the SOAP format on the nursing progress notes, (2) a discharge summary, and (3) the use of flow sheets for repetitive components of care.

The SOAP Format

Problem #: _____
Problem Name: _____
S: Subjective information: Includes what the patient says. Use quotation marks; or note that patient stated something, and what he communicated.

O: Objective information: Firsthand observations made by nursing personnel.

A: Assessment: Based on subjective and objective information. This is the conclusion the nurse makes.

P: Plan of action.

The use of the SOAP format requires ability in communication, especially listening and observing; skill in the analysis of data; knowledge of clinical information and appropriate terminology; planning and organizing of information; and appropriate action. Learning the skills requires practice and patience. Some nurses question the need for using all of the four SOAP components all of the time. Common sense, observed practice, and judgment indicate the need for including each step each time. However, the entry for one or another of the SOAP items may be simply "none," "no change," or a dash to indicate no new data available. Mazur provides in his manual *The Problem-Oriented System in the Psychiatric Hospital* some of the best examples of the flexibility of the SOAP format, as well as some examples of SOA, OAP, and SAP notes (Mazur, 1974).

Flow Sheets

Flow sheets provide an efficient and timesaving way to record information that must be obtained repeatedly at regular and/or short intervals of time. Usually such necessary information, accumulated without suitable flow sheets, clutters the progress notes and defeats the purpose of the SOAP format. The nursing care flow sheet does not substitute for progress notes, but is used to supplement them.

Flow sheets can be used to record information on such things as vital signs, intake and output, treatments, postoperative care, postpartum care, and diabetic regimen—to mention only a few. The rule of thumb is to use a flow sheet whenever information needs to be documented repeatedly, and can be done adequately by numbers or check marks.

Discharge Summary

The nursing discharge summary is more than the conventional recording of the date, time, and mode by which the patient leaves a healthcare facility—as pertinent as these may be upon the occasion of actual discharge. The nursing discharge summary is the direct result of planning for discharge that begins soon after the person is admitted to a healthcare agency. Evidence of discharge planning should be documented throughout the patient's stay. It should be in evidence and recognized by the patient and the patient's family. It should be retrievable from the documentation in the nursing care plan, the progress notes, and flow sheets.

The actual discharge summary of a patient should include: (1) the state of health now compared with the state at the time of admission; (2) the patient's activity level; (3) the patient's knowledge and feelings about his state of health, medications, diet, activity, equipment and supplies, referral, follow-up care, and resources available in the community. Patients, upon discharge, require information that is highly specific to them. The kind, amount, and detail of the information depends upon each patient's own unique needs in a given situation. It also depends on other variables such as the person's knowledge, feelings, values, prejudices, life style, and experiences in living and working, as well as the amount and kind of intrusions upon the patient's health status. Patient teaching, based upon these variables and on standards of care for specific illnesses, helps each individual to learn what he or she needs to know at the time of discharge. The discharge summary is intended as a final entry by the nurse in the patient's record. It may be a part of the progress notes, or it may be a more extensive summary on a separate form.

Discharge planning requires a collaborative effort on the part of all members of a healthcare team. Doctors, nurses, therapists, nutritionists, and many others may need to pool their efforts to provide good continuity of care from one healthcare setting to another and into the patient's home. The nurse can and should play a pivotal role in coordinating the efforts of all those involved, including the patient and the patient's family. Since the discharge summary is prepared on the patient's behalf, each patient should receive a copy of the discharge summary.

THE NURSING AUDIT AND PONS

Nursing audit is the fourth component of the problem-oriented nursing system. Audit plays an essential role in the system. It is the inspection function. It is part of the quality assurance program. Nursing audit is defined as a method for assuring documentation of the quality of nursing care in keeping with the standards of the agency, the nursing department, and the professional, governmental, and accrediting groups.

Among those who are concerned with quality control in industry, there is a familiar statement that rings true: "You cannot inspect quality into a product; quality must be built into the product or service." So it is in nursing and the other helping relationships within healthcare agencies. The level of quality is determined at the point of service. People provide service to and for patients. People determine the quality level of the care being provided. This level of care, however it is experienced and perceived by the patient, may or may not be so reflected in the audit results. Part of the reason for PONS is to assure that patient needs are met with an appropriate level of care which is reflected accurately in the audit reports.

Too often in the past the patient's record has not reflected, accurately and completely, the excellence of the nursing care actually provided to the patient. Nursing care plans maintained conscientiously from day to day in the open chart, have (in some hospitals) been removed and destroyed by nursing service as a regular practice when the patient was discharged. This action effectively eliminated from the closed chart vital evidence of the quality of nursing care provided to the patient. An organized audit procedure will lead to corrective action in such cases, and assure preservation of the necessary data in an appropriate way.

Here are the major purposes and benefits of a systematic nursing audit procedure. Nursing audit:

1. Necessitates adequate documentation of the nursing care provided to the patient through the entire nursing process.
2. Directs attention to the design and utility of the charting records.
3. Encourages use of the Problem-Oriented Nursing System.
4. Supports, and becomes an integral part of, the Nursing by Objectives Program.
5. Facilitates the cooperative planning and delivery of patient care by physicians and nursing personnel.
6. Increases the priority for a Results-Oriented Performance Evaluation Program for nursing service employees.
7. Enriches and provides direction to inservice education efforts.
8. Provides a specific management technique to aid nurse managers in carrying out their evaluation and control function.
9. Identifies ways to improve patient care, both short range and long range.
10. Provides a meaningful way for nursing staff members to participate and achieve career growth.

Nursing Audit and the Problem-Oriented Nursing Record (PONR)

Nursing audit, like any other management technique, works best when it is used as part of an integrated system. Before beginning an audit program, it is worthwhile to examine the components of the patient care system within which nursing audit is to be introduced. In order to do this, it is helpful to have a frame of reference from which to begin. The problem-oriented nursing system, inclusive of the nursing process, provides such a frame of reference.

The audit procedure is an aspect of the evaluation phase of the ongoing nursing process. Implementation of the audit procedure is greatly facilitated when a problem-oriented charting system is used. The very nature and purpose of problem-oriented charting is to provide for reliable evaluation of a patient's problems, progress, and treatment results. A more complete presentation of nursing audit as a nursing management technique is provided in Part III.

As a management technique, nursing audit is part of the evaluating and planning phases of the management process. It is ongoing rather than sporadic. Monthly and quarterly comparisons of results provide a way to determine the efficacy of the audit program.

The retrospective audit procedure may focus on either an outcome audit or a process audit. The outcome audit identifies patient outcomes that are unsatisfactory, and is intended to identify the patterns of nursing care that appear to be responsible. The process audit is a deeper probe of problems already recognized (or suspected) in the nursing care process.

SUMMARY

The problem-oriented nursing record offers nurses the particular opportunity to integrate the care they give with a way of documenting that care. We know that, for nurses accustomed to traditional practices, much time and effort is required to change long-standing habit patterns. But we also believe that the effort is worth it. Nurses cannot rely upon sketchy notes supplemented by memory and share it all verbally. The complexity of healthcare today no longer encourages or permits such practices. They are neither safe nor efficient. Random-style charting and traditional narrative notes fall into the same category.

The problem-oriented record as part of an entire problem-oriented system is no panacea—but it has been well tested; it works well; it holds great continuing promise for patients and for nurses. We believe strongly that nurses can and will bring that promise into full realization.

The quality of nursing care is becoming more measurable and quantifiable. It can be and is being translated into numbers. While this trend may not be easy for some nurses to accept or comprehend, for other nurses it is most welcome. Experience in every field of human endeavor indicates that when quality or performance standards are established and results are measured against such standards, the results improve. There is every reason to believe that this ongoing process in patient care will contribute to greater, not less, satisfaction among nursing personnel.

PONS is a patient-centered system with the focus on the needs and problems of the individual patient. Five interrelated components make up the complete system. If one of the components is missing, the system is incomplete. These components include a foundation (principles of nursing practice) on which to build the nursing process and document that process on a problem-oriented nursing record which is audited to determine quality and identify the educational needs of patients and nursing personnel.

NOTES

Combs, A. W., Avila, D. L., & Purkey, W. W. *Helping relationships: Basic concepts for the helping professions.* Boston: Allyn and Bacon, 1971, p. 166.

Cook, G. Rx for the maladies of health care; A medical revolution in the making. *The Futurist,* June 1979, pp. 179–189.

Durant, W. *The mansions of philosophy.* Garden City, N.Y.: Garden City Publishing, 1927. (Newer publication available by the title *The pleasures of philosophy*, Simon & Schuster, 1953.) Reprinted with permission of Simon & Schuster, Inc. © 1953.

Herzberg, F. One more time: How do you motivate employees? *Harvard Business Review,* January-February 1968, *46*, 53–62.

Herzberg, F., Mausner, B., Peterson, R. O., & Capwell, D. F. *Job attitudes: Review of research and opinion.* Pittsburgh: Psychological Service of Pittsburgh, 1957.

Joint Commission on Accreditation of Hospitals. *Accreditation manual for hospitals* (1980 ed.). Chicago: Author, 1979.

Kraegel, J., Mousseau, V. S., Goldsmith, C., & Arora, R. *Patient care systems.* Philadelphia: J. B. Lippincott, 1974.

Mazur, W. P. *The problem-oriented system in the psychiatric hospital.* Garden Grove, Ca.: Trainex Press, 1974, pp. 6, 15–16.

Roy, C. *Introduction to nursing: An adaptation model.* Englewood Cliffs, N.J.: Prentice-Hall, 1976.

Walker, H. K. The problem-oriented medical record. In *Applying the problem-oriented system* (H. K. Walker, J. W. Hurst, & M. F. Woody, Eds.). New York: Medcom, 1973.

Yura, H., & Walsh, M. *The nursing process.* Washington D.C.: Catholic University of America Press, 1967, p. 23.

Zander, K. *Primary nursing: Development and management.* Germantown, Md.: Aspen Systems Corp., 1980.

Reading List

Books

Bradt, D. The nursing process. In N. Chaska (Ed.), *The nursing profession: Views through the mist.* New York: McGraw-Hill, 1978.

Cantor, M. M. *The JCAH standards.* Wakefield, Mass.: Contemporary Publishing, 1974.

Carter, J. H., Hilliard, M., Castles, M. R., Stoll, L. D., & Cowan, A. *Standards of nursing care: A guide for evaluation* (2nd ed.). New York: Springer, 1976.

Documenting patient care responsibility. Nursing Skillbook. Horsham, Pa.: Nursing 78 Books, 1978.

Easton, R. *Problem-oriented medical record concepts.* New York: Appleton-Century-Crofts, 1976.

Enslow, A., & Swisher, S. *Interviewing and patient care.* New York: Oxford University Press, 1972.

Epstein, C. *Effective interaction in contemporary nursing.* Englewood Cliffs, N.J.: Prentice-Hall, 1974.

Froebe, D. J., & Bain, K. J. *Quality assurance programs and controls in nursing.* St. Louis: C. V. Mosby, 1976.

Futtrell, M., & Kelleher, M. *The nurse's guide to health services for patients.* Boston: Little, Brown, 1973.

Ganong, J., & Ganong, W. *HELP with the problem-oriented nursing system.* Chapel Hill, N.C.: W. L. Ganong Co., 1975.

Gorton, J. *Behavioral components of patient care.* New York: Macmillan, 1970.

Gosnell, D. J. *HELP with the nursing process.* Chapel Hill, N.C.: W. L. Ganong Co., 1980.

Joint Commission on Accreditation of Hospitals. *Accreditation manual for hospitals.* Chicago: Author, 1979.

Marriner, A. *The nursing process: A scientific approach to nursing care.* St. Louis: C. V. Mosby, 1975.

Mayers, M. *A systematic approach to the nursing care plan.* New York: Appleton-Century-Crofts, 1972.

Mayers, M. *Standard nursing care plans,* Palo Alto, Ca.: R/P Co., Medical Systems, 1974 and 1975.

Mazur, W. P. *The problem-oriented system in the psychiatric hospital.* Garden Grove, Ca.: Trainex Press, 1974.

Neelon, F. A., & Ellis, G. J. *A syllabus of problem-oriented patient care.* Boston: Little, Brown, 1974.

Nursing Clinics of North America. *I. The problem-oriented record. II. Quality assurance.* Philadelphia: W. B. Saunders, 1974.

Phaneuf, M. C. *The nursing audit: Profile for excellence.* New York: Appleton-Century-Crofts, 1972.

Riehl, J., & Roy, C. *Conceptual models for nursing practice.* New York: Appleton-Century-Crofts, 1974.

Sherman, J., & Fields, S. *Guide to patient evaluation.* New York: Medical Examination Publishing Co., 1974.

Vasey, E., & Riley, M. *Quality assurance: Peer review for nursing.* Pittsburgh: Western Pennsylvania Regional Medical Program, 1975.

Walker, H. K., Hurst, J. W., & Woody, M. F. (Eds.). *Applying the problem-oriented system.* New York: Medcom Press, 1973.

Weed, L. L. *Medical records, medical education, and patient care.* New York: Appleton-Century-Crofts, 1972.

Weed, L. L. *Your health care and how to manage it.* Burlington, Vt.: Promis Laboratory, 1975.

Wooley, F. R., Warnick, M. W., Kane, R. L., & Dyer, E. D. *Problem-oriented nursing.* New York: Springer, 1974.

Yura, H., & Walsh, M. *The nursing process.* Washington, D.C.: The Catholic University of America Press, 1967.

Yura, H., & Walsh, M. *Human needs and the nursing process.* New York: Appleton-Century-Crofts, 1978.

Articles

Harris, R. J. Facilitating change to the problem-oriented medical record system. *Journal of Nursing Administration,* August 1978, *8*(9), 35–38.

Hushower, G., Gamberg, D., & Smith, N. The nursing process in discharge planning. *Supervisor Nurse,* September 1978, *9*(9), 55–60.

Lewis, E. P. The care of the sick. *Nursing Outlook,* October 1974, *22*, 625.

Reines, M. O. A visiting nurse in a problem-oriented group practice. *The American Journal of Nursing,* July 1979, *79*, 1225–1226.

Vasey, E. K. Writing your patient's care plan ... efficiently. *Nursing 79,* April 1979, *9*(4), 67–71.

Chapter 4

Primary Nursing

INTRODUCTION

Primary nursing is one modality available for the delivery of nursing care. It offers to patients a registered nurse with whom they can relate on a one-to-one basis.

In just over a decade of efforts to implement primary nursing, the results have been mixed. This is partially because some nursing administrators, seeing its true potential, have attempted to introduce it by edict. In one fine hospital recognized for its high caliber of patient care, the head nurses rebelled at being told to adopt primary nursing and make it work. Their independent, hardheaded investigation of how it was actually working at a respected local university hospital only confirmed their reasoned opinion that primary nursing—with its low patient-nurse ratio—was not for them, at least not yet, because of inadequate staffing. And they prevailed.

The trend toward primary nursing has led to a wide variety of results: blind acceptance; failed application attempts; judicious exploration and successful implementation. Primary nursing is no panacea. It is an appealing concept; it deserves serious consideration and can be used with great satisfaction in some situations.

A key feature of primary nursing is the way in which it places on the registered nurse full 24-hour responsibility and accountability for assessing, planning, implementing, and evaluating nursing care for a reasonable caseload of patients. It emphasizes professional clinical practice and encourages every registered nurse to perform the essential roles of practitioner, teacher, and manager of patient care and services in a hospital or related healthcare setting.

Primary nursing is an alternative to the case, functional, and team modalities used in varying degrees and combinations in hospitals and healthcare agencies. These modalities, derived in part from the military and religious heritage of nursing, are entrenched by custom and habit. They have become common practice throughout the United States. In their time they served nurses and patients well. Some, however, have become outdated and are in need of review, revision, and innovative updating.

DEFINING PRIMARY NURSING

Primary nursing as a patient care modality includes the following characteristics (Ganong and Ganong, 1977):

- Professional nurses are identified as *primary* or *associate nurses*. LPNs may be associate nurses.
- Each professional nurse is assigned a relatively small caseload (from four to eight patients).
- The nursing process is used.
- The focus is on the one-to-one relationship of *my patient/my nurse* from admission to discharge.
- Care is based on patient needs and patient problems.
- A decentralized patient unit organizational structure is used, with responsibility and authority vested in the head nurse or patient care coordinator for integrating hospital-wide patient care.
- The primary nurse is *accountable* for assigned patients 24 hours a day, 7 days a week. In the absence of the primary nurse, the written nursing care plan prepared by the primary nurse is used by the associate nurse on every shift.
- The emphasis is on professional clinical practice rather than on the performance of routines and tasks.
- There is a *problem-solving, nursing-by-objectives* approach to patient care management based on sound clinical knowledge and skills.
- Newly defined roles are identified for LPNs, aides, technicians, and secretary/clerks. The roles of evening and night "house supervisors" also need clarification.

Here are some examples of attempts by groups of experienced nurses to translate their understanding of primary nursing into written definitions.

Example 1

In primary nursing, the primary nurse is a professional nurse who assumes accountability for the nursing care of the patients in his/her caseload throughout the entire hospitalization. When the primary nurse is off duty, an associate (who is also a professional nurse) has the responsibility for the care of these patients. Continuity of care is ensured by a written nursing care plan based on the total needs and problems of the patient as a unique human being.

Example 2

Primary nursing is a system of patient care based on a problem-solving process, with the main concern being the patient's needs and problems. The primary nurse is accountable for and responsible for his/her patients and their care. This concept emphasizes professional clinical practice instead of routines. The head nurse functions as care coordinator and resource person. The professional nurse functions either as a primary nurse or an associate nurse; the practical nurse functions as an associate nurse; the clerk handles clerical duties such as admission sheets; and the aide serves as an aid to the nurse. Primary nursing fosters the "my nurse/my patient" concept and facilitates communications of the entire health team.

Example 3

Primary nursing is a method of managing patient care in which one nurse, the primary nurse, assumes 24-hour accountability for a caseload of patients by implementing the nursing process from admission to discharge or transfer. The primary nurse coordinates the varied patient services by utilizing appropriate members of the healthcare team.

Example 4

Primary nursing is professional nurses executing the nursing process, with emphasis on patient care management, effectively utilizing LPNs, nursing assistants (NAs), and clerical personnel on a 24-hour basis.

Ciske highlights a significant aspect of primary nursing by stating that:

> Primary nursing fosters a therapeutic relationship with the patient in which his needs for nursing care are most important, not the nurse's need to feel liked and successful. The relationship is not social, nor is it psychotherapy (Ciske, 1979, p. 893).

It is important to define primary nursing so that the nursing staff has a clear understanding of the concept. Keep in mind the characteristics mentioned earlier in this chapter, and build a meaningful definition without sacrificing *any* of the characteristics. A well stated definition, which the nursing staff has helped develop, provides a uniform way of explaining to nurses, doctors, patients, and others what primary nursing means. Nurses must be able to answer questions about primary nursing as often as these questions arise.

The day may come when nursing does not need special qualifying names or adjectives. Some day instead of *team* nursing, *functional* nursing, or *primary* nursing, there will be one recognized field of endeavor—*NURSING*. We hope to speed the arrival of that day. It will come when nurse educators, administrators, practitioners of nursing, and nurse managers work together to make it happen.

EVALUATING YOUR READINESS FOR PRIMARY NURSING

Exhibit 4-1 is a form entitled "Primary Nursing Readiness Evaluation." You will find it helpful as you begin to consider introducing primary nursing. It can also function as a periodic audit of how well primary nursing is being practiced on specific units. Much of the ensuing discussion follows the outline of Exhibit 4-1. (A more extensive audit form, "Nursing Organization Inventory Checklist: An Audit of Where We Are Now in Our Departmental Workworld," is included in Chapter 13 as Exhibit 13-1.)

Before you begin to implement primary nursing, you must first understand and be able to describe the way you are practicing nursing now. In Chapter 2 we reviewed two contrasting perceptions of the nurse's role: the *Nursing Workload Concept* (Concept A), and the goal-oriented *Patient Care Management Concept* (Concept B). Primary nursing requires a Concept B approach. It presumes a willingness to structure one's work day around patient needs and goals rather than around an assigned workload of procedures, tasks, and routines. The emphasis in primary nursing is problem solving to meet patient needs. It shifts the focus from "getting things done" to helping the patient meet certain objectives. It involves taking a critical/analytical look at the many routines carried out for all patients regardless of need, and replacing such routines with individualized problem solving through meaningful patient care planning. Yes, procedures and need-oriented tasks are necessary—but as a part of the implementation phase of the nursing process, not as slavish routines. For example, it may be necessary to establish a routine for an individual patient if that patient is unconscious or just too sick to participate.

One way to determine your own state of readiness for primary nursing is to identify those work routines that can be eliminated with no negative impact on the quality of patient care. Consider these nursing routines in the context of value analysis, cost/benefit ratios, and quality control—the way a management engineer or a good nurse manager has to evaluate such activities.

Exhibit 4-1 Primary Nursing Readiness Evaluation

Which of your patient care units (or service clusters) are most ready for primary nursing? List the most likely units at the top of columns. Evaluate their degree of readiness against the primary nursing components. Use your own scoring method. Results will help decide priorities for progress.

Primary nursing components / Patient care units					
Clinical knowledge and skills					

Nursing process:
  Assessment
  Plan
  Implement
  Evaluate					

Problem-oriented nursing
● The foundation:
  Philosophy
  Goals
  Objectives
  Functions
  Definitions
  Education
  Research					

● Nursing record:
  Data base
  Problem list
  Nursing care plan
  Progress notes
  Flow sheets
  Discharge summary					

● Nursing audit
● Education:
  Patients
  Staff and personnel					

Performance responsibilities and leadership:
  Head nurse
  Primary nurse
  Associate nurse
  LPN
  Nursing assistant
  Unit secretary					

Source: Ganong, J. and Ganong, W. *HELP with primary nursing*. Chapel Hill, N.C.: W. L. Ganong Co., 1977, p. 40.

You may be surprised to discover ways to offset some of the start-up costs related to primary nursing.

A Foundation for Primary Nursing

Primary nursing requires a problem-oriented approach to patient care. Chapter 3 presents one such approach—a Problem-Oriented Nursing System (PONS). The great numbers of nurses with whom we have regular contact want to *nurse*, and want to do it well. The existing healthcare system offers them that opportunity, provided they have adequate leadership—in the clinical, operational, and developmental aspects of nursing—recognizing that nursing is one of many disciplines involved in patient care.

Here are elements of a foundation for primary nursing. These are adapted from PONS in Chapter 3.

A. Philosophy
   We believe in:
   1. Each patient's human right to the best possible individualized care consistent with his/her own needs and objectives, as related to available resources.
   2. Responsibility and accountability by each professional nurse, as well as by every other member of the patient care team as appropriate to each one's identified function.
   3. The use of a problem-oriented system, with a problem-oriented nursing (or medical) record.
   4. The use of the nursing process by every nurse as a basis for nursing actions, rather than dependence upon routines.
   5. Decentralization of the nursing department for optimum patient care, employee care, and cost-effectiveness.
   6. The dignity and worth of each patient, family member, and healthcare team member.
B. Goal
   To utilize the primary nursing concept in a way that is consistent with our philosophy to help patients resolve their healthcare problems and meet their identified needs.
C. Current Objectives
   1. Identify patient care routines that can be modified or eliminated by (target date).
   2. Begin use of the complete nursing process by selected professional nurses for identified patients by (target date).
   3. Expand use of the complete nursing process to include more patients and more professional nurses by (target date).

4. Introduce a complete problem-oriented system on selected units by (target date).
5. Expand the problem-oriented system to include more units by (target date).
6. Begin primary nursing as a modality on selected units by (target date).

D. Definitions for Each Unit (your "unit profile")
   1. Patient population: source (where do they live?), sex, age group, life style, educational level, income level, family unit, expectations, and so on.
   2. Our concept of care: patient care, nursing care, patient needs, patient involvement, employee care considerations, etc.
   3. Interpersonal and interdepartmental relations: support, coordination, cooperation, communications.

E. Functions of Nursing Staff
   This means role clarification through performance descriptions (to include job purpose as related to unit goals, major performance responsibilities, for whom performed, standards of performance) prepared jointly by and with head nurse/patient care coordinator, primary nurse, associate nurse, LPN/LVN, nurse aide, nurse technician, unit secretary/clerk. (See also Chapter 6.)

F. Education and Research
   1. Scheduled inservice and continuing education to:
      a. develop skill in using the elements of the nursing process.
      b. develop managerial skills at the unit level.
   2. Implement a study of the effectiveness of primary nursing as compared with the existing nursing care method.

All of the foregoing appears to entail a considerable amount of work. It does. It is all necessary—if you wish to consider primary nursing as a means of improving the kind of nursing you have now. And there is more work to come. The fact is, such work by nurse managers and the nursing staff is important regardless of what type of nursing care you wish to deliver. It is all part of carrying out the nurse manager functions of planning, doing, and controlling in the three major areas of responsibility: clinical management, operational management, and human resources management.

Quite possibly you already have available, in various states of completion, many of the elements described in the foregoing outline. Many nurse managers (head nurses and others) find great satisfaction in thinking through these matters with the unit nursing staff members, putting it all in writing, and then using the resulting sense of agreement as a valid base from which to examine primary nursing. As a beginning, assemble those elements of PONS that already exist; redefine them as necessary; complete the missing components. Only then are you adequately prepared to answer the question, "Do we want to adopt primary nursing?"

Expanding on the Principles

The practical application of a problem-oriented nursing system using a primary nursing approach requires a focus on the direct care one nurse gives to one patient. A management-by-objectives approach (call it nursing by objectives—NBO—if you wish) facilitates the setting of patient care goals with the patient and family. In addition to the goals and objectives of the patient's doctor, there are three other aspects of nursing goals and objectives:

1. your own, as the patient's primary nurse.
2. the patient's, as a person.
3. the family's or significant others', as healthcare consumers.

Here is an example of four short-range goals for a married female patient, age 40, who has successfully undergone surgery and initial recovery for an abdominal hysterectomy.

Patient's Goal	Husband's Goal	Nurse's Goal	Doctor's Goal
To move about without pain.	To reassure wife that she is still loved and needed.	To prevent circulatory complications.	No complications.

Note that each goal is set by the individual involved: the patient, the husband, the nurse, and the doctor. All are meaningful goals that require attention. The nurse must be aware of all four goals and understand that, while each person can set objectives to meet parts of each goal, no one person can meet *all* of the goals. Successful recovery will require the patient, husband, doctor, and nurse—working together. For patient care objectives to be practical at the direct care level, it is necessary to determine which *components of an objective* are appropriate and useful in a given situation. These components are (1) What will be done? (2) How much will be done how well? (3) When will it be done? (4) Who will do what, where? and (5) What will it cost? (See Chapter 5.)

The Nursing Process and Primary Nursing

The nurse, as a key member of the helping professions, is in a unique position to lead, coordinate, and integrate efforts in meeting patient needs. Skillful use of the nursing process, as an essential component of a problem-oriented approach, is necessary. The process is enhanced when the nurse recognizes and uses both the technical mode and the human mode to get results. This is especially true in primary nursing. The primary nurse and associate nurse must have a sound grasp of the nursing process or true primary nursing cannot happen.

Chapters 1 and 3 present the nursing process as compared with the management process and as part of a problem-oriented nursing system. Figure 4-1 provides a graphic summary of the Doing and Documenting aspects of the nursing process. (See also Chapter 3 and Chapter 7.)

"The nursing process is the core process for the practice of nursing," say Yura and Walsh. They go on to state that the "basic human needs—their maintenance, their fulfillment, their integrity—are the territory of nursing" (Yura & Walsh, 1978). We heartily agree.

ORGANIZING FOR PRIMARY NURSING

Primary nursing can become an asset only when it is integrated carefully into existing organizational structures. Primary nursing involves a new way of staffing, of defining role relationships among personnel, of managing patient care, of establishing accountability, of computing the costs of patient care, of delineating doctor/patient/nurse/administrator relationships.

Tampering with such matters is no business for amateurs. It is sad but true: some of the best-intentioned nurses at all levels have the least organizational sense. Such nurses may have little or no broad comprehension of the existing agency's mission or complex organizational structure. Primary nursing requires a cautious, well-planned approach. Nurse managers should anticipate the booby traps ahead and learn how to avoid them.

Changing Organizational Concepts to Support Primary Nursing

Organizations are living, dynamic entities. To remain healthy they must react to and adjust to their environment. For primary nursing, this may mean making the design of the organization flexible to adapt to changing conditions. (See also Chapters 2 and 10.)

Organization design is defined as:

> The ways, formal and explicit, used by management to indicate to organization members what is expected of them. The *elements* include organization structure; planning, measurement, and evaluation schemes; rewards; selection criteria; training. *Situational theory* provides managers with a way to think about organization

Figure 4-1 The Nursing Process

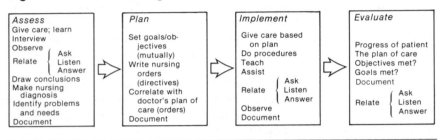

design issues in relation to the environmental and human characteristics of their situation; and to understand the complex causes of organization problems; and help managers use their own creativity to invent new designs uniquely suited to their situation (summarized from Lorsch, 1977).

Structure in this context refers to "the interrelation of parts or the principle of organization in a complex entity" (American Heritage Dictionary, 1973).

Primary nursing needs an organizational structure in which it can flourish. Spitzer says it well:

> "Primary nursing is a commitment. It cannot succeed in the traditional hierarchical structure. It requires a support system for professional practice, a system that will promote the development of the potential of each individual providing direct care. Only through this type of approach can a mutually beneficial environment evolve for the patient and the practitioner" (Spitzer, 1979, p. 14).

A support system such as Spitzer refers to is possible through a decentralized organization where responsibility and authority are delegated to nurses at the patient unit level. (See Chapter 2 for six models of decentralized versus centralized organizational structures.) The nurse manager at the unit level must have decision-making authority and be able, in turn, to delegate authority to the primary nurses who make decisions regarding direct patient care.

The primary nurse must act as a manager of direct clinical patient care. The head nurse or coordinator then assumes the important role of manager of the entire unit and acts as a resource person who facilitates the actions of the primary nurses. Mutual respect and trust among the nurses is essential if primary nursing is to succeed. Whatever the organizational structure, the primary nurse must be free to practice *clinical* nursing with administrative support.

Focus on Clinical Nursing

Essential to the success of primary nursing is adequate clinical knowledge by the primary nurse. The ability to translate that knowledge into active care is achieved through effective use of the nursing process. The primary nurse needs to know the normal and abnormal aspects of anatomy, physiology, psychology, sociology—and to know these in enough depth to be able to assess problems and needs, work with the patient to create a plan that addresses these identified problems and needs, implement the plan, and evaluate patient outcomes.

This implies a background of current information about wellness, illness, various disease processes, and human behavior. It is not enough for the primary nurse simply to be able to cite chapter and verse of a particular disease, or be skillful at performing a specific procedure. It is the combination of these—knowing, understanding what is known, and using that knowledge skillfully with patients—that makes the primary nurse different.

Admittedly, it is difficult to keep up with advances in medical and nursing technology. Changes are frequent in both software and hardware. New medicines come on the market constantly. Disposable products change frequently. New techniques and procedures are introduced regularly. The detail men, representing an ever-widening number of companies anxious to compete for a piece of the healthcare market, bombard our healthcare agencies through staff members, administrators, and even members of the board of trustees.

When clinical advances come at such a rapid rate, primary nurses find themselves in a constant state of transition with few periods of stability. Since there are only so many hours in a day, something suffers. Frequently, in the press of time, clinical learning falls lower and lower as a priority.

The primary nurse must plan carefully in order to keep up to date. Retraining is both necessary and costly. The nurse manager can help by making available the following:

- Patient-oriented interdisciplinary conferences
- Inservice programs at the patient unit level—all shifts
- Use of resource people: head nurse, clinical specialist, coordinator, nurse consultants, nurse practitioner, nurse clinician, physician, surgeon, pharmacist, nutritionist, therapists, quality assurance nurse
- Staff development programs as part of career ladders (wide-track careers programs)

- Telelecture programs sponsored by universities, available during day shift, usually at selected hospital sites
- Internships and residencies.

It is the responsibility of individual primary nurses to avail themselves of the following:

- Articles and books—written with the busy nurse in mind
- Closed-circuit TV programs
- Dial-A-Question systems
- Taped audio programs on clinical topics
- Self-study packaged programs; continuing education programs
- Workshops, seminars, institutes
- The opportunity to ask questions
- Courses at colleges and universities
- Reading promotional and informational materials on products, drugs, etc.
- Regular use of the Physician's Desk Reference (PDR); nursing, medical, and regular dictionaries; diagnostic findings; books
- Use of learning labs where available
- Filmstrips and films
- Advanced degree preparation
- Independent study programs.

Primary nursing provides nurses with a unique, long-sought opportunity to get back to the patient in a meaningful, goal-oriented way. Individual nurses and nurse managers can make the most of this opportunity only if they maintain their clinical knowledge, understanding, and skills at suitably high levels.

IMPLEMENTING PRIMARY NURSING

Introducing primary nursing entails considerable change. It should be remembered that people don't resist change quite as much as they resist *being* changed. Each staff member will experience the three phases of change: initial impact, recoil/turmoil, and adjustment and reconstruction (see Chapter 10). Here are some things that can help during a period of change to primary nursing.

- Give people the information they want and need about primary nursing.
- Involve those whose lives will be affected in any way by the change to primary nursing.

- Give reassurance and support. Let people know you care. Give them feedback on how they are doing during the change to primary nursing.
- Give enough guidance to help people learn about primary nursing and the new skills involved.
- Be available to the people who need reassurance.
- Encourage people—nursing and medical staffs, patients—to talk about all aspects of primary nursing: how they feel, what they fear.
- Clarify role expectations involved in primary nursing.
- Show respect for people's values and sense of self-worth.
- Hold out hope for the success of the change to primary nursing through supportive leadership.

A Management-by-Objectives Approach

Management by Objectives (MBO) works well for introducing a program such as primary nursing. "Because MBO is an employee-involving process that places high priority on change and progress (as opposed to ritual and crisis), its methodology is more conducive to primary nursing than any other management system" (Zander, 1980).

Once your nursing department decides to proceed with a study and a trial of primary nursing, here is an outline of possible steps following the MBO pattern:

Goal: Implement primary nursing

Objective: After exploration and decision, initiate primary nursing for a trial period of one year on two patient units by September 30, 19__, with operating expenses not to exceed present unit costs per patient day on each unit.

Program Steps

(A specific target date is to be set for the completion of each step.)

Phase I: Exploration

1. Establish task force to carry out exploration.
2. Review current nursing care program philosophy, goals, objectives, policies, and procedures; identify those requiring revision.
3. Review the literature on primary nursing.
4. Visit and consult with selected hospitals using primary nursing to identify strengths, weaknesses, problems, suggestions, cost, and results.
5. Attend workshops and seminars throughout exploration phase.

6. Develop an initial plan for implementing primary nursing as an alternative to the present nursing care program, including projected costs. This plan is subject to review by nursing staff.
7. Complete nursing staff information program about the concept and the suggested plans in order to elicit their support and recommendations.
8. Secure staff decision on implementing primary nursing.
9. Identify learning needs of nursing personnel on the two selected units on the subjects of the nursing process and the problem-oriented nursing system.

Phase II: Implementation

1. Complete primary nursing program philosophy, goals, objectives, policies, procedures, and functions.
2. Identify methods for evaluating results of trial period.
3. Conduct classes in the nursing process and PONS for personnel on the two units.
4. Orient all personnel to the agreed-upon primary nursing program on the two nursing units.
5. Present program to hospital administration, department heads, and medical staff to elicit their cooperation.
6. Clarify the role expectations and responsibilities of staff members on the two units.
7. Initiate trial period of primary nursing on the two units.
8. Evaluate progress throughout trial period and upon completion.

Involvement in the MBO approach needs to take place at all levels among all groups, but especially in *small* groups at the patient unit level, in *brief* time frames, *frequently* enough to lower frustration levels, encourage open sharing of feelings and concerns, and identify and resolve needs and problems.

Making primary nursing work is part of every nurse manager's responsibility, at every organizational level. From nursing administrator to head nurse, nurse managers need to take the lead in using and guiding primary nursing. Their leadership is especially important in hospitals, extended care facilities, and public health agencies since so many projects initiated here involve the participation of other hospital or agency department heads. The expansion or withdrawal of patient care programs such as primary nursing have impact throughout the entire organization, and often throughout the community, because of their relation to hospital goals and to competing demands for resources—personnel, money, facilities, and equipment.

Bloom conducted a study to determine if head nurses manifest the six general categories of role behavior recommended in the literature on primary nursing. The six general categories of role behavior were as follows:

1. The head nurse is a clinical role model.
*2. The head nurse is a validator and evaluator of the primary nurses' ability to carry out their nursing care responsibilities.
*3. The head nurse facilitates and encourages primary nurses to be the "primary" communicator, coordinator, and planner of nursing care for their patients.
4. The head nurse facilitates and encourages professional staff development.
*5. The head nurse utilizes leadership skills and is the nursing administrative manager of the nursing care of all the patients on the unit.
*6. The head nurse encourages primary nurses to be independent problem solvers who will feel free to learn, to risk, and to seek guidance when necessary.

The findings in this study indicate that staff nurses *often* perceive that their head nurses manifest four of the six categories of behavior, as noted by the asterisks (Bloom, 1978).

The organizational climate is important to the implementation of primary nursing. And it is the nurse managers themselves who, more than anyone else, influence the organizational climate, employee morale, and motivation.

The intended ultimate result of primary nursing is a better quality of care for the patient. Unless this goal is realized, little will have been achieved by changing to primary nursing.

Ongoing evaluation must be built into the primary nursing program through:

- retrospective outcome and process audits
- day-to-day coaching of staff members
- regular performance evaluation
- patient satisfaction questionnaire
- nursing staff and personnel satisfaction surveys
- cost/benefit analyses
- nursing management audits.

The decision to go into primary nursing requires a personal commitment by the individual nurses who are working as a group, a commitment to become involved with patients, a commitment to put oneself in a therapeutic relationship with patients. This is not something that should be decided by one person for another .... For primary nursing to succeed it has to be done in an atmosphere where risk taking and judgment making are supported, where everything isn't done according to rules and regulations, but where a nurse is expected to use clinical judgment in this or that precise situation. Now that is the tough part in implementing primary nursing (Manthey, 1978, p. 426).

NOTES

Bloom, J. *Primary nurses' perception of their head nurses' role behavior.* Unpublished masters thesis, Boston University School of Nursing, 1978. Reprinted with permission.

Ciske, K. Accountability—The essence of primary nursing. *American Journal of Nursing*, May 1979, *79*, 890–894.

Ganong, J., & Ganong, W. *HELP with primary nursing.* Chapel Hill, N.C.: W. L. Ganong Co., 1977.

Lorsch, J. W. Organization design: A situational perspective. *Organizational Dynamics*, Autumn 1977, pp. 2–14.

Manthey, M. If you are instituting primary nursing. *American Journal of Nursing*, March 1978, *78*.

Spitzer, R. Making primary nursing work. *Supervisor Nurse*, January 1979, *10*(1), 12–14.

Zander, K. S. *Primary nursing: Development and management.* Germantown, Md.: Aspen Systems Corp., 1980.

Reading List

Books

Gosnell, D. J. *HELP with the nursing process.* Chapel Hill, N.C.: W. L. Ganong Co., 1980.

Marram, G. D., Barrett, M., & Bevis, O. *Primary nursing: A model for individualized care* (2nd ed.). St. Louis: C. V. Mosby, 1979.

Marram, G. D., Flynn, K., Abaravich, W., & Carey, S. *Cost effectiveness of primary and team nursing.* Wakefield, Mass.: Contemporary Publishing, 1976.

Marram, G. D., Schlegel, M. W., & Bevis, E. O. *Primary nursing: A model for individualized care.* St. Louis: C. V. Mosby, 1974.

Marriner, A. *The nursing process: A scientific approach to nursing care.* St. Louis: C. V. Mosby, 1975.

Murchison, I. A., Nichols, T. S., & Hanson, R. *Legal accountability in the nursing process.* St. Louis: C. V. Mosby, 1978.

Nicholls, M. E., & Wessels, V. G. (Eds.). *Nursing standards and nursing process.* Wakefield, Mass.: Contemporary Publishing, 1977.

Yura, H., & Walsh, M. B. *The nursing process: Assessing, planning, implementing, evaluating* (2nd ed.). New York: Appleton-Century-Crofts, 1973.

Yura, H., & Walsh, M. B. (Eds.). *Human needs and the nursing process.* New York: Appleton-Century-Crofts, 1978.

Articles

Beltran, H., Covey, D., Koban, B., Lopez, J., Peerson, B., Sterling, S., VanderWal, V., & Witthoft, G. An adaptation of primary nursing. *Supervisor Nurse*, July 1979, *10*(7), 16-19.

Carey, R. G. Evaluation of a primary nursing unit. *American Journal of Nursing*, July 1979, *79*, 1253-1255.

Dahlen, A. L. With primary nursing we have it all together. *American Journal of Nursing*, March 1978, *78*, 426-428.

Forman, M. Building a better nursing care plan. *American Journal of Nursing*, June 1979, *79*, 1086-1087.

Hegedus, K. A patient outcome criterion measure. *Supervisor Nurse*, January 1979, *10*(1), 40-45.

Hegyvary, S. T. Symposium on primary nursing. *The Nursing Clinics of North America*, June 1977, *12*(2), 185-255.

Mayer, G. G., & Bailey, K. Adapting the patient care conference to primary nursing. *Journal of Nursing Administration*, June 1979, *9*(6), 7-10.

McCarthy, D., & Schifalacqua, M. M. Primary nursing: Its implementation and six month outcome. *Journal of Nursing Administration*, May 1978, *8*(5), 29-32.

Moritz, D. A. Primary nursing: Implications for curriculum development. *Journal of Nursing Education*, March 1979, *18*(3), 33-37.

Osinki, E., & Morrison, W. The all-RN staff. *Supervisor Nurse*, September 1978, *9*(9), 66-74.

Zander, K. S. Primary nursing won't work . . . unless the head nurse lets it. *Journal of Nursing Administration*, October 1977, *7*(8), 19-23.

Part III

Operational Management

Chapter 5

Management by Objectives: A Systems Approach

HISTORICAL PERSPECTIVE

Setting goals and objectives in human endeavor is not new. From time immemorial farmers have set daily and yearly goals for themselves in terms of size and quality of crops. Seafarers have set trip goals and daily objectives, and measured their performance accordingly. Salesmen have traditionally set (or had set for them) sales quotas and have been rewarded for exceeding those quotas.

Task-oriented quality and quantity standards for all kinds of work have been used commonly for measuring performance results. Organizationally, the amount of profits (and/or the quality of services) has been accepted as the performance measure.

Only in fairly recent times, however, has there been a meaningful productive effort to develop and implement a system of performance objectives and standards especially for managers in our organizations and institutions. In 1954 Peter Drucker's management classic *The Practice of Management* first coined the term "management by objectives" (MBO). Drucker wrote:

> What business enterprise needs is a principle of management that will give full scope to individual strength and responsibility, as well as common direction to vision and effort, establish team work, and harmonize the goals of the individual with the commonweal. Management by objectives and self-control makes the commonweal the aim of every manager. It substitutes for control from outside the stricter, more exacting, and more effective control from inside. It motivates the manager to action, not because somebody tells him to do something or talks him into doing it, but because the objective task demands it. He acts not because somebody wants him to but

because he himself decides that he has to—he acts, in other words, as a free man.

I do not use the word "philosophy" lightly; indeed I prefer not to use it at all; it's much too big a word. But management by objectives and self-control may properly be called a philosophy of management. It rests on an analysis of the specific needs of the management group and the obstacles it faces. It rests on a concept of human action, behavior, and motivation. Finally, it applies to every manager, whatever his level and function, and to any organization whether large or small. It insures performance by converting objective needs into personal goals. And this is genuine freedom (Drucker, 1974, pp. 441–442).

During the fourth and fifth decades of this century, great progress was made in the behavioral sciences. The names of many persons who contributed to this progress became familiar to managers everywhere—names such as Argyris, Bakke, Bennis, Brown, Drucker, Etzioni, Gellerman, Herzberg, Jourard, Lewin, Likert, Maslow, Mayo, McClelland, McGregor, Myers, Perls, and Rogers. The prodigious output of these researchers, teachers, and writers was combined with the great work of earlier management consultants and practitioners, such as Barnard, Fayol, Follett, Gantt, Gilbreth, Roethlisberger, Taylor, Urwick, and Wiener. MBO was one outgrowth of this evolution of theory, thought, research, and practice.

UNDERLYING CONCEPTS AND PHILOSOPHY

Marie DiVincenti, a highly respected nurse educator and nursing administrator, presents an excellent overview of management by objectives and its relationship to other aspects of nurse management, including the need for administrative support. "Providing a supportive environment assures a maximum probability that each staff member, in the light of his background, values, desires, and expectations, will view each experience and interaction as supportive—as something which builds and maintains his sense of personal worth and importance" (DiVincenti, 1977, p. 75). Yes, it is important that a supportive environment exist for MBO to help all employees satisfy their personal needs and goals and to help the entire staff meet the immediate needs and objectives of the people who come to them as patients and clients.

Since MBO is an outgrowth of the historical developments described earlier in this chapter, it is a technique that is based upon some of the findings about people that reflect a different view of the nature of man from the views commonly held by many managers in years past—and still retained by some. Theory X and Theory Y, as propounded by McGregor (1960), show the contrasts between the assumptions and propositions that form the basis of the attitudes held by old-school managers and research findings about the real nature of people (see Table 5-1).

Table 5-1 Comparison of Theories X and Y

Assumptions and Propositions	Theory X (Direction & Control)	Theory Y (Participation & Self-Control)
1. Management is responsible for organizing the elements of productive enterprise—money, materials, equipment, people—in the interest of economic ends.	Yes	Yes
2. With respect to people, this is a process of directing their efforts, motivating them, controlling their actions, modifying their behavior to fit the needs of the organization.	Yes	Yes—but with an enlightened interpretation of what these words mean.
3. The average man has an inherent dislike of work and avoids it if he can.	Yes	No—Physical and mental effort are as natural as play or rest.
4. He lacks ambition, dislikes responsibility, prefers to be led.	Yes	No—The evidence of these are generally the consequences of experience, not inherent human characteristics.
5. He is inherently self-centered, indifferent to organizational needs.	Yes	No—He is concerned with organizational needs when they can be identified with his own needs.
6. He is by nature resistant to change.	Yes	No—He may have learned to appear this way for reasons of self-protection.
7. He is gullible, not very bright, the ready dupe of the charlatan and the demagogue.	Yes	No—Imagination, ingenuity, and creativity are capacities which are widely, not narrowly, distributed in the population.
8. People must be coerced, controlled, directed, threatened with punishment to get them to put forth adequate effort toward the achievement of organizational objectives.	Yes	No—These are not the only means for bringing about effort toward organizational objectives. Man will exercise self-direction and self-control in the service of objectives to which he is committed.

Source: Adapted from McGregor, D. *The Human Side of Enterprise.* New York: McGraw-Hill, 1960. Reprinted with permission.

Simplified for purposes of comparison, Theory X represents the view that people require authoritarian direction and control by managers to achieve organizational goals. Theory Y supports the view that the true nature of people is such that, with managerial leadership that permits a high degree of involvement and participation, employees will direct their own efforts toward organizational goals as a means of meeting their own needs and objectives. Here is the message of Theory Y in its positive assumptions and propositions about people:

1. Physical and mental effort are as natural as play or rest.
2. Ambition and acceptance of responsibility are traits which come naturally to people. When they seem to be lacking, it is generally the consequence of experience.
3. People are concerned with, and will work toward accomplishing, organizational needs when they can be identified with their own needs.
4. People do not resist change; they resist being changed. People may have learned to appear resistant to change for reasons of self-protection.
5. Imagination, ingenuity, and creativity are capacities which are widely distributed in the population.
6. People will exercise self-direction and self-control in the service of objectives to which they are committed.

ACHIEVING MUTUAL GOALS

The achievement of mutual goals is the anticipated outcome of management by objectives. People who work within the same organization usually have many similar goals. Nurse managers and nursing staff members serve as a case in point. One mutual goal held by both groups is the delivery of high quality care to patients. According to Douglas McGregor, mutual goal achievement requires a participative approach on the part of management acting on the "Y" assumptions about people. Management can arrange organizational conditions so that people can achieve their own goals by directing their efforts toward the goals of the organization within which they work. McGregor points out that this can be done best when management creates opportunities, releases potential, removes obstacles, encourages growth, and provides necessary guidance. It is management by objectives rather than management by control.

The integration of hospital and nursing department goals with the needs and goals of individual nursing staff members—through mutual understanding, mutual trust, cooperative effort, and leadership skill—can achieve meaningful results for all: the hospital administrator, the doctor, the nurse manager, the nursing staff members, and the patients.

Dr. E. Wight Bakke in *Teamwork in Industry* pointed out that people want progress toward and security with respect to certain goals. The first of these is "the respect of their fellows," to be considered important and respectable by the people with whom they associate. Another goal Bakke refers to as "creative sufficiency," or the desire to have the amount of food, clothes, shelter, health which compares favorably with associates. People want "increasing control over their own affairs." They want their own decisions to be effective in shaping their lives, and to reduce the amount of control exercised by others over them. Bakke notes "understanding" as a goal. People want to know the score, to know the relation between what happened and what caused it to happen. They also want to be able to use the full range of their abilities, to have the chance to do the things they think they can do. Lastly, Bakke mentions "integrity" as a goal. This he describes as the desire of people to feel that their actions and principles are consistent, to feel that they are a significant part of the world about them (Bakke, 1948).

People express their wants in diverse ways. These modes of expression vary from person to person, from group to group, from time to time—even from decade to decade. The *new breed* of every generation invents its own ways of expressing its needs. These reflect the environmental factors discussed in Chapter 2, as well as the interpretations of research findings as summarized by educators, researchers, and other writers. For example, Table 2-2 in Chapter 2 presents a comparison of how the people's wants identified by Bakke (characterizing the late 40s, the 50s, and into the 60s) were translated into the new-breed desires described by Peterfreund (exemplifying the 70s and beyond). Nurse managers can use this kind of information to check out their own understanding of their experiences with people (as employees and as patients), and as a basis for MBO goal setting.

People working in healthcare settings have many similar goals regardless of their job titles. The goals referred to by Bakke can be identified among Maslow's hierarchy of five human needs. And we know that the unmet goals and needs serve as motivators for people. The nurse manager who understands the relationship between needs and self-motivation can use motivational methods and leadership techniques that lead to satisfaction of personal needs and goals while working in harmony with the goals of the organization. This is mutual goal setting at its best.

ACCOUNTABILITY AND CONTROL

The management process has control as one of its components. In the traditional approach to accountability described by McGregor, control systems have been used in which management sets performance standards and measures the results, and then rewards employees who meet the standards and punishes those who fail to do so. The consequences of such a system may be identified as follows:

- The system works—but not as well as desired.
- There may be widespread antagonism to the controls and to those who administer them.
- Employees at all levels may offer successful resistance and noncompliance to administrative controls.
- Performance information may well be unreliable due to the negative effect of resistance and noncompliance.
- There is a need for close surveillance of employees which dilutes delegation, impinges on the manager's time, and impedes employee development.
- It creates high administrative costs.

Such an approach has a tendency to generate and accentuate noncompliance. When the pressure to comply is coupled with lack of trust and support, the end result may be perceived as a threat. People often respond to threats through the use of defensive, hostile, and protective behavior. A more productive approach to the control element of the management process is described by McGregor:

> When members of an organization are committed to the organization's goals, surveillance in the usual sense becomes largely unnecessary. The problem is not one of obtaining passive compliance but of enabling all parts of the organization to achieve the goals to which they are committed. Each unit down to the individual level has a degree of control over its own fate. The total process, from the initial exploration of reality to the solution of problems arising in the day-to-day attempt to meet goals and standards, provides ample opportunity for intrinsic rewards and for the motivational effects of intrinsic punishments arising from mistakes and failures (McGregor, 1967, p. 12).

The nurse manager can apply a sound strategy that will assist with accountability and control. The strategy is based upon two principles: (1) people's response to information about their performance varies with their commitment to goals, and (2) to cope with reality requires open communication, mutual trust, mutual support, and mutual working through of conflicts. The strategy includes the following steps:

1. An open presentation and discussion of the nurse manager's requirements for successful goal accomplishment at any given point in time;

including review of external forces and internal problems shown by past performance.

2. A broad analysis of changes in performance required to meet the demands of reality.
3. An analysis of how everyone in the department can contribute best to the organization effort—carried out face-to-face at all levels.
4. Statements from each patient unit of the goals and standards to which it commits itself. This includes an analysis of the help the unit feels is needed to accomplish the goals such as information feedback, staff resources, policy or procedure changes, and equipment and manpower needs.

The success of the strategy is dependent upon the intent and thoroughness with which it is used as well as the involvement of people at all levels. Properly implemented, this strategy leads to a type of self-control and accountability consistent with a Theory Y philosophy.

These concepts and beliefs about people can be translated into daily productive action through appropriate use of management functions, techniques, and skills. MBO is one such technique. The three basic steps of MBO (set objectives, perform, measure results) are, like the management functions, a cyclical process. Each phase builds upon the input from the one preceding. Each phase provides the feedback or output for the one that follows.

People who think together stay together. This paraphrase of a familiar slogan carries much meaning for those who use MBO. Much thinking together—using the variety of performance skills in communicating, conceptualizing, perceiving, discussing, problem solving, understanding, compromising, decision making—is desirable at the outset of an organization-wide MBO program. This is because goals and objectives at the departmental or unit level of a healthcare agency need to be related to the broader divisional and organizational goals and objectives. Staying together, literally and figuratively, is then possible. A sequential plan of action follows in Figure 5-1. (See also Appendix F for a pertinent example of the goals and annual objectives for Nebraska Methodist Hospital.)

THOUGHT PRECEDES ACTION

Combs, Avila, and Purkey wrote in *Helping Relationships*, "A helper's conceptions of the goals he is seeking to accomplish have inexorable effects upon his behavior . . . . Goals and purposes determine action" (Combs et al., 1971, p. 165). These words provide a useful transition from the concepts and

Figure 5-1 Plan for MBO

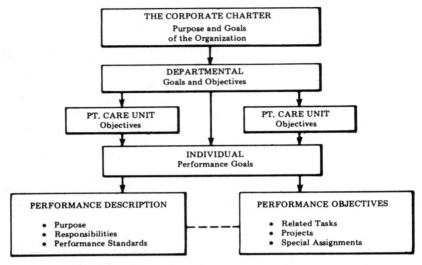

The Corporate Charter (Purpose of the Organization)

Every organization exists for some purpose. This is
stated in the articles of incorporation. The purpose is
often elaborated in the form of a number of specific
goals with specific objectives identified annually.

Departmental Goals and Objectives

Each division, section, department and unit exists to
help achieve the purpose of the organization. Thus
departmental goals and objectives need to be identified
in writing, consistent with the organizational purpose,
but departmentally distinctive as related to the department's special function. Specific objectives for each
patient care unit are essential.

Job Purpose, Responsibilities, and Objectives

Within each department, people work at jobs to help
achieve departmental goals and objectives. Thus a
performance description identifies for each person the
purpose, responsibilities, and measures of satisfactory
performance to be met.

Beyond the normal performance responsibilities,
however, are related tasks, projects, and special
assignments. These are the short or longer-term
activities necessary to attain identified objectives
that are steppingstones to goal achievement.

Source: Ganong, J., & Ganong, W. *HELP with management by objectives.* Chapel
Hill, N.C.: W. L. Ganong Co., 1975, p. 16.

philosophical considerations of the foregoing paragraphs to the pragmatic aspects of MBO in healthcare settings.

The steps in the Plan for MBO may appear to be a logical, necessary sequence of events leading from the translation of the purpose and goals of the corporate organization (hospital, nursing home, school) to the development of departmental and unit goals and objectives, and thence to the development of the performance goals and objectives for individual employees. But too often the process does not work this way. Sometimes one or more of the initial steps are not carried out, or receive only cursory attention. What then? Can department heads, the nursing administrator, patient care coordinators, or head nurses still proceed to use MBO in their own areas? Yes! Sometimes, for identifiable reasons, the only way to begin is at the departmental or unit level. In such cases, the person initiating the program will certainly need to do so with the knowledge and approval of his or her own manager, using whatever broad statements are available, written or understood, of institution-wide and/or department-wide goals.

Assume that you plan to take the initiative to begin using MBO for your own area of responsibility, whatever your position title in your hospital. Insofar as you know (and you have inquired) there are no available written statements of the goals and objectives of the larger organizational unit (such as maternal and child care, nursing service department, or the entire hospital) of which you and your co-workers are a part. So you write down, to the best of your ability, what you think are the philosophy, goals, and objectives for the organizational unit supervised by your own manager.

For your next step, you have several options. The order in which you do them depends upon your own inclination, your knowledge of your own boss and subordinates, and how you size up the whole situation. Whatever the sequence, all of these steps will need to be carried out:

1. Discuss with your own personnel the philosophy and goals (as you understand them) of the entire organization unit of which you all are a part.
2. Develop with your own people a simple statement of the philosophy and goals of your own unit. (If such a statement already exists, review it with your employee group to determine what each one thinks it means in relation to his/her own job.)
3. Develop with your own people a series of specific objectives for the months ahead. These should relate, insofar as possible, to your understanding of the objectives for the entire department or hospital.
4. Take to your boss, for discussion and approval, the list of written objectives you have developed with your people. Review what you have been doing. Say something like this: "We have based our own statements upon the philosophy, goals, and objectives of the hospital (or institution

or agency) and of the department (nursing service, maternal and child care, or whatever) as we understand them. We used these statements as our guide for these."

Show and discuss what you have available for the philosophy, goals, and objectives of the larger organizational unit. Obtain agreement, modified as necessary, that your statements of the foregoing are adequate as a starting point for what follows. Then say:

"Here are the statements we have developed for our own philosophy, goals, and objectives. You will note that the philosophy and goals are the same as, or only slightly modified from, the larger goals and philosophy we have just discussed. Our objectives are specific to our own area of responsibility, and relate directly to the broader institutional and departmental objectives. We will appreciate your comments and suggestions."

The outcome of such an effort on your part depends upon a number of factors. One of the most important of these factors is the motive force at work in your relationship with your boss. Thus what happens as a result of your initiative in taking the foregoing steps may be surprisingly satisfying or predictably disappointing. Regardless of the outcome, however, you will have established a new base from which to build toward what you want to accomplish as manager of your unit.

THE BIG PICTURE

A few pages back we quoted McGregor (writing about a productive approach to the control function of the management process) as follows: "Each unit down to the individual level (*each person*) has a degree of control over its own fate." Figure 5-2 portrays how all employees on all shifts of every unit of every department in the entire organization are a vital part of implementing objectives that have their focus on the goals of the organization—its purpose and reason for existing. Your examination of this diagram will help in comprehending the significance of an MBO program in relation to your role in patient care and in making PONS work well in your agency. Note that the arrows on the vertical and horizontal dash lines show the flow of the *implementation* of the objectives and goals. From a *planning* standpoint, reverse the direction of the arrows so that the flow is from the hospital goals to the goals of the other units of organization, and thence to the relevant objectives. In this connection, the value of MBO and the other management techniques will become clearer as we examine the ways you can use these techniques.

Figure 5-2 The MBO Schematic Organizational Plan

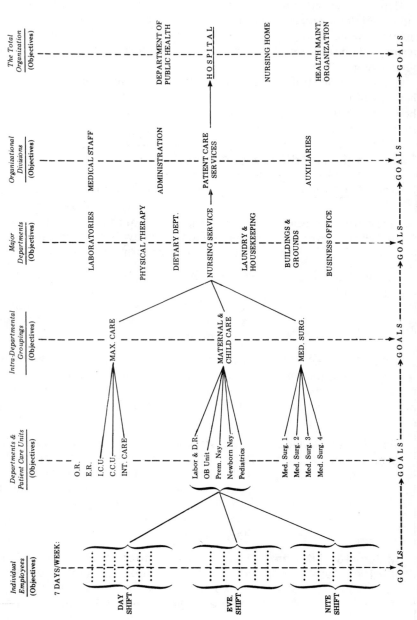

Source: Ganong, J., and Ganong, W. *HELP with management by objectives.* Chapel Hill, N.C.: W. L. Ganong Co., 1975, p. 19.

Here is an example of a program performance plan that relates the individual employee and unit objectives to those of the larger organizational segments. The hospital goal is: Provide a complete range of emergency, short term, acute healthcare services at optimal cost for the community within our service area.

Exhibit 5-1 illustrates that MBO is a systematic, well organized process. It is a way of managing well—of planning, doing, and controlling what has to be done. It will work best when the people in an organization make it work that way for them.

Exhibit 5-1 An MBO Program Performance Plan

Unit of Organization	A Sequence of Related Objectives
Hospital (President or Administrator)	Expand the scope of maternal and child care services to provide a complete family-centered program by June 30, 1981.
Medical Staff (President)	Present by September 1, 1979 the outline of an expanded patient care medical program in maternal and child care consonant with the goal of a complete family-centered emphasis.
Department of Nursing Service (Nursing Administrator)	Present by October 30, 1979 an expanded nursing care program in maternal and child care consonant with the goal of a complete family-centered emphasis.
Patient Care Services (Associate Administrator)	Integrate the planning of the OB/GYN/Peds section of the medical staff with the budget committee of the board of trustees, the facilities planning group, and the director of nursing service; complete program performance plan by March 1, 1980.
Maternal & Child Care (Patient Care Coordinator)	Prepare specifications for the necessary equipment, facilities, supplies, and staffing to implement a complete nursing service program for family-centered maternal and child care by December 31, 1980.

Obstetric Unit (Head Nurse) Labor & Del. (Head Nurse) Premy Nursery (Head Nurse) OB Nursery (Head Nurse) Pediatrics (Head Nurse)	Plan the details of initiating the expanded family-centered program as it affects the day to day operation of the unit; recruit and train additional personnel as required; reorient present staff to the concept and changed nursing requirements; schedule necessary implementation steps; complete plan by March 1, 1981.
Individuals (Nursing Staff) (Supervisors and/or Associate Directors of Nursing Service; Evenings, Nights, Weekends) (Employees of other affected hospital services)	Participate in planning as appropriate; assist in updating own performance description; contribute own suggestions; participate in reorientation program activities.

HELP WITH WRITING OBJECTIVES

A systems approach to MBO means more than just the *writing* of objectives. Anybody can write objectives. But objectives have not been *set* until they have been thoroughly discussed, mutually understood, modified as necessary, and then agreed upon by all parties. At the patient unit level, this means that objectives for the unit must be mutually agreed upon by the staff, nurse manager, and patient care coordinator. This is because these objectives are part of the bigger agency-wide plan (mission, purpose, goals); and objectives cost money. This vital objective-setting process begins with the identification and writing of appropriate objectives.

An objective is a specific task-oriented statement of results to be achieved in order to accomplish a goal. *Our objective in writing this section is to provide you with a model for writing objectives and with practice exercises so that when you have finished your reading and have done the exercises, by a date you set for yourself, you will have acquired the skill to write meaningful objectives for your own work setting.*

You have just seen one example of a program performance plan with a series of objectives, written by employees in a hierarchy of job levels, all per taining to the same organizational goal. Here are three additional examples of objectives that fulfill the requirements for the inclusion of necessary components:

A. By an Inservice Education Director
Provide training and orientation for all newly hired groups of nursing school graduates so that they will be prepared to assume their job performance responsibilities by June 1.

B. By a Nursing Administrator
Institute an effective problem-oriented system of charting on two selected patient care units by October 6, at a cost not to exceed the present unit cost per patient day for nursing service on these units.

C. By a Head Nurse
Adjust the staffing pattern and practices on my unit by January 1, so that the nursing hours per patient day, regardless of the patient census, do not vary more than plus or minus 5 percent from the established standard developed for my unit; and maintain my flexibility to change the mix of nursing personnel classification if significant changes occur in the level of care required by a changing patient mix.

We find that in spite of so much emphasis on MBO during recent years, very few nurses have received instruction in how to write an objective. The following guidance will be of assistance. A meaningful written objective meets several important criteria. The written statements should include the following components: (1) What will be done? (2) How much will be done how well? (3) When will it be done? (4) Who will do what, where? (If pertinent) and (5) What will it cost? (If pertinent).

A useful exercise is to examine the second paragraph at the beginning of this section. Identify how our statement of objective for this section (shown in italics) includes the foregoing components. Note any ways you would improve the statement so that it presents the components more clearly. This is a step toward helping you remember the components. Next review the three examples of objectives by the inservice director, nursing administrator, and head nurse. For each example identify the components by marking them with key words such as "what," "how much," and "how well" over the appropriate portion of each objective. Compare your results with those of someone else. Now review again each of the components. Additional explanation of each one follows.

What will be done? The "what" portion of the objective begins with an active verb—provide, institute, adjust. The form of the statement is a simple declarative sentence: "Somebody does something." In the three examples, the "somebody" is understood; it is the "I" of the person in the job title. The "something" is the predicate. In example A, it is "training and orientation." In B, it is "an effective problem-oriented system of charting." In C, it is "the staffing pattern and practices."

How much will be done? This is the quantitative and qualitative component. This is frequently significant since it provides a way to measure if the objective has been attained.

In A: *All* new groups; will be *prepared*
In B: On *two* units; *no* increase in cost
In C: On *my* unit; *within plus or minus 5 percent* of standard; *flexibility* in mix of personnel categories.

When will it be done? This is the target date for completion. It is an essential item in every objective; it provides the basis for integrating a series of objectives (see examples of program performance plans). The target dates are necessary also for cash-flow planning.

In A: June 1 (of each year)
In B: October 6
In C: January 1

Who will do what, where? (Optional) Include names and places when the who and where are pertinent, as this will avoid later confusion and misunderstandings. These will be helpful too in preparing the program performance plan which needs to include identification of who will do, or help with, each implementation step.

In A: "I" implied; "In-house" implied
In B: "I" implied; two selected units
In C: "I" implied; my unit

What will it cost? (Optional) Every objective carries a cost that can be calculated. A cost effectiveness study in relation to an objective (or series of objectives) is simply an estimate of the financial cost of achieving the objective compared with the expected financial benefits (income, savings, lowered expense). Reference to cost may be included in the written statement when pertinent or required.

In A: None cited
In B: Not to exceed present unit cost/patient day (in operating cost)
In C: No installation cost; better control of wage cost (plus or minus 5 percent of standard) implied

In your own planning you undoubtedly have some goals you want to achieve. What project do you want to get done in your unit that will contribute directly to the quality of patient care, better working conditions, or better control of expenses? Write a realistic, meaningful statement for a single objective in one of these three categories. Use each of the first three basic components, and include numbers 4 and 5 if appropriate. Identify and mark the components you have included, just as you did earlier for the examples.

THE NURSE MANAGER'S ROLE IN MBO

Making MBO work is a part of every manager's responsibility in every department, at every organizational level. Nurse managers are no exception. From nursing administrator to head nurse, the nurse managers need to take the lead in using and guiding MBO. Their roles are especially important in hospitals, nursing homes, and public health agencies since so many projects and objectives initiated in nursing service necessarily involve the participation of other hospital or agency department heads if the objectives are to be met successfully. The expansion or withdrawal of patient care programs has impact throughout the entire organization and often throughout the community, because of their relation to hospital goals and the competing demands for resources—personnel, money, facilities, and equipment.

The organizational climate and its influence upon the motivation of all personnel is as important to the implementation of MBO as to other management-initiated programs. And it is the managers themselves who, more than anyone else, influence the organizational climate, employee morale, and motivation. Myers presents a concept of job enrichment that permits each employee the maximum possible degree of planning and control of his work (Myers, 1970). This is highly relevant as a useful concept to aid managers in using MBO. It influences the managerial style of managers and how they use their leadership skills. Consider how the performance results of your people reflect the degree of success you achieve in the leadership behaviors listed in the goal-oriented column of Figure 5-3. Evaluate yourself for your level of ability in performing, regularly, each of the eight items using a scale with a plus for "very well," a check mark for "OK, as well as I'd expect," and a dash for "less satisfactorily than I'd like." Relate this self-evaluation to your own level of motivation for using MBO as part of your nurse-manager responsibilities and functions.

DEVELOPING A PROGRAM PERFORMANCE PLAN

A program performance plan (PPP) is a long-range schedule of interrelated steps required to effect a desired result, objective, or goal. It is a plan-

Figure 5-3 The Role of the Manager

Authority-Oriented

Set goals for subordinates, define standards and results expected.

Give them information necessary to do their jobs.

Train them to do the job.

Explain rules and apply discipline to ensure conformity; suppress conflict.

Stimulate subordinates through persuasive leadership.

Develop and install new methods.

Develop and free them for promotion.

Reward achievements and punish failures.

Goal-Oriented

Participate with people in problem solving and goal setting.

Give them access to information which they want.

Create situations for optimum learning.

Explain rules and consequences of violations; mediate conflict.

Allow people to set challenging goals.

Teach methods improvement techniques to job incumbents.

Enable them to pursue and move into growth opportunities.

Recognize achievements and help them learn from failures.

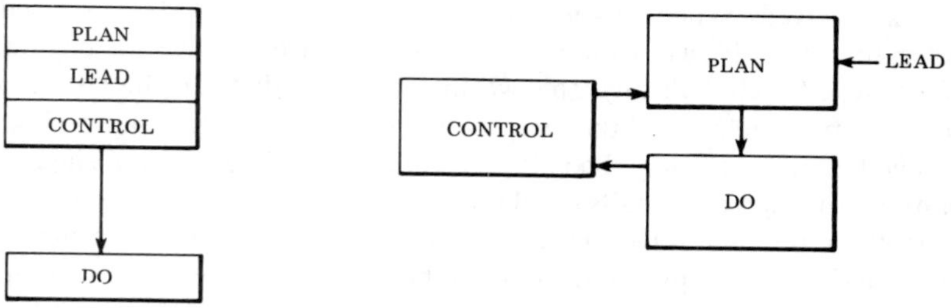

Source: Myers, M. S. *Every employee a manager.* New York: McGraw-Hill, 1970, p. 99. Used with permission from McGraw-Hill Book Co.

ning tool. "Planning" is thinking ahead, determining what shall be done; it is the management function of establishing goals, setting objectives, defining problems and opportunities, and developing strategy and tactics for achieving objectives.

A graphic portrayal of a PPP is shown in Figure 5-4. The first example is one we prepared for an operations appraisal project within a large county Board of Health. You may wish to construct your own plan using the sequence of objectives found in Exhibit 5-1. There are many advantages to using a graphic chart showing weeks and months of the year. The benefits of this format are that it:

1. permits seeing at a glance the timetable for beginning and completing each step.

2. shows the interrelationships of the steps (and objectives) with other scheduled events (holidays, budget submission, vacations, etc.).
3. provides (in column at right margin) for including names of who will do or help with each step.
4. emphasizes the variety of demands upon manager's time, and helps to avoid overly optimistic target dates for completion.
5. communicates the schedule to others in a form easy to understand.
6. is highly flexible and adaptable to inclusion of other dates, color coding, revisions, progress notes, and symbols.

Here are some tips to remember in connection with establishing the target dates for each step. A person inexperienced in setting up such a schedule is inclined to begin from today's date with the first step and plan forward with each succeeding step. A better plan is to use a worksheet, and start by listing the last step you visualize prior to the target date for completing the objective. Then, working backwards to the present time of year, list each preceding step with its beginning and ending date based upon your best estimate of the work involved. When this is done realistically, you may be surprised to discover that already, as of the present date, you are overdue for beginning the first step. Psychologically, this working backwards from the last step to the first seems to help avoid the temptation of unrealistically compressing the time schedule for each step. Too often the end target date is established prior to thinking through the details of all the work involved in carrying out the objective. When the final schedule is transferred to the PPP form, the steps will be listed in calendar sequence from top to bottom for ease of use and comprehension.

Another approach is to write on separate cards all of the steps you can visualize as they occur to you, in no particular order. Then arrange the cards in the sequence in which you think the steps should be taken. Finally, assign the projected starting and ending dates for each step.

MBO AND NMBO

NMBO is Nursing Management by Objectives. It is MBO as applied by nurse *managers* as part of their management responsibilities for personnel, facilities, patient care, budgetary planning and control within their own segments of the nursing department. The term NMBO is used herein to distinguish it from NBO—Nursing by Objectives—which is the application of MBO to the management of direct patient care by individual RNs and team leaders, the *nurse* managers.

To clarify the emphasis of NMBO, a review of the scope of nurse manager responsibilities will be helpful. These are presented in Part 1 where the

Workworld of the Nurse Manager shows the three major areas of responsibility as patient care management, operational management, and human resources management. These are not three distinct, separate areas of responsibility. They necessarily overlap, merge, and harmonize in the interests of nursing, patient care, and organizational goals.

Management by objectives is simply one of several techniques used by nurses at all organizational levels to assist in bringing about this harmony of

Figure 5-4 Sample Operations Appraisal Program Performance Plan

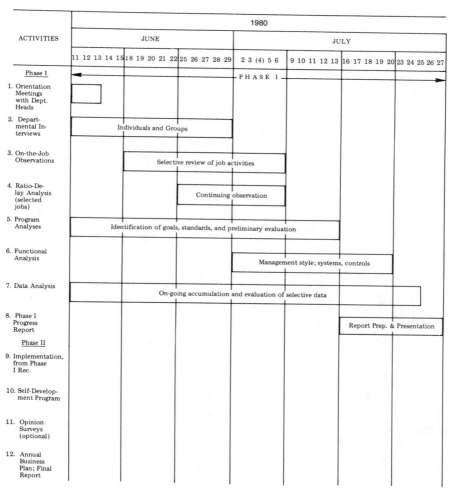

Figure 5-4 continued

1980							
JULY	AUGUST					SEPTEMBER	
30 31	1 2 3	6 7 8 9 10	13 14 15 16 17	20 21 22 23 24	27 28 29 30 31	(3) 4 5 6 7	10 11 12 13 14

PHASE II (OPTIONAL)

PHASE II

Follow-through with more of Steps 1 through 7 as may be helpful or requested.

Initiate self-development program as agreed upon.

Carry out personnel and consumer opinion surveys (optional; based on Phase I).

Development of Annual Business Plan; Final Report.

effort toward achieving mutual goals. The scope of the nurse manager's application of NMBO, therefore, is greater and for a wider variety of purposes than the applications to be made by a staff nurse. All nurses, however, are expected to use the elements of the management process as they pertain to each nurse's performance responsibilities (see Appendices A and G).

ROPEP AND MBO

One of the other management techniques that works hand-in-hand with NMBO is a results-oriented performance evaluation program (ROPEP).

"Plan for MBO" (Figure 5–1) shows the sequence of steps in translating the hospital (or organization-wide) goals and objectives into performance responsibilities and objectives for individual employees. That diagram is expanded in Figure 5–5 to show how the techniques of MBO and ROPEP combine to produce the desired performance results and goal achievement. The ROPEP cycle involves: first, Identifying for Whom Major Performance Responsibilities are Performed; second, Writing the Segments of Performance Responsibilities; and third, Developing the Performance Standards for each Segment. The MBO cycle involves: first, Setting Mutual Goals and Objectives; then, Performing the Necessary Activities to Achieve the Objectives; and finally, Reviewing Progress and Evaluating Achievements. Note the significance of the continuation of the sequence. This emphasizes the importance of developing the individual performance descriptions before setting mutual goals and performance descriptions with those individuals who will participate. Objectives are carried out by people as part of their regular performance responsibilities. Thus the measure of achievement in meeting objectives is not an evaluation exercise separate from regular performance evaluation. Successful carrying out of individual performance responsibilities leads to successful achievement of objectives—and of the goals to which such objectives are related.

The foregoing is true even in those cases when out-of-the-ordinary projects and special assignments are necessary. Some projects and assignments may be agreed upon for the purpose of challenging or expanding the capabilities of the person involved. It may be a part of that person's growth and development program in connection with both individual and organizational goals. Even when such assignments are part of a person's preparation for assuming a position of greater responsibility, the activities related to such projects are necessarily a part of a person's current performance responsibilities.

The shaded area marked "Revisions" in Figure 5–5 indicates where the ROPEP/MBO cycles overlap. It is that portion of the introductory/implementation/follow-through phases of performance evaluation and MBO which provides for making necessary revisions in the tools and procedures. Performance requirements change; statements of satisfactory performance have to be updated; objectives have to be modified, eliminated, expanded, or replaced. Such revisions are essential and must be made as soon as their need is identified, rather than being accumulated for an annual or semiannual updating process. ROPEP and MBO provide nurse managers with important

Figure 5-5 ROPEP & MBO: A Functional Diagram

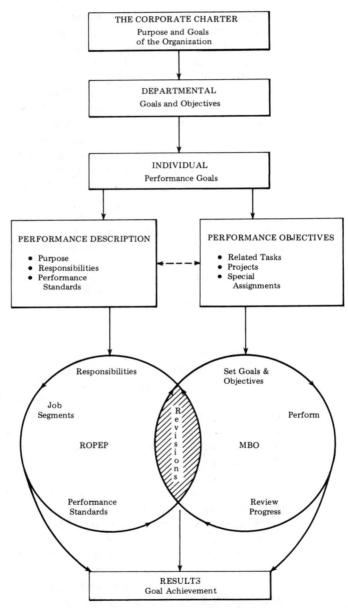

Source: Ganong, J., and Ganong, W. *HELP with management by objectives.* Chapel Hill, N.C.: W. L. Ganong Co., 1975, p. 57.

tools and techniques for daily use in their managing process. Most tools require regular maintenance, whether they are clinical tools (stethoscopes, monitors, blood pumps) or management tools (performance description, written objective, program performance plan). If they do not receive regular care and maintenance, they do not work well and impair the nurse manager's performance.

In short, the lower portion of the diagram shows both ROPEP and MBO as management techniques being used by nurse managers in carrying out their management functions of planning, doing, and controlling. Thus a performance evaluation discussion by a nurse manager and a staff worker involves not only a review of the performance results of the employee in carrying out the regular performance responsibilities, but also a review of progress and results on previously agreed-upon objectives.

Results are produced by people. Some results are achieved through efforts and activities that are part of a person's regular day-to-day performance responsibilities in the job. Other results are attained primarily through an extra quota of effort and the effective performance of special projects and task assignments. (See "Matrix Organization," Johnson & Tingey, 1976.) ROPEP and MBO, together, provide the techniques, stimulus, and evaluative methods for securing optimum results through both types of individual effort.

The expected outcomes of this process are results that contribute to achievement of the purposes of the individual employee, the department, and the organization. In hospitals and other healthcare agencies, the expected beneficiaries are the consumers themselves.

The Objectives Worksheet

Another tool for use with both MBO and ROPEP is the Objectives Worksheet (Figure 5-6). This form supplements the program performance plan and the performance description. It can be used to plan and evaluate the performance of special tasks and assignments that are part of carrying out a specific objective. The objectives worksheet can be used also to plan and evaluate objectives that are generated as a follow-through to a discussion of job-connected performance results that are less than satisfactory.

An examination of the Objectives Worksheet shows that it is a larger and different version of the MBO cyclical diagram, expanded to serve as an 8½ inch × 11 inch worksheet. One of these worksheets prepared for each objective serves as a planning and evaluative tool in connection with discussions between a person and that person's boss. Each worksheet remains active for the life of the objective to which it pertains. It is revised as required or when target dates have to be extended. When an objective is terminated for what-

Figure 5-6 Objectives Worksheet

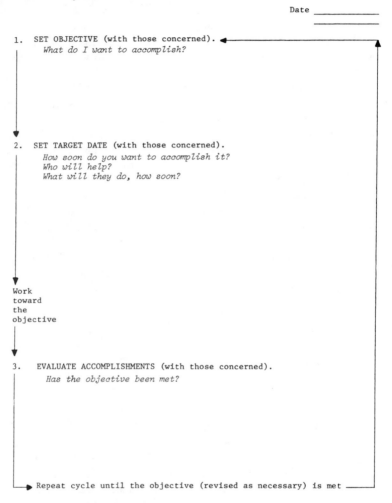

Date _____
                 _____

1. SET OBJECTIVE (with those concerned).
    What do I want to accomplish?

2. SET TARGET DATE (with those concerned).
    How soon do you want to accomplish it?
    Who will help?
    What will they do, how soon?

Work
toward
the
objective

3. EVALUATE ACCOMPLISHMENTS (with those concerned).
    Has the objective been met?

Repeat cycle until the objective (revised as necessary) is met

ever reason (successful completion, cancelled due to budgetary curtailment, phased out, or merged with another project), the related worksheet, properly annotated, becomes a historical record for follow-through purposes.

NMBO and Other Management Techniques

Nurse managers who develop familiarity and skill with NMBO quickly learn its value as a kind of master coordinating tool for other aspects and techniques of nurse management. These include patient care program development, nursing audit, problem-oriented nursing system, wide-track careers planning, handling complaints and grievances, motivational management, personnel development, and annual budgetary planning and control.

Annual budgetary planning (ABP) is used here as an example which, like ROPEP and MBO, reflects the cyclical three steps of plan, do, and control. From some points of view, budgetary planning represents the ultimate application of MBO. This is because the budgetary planning process, when properly carried out, necessarily:

- builds upon the short- and long-range program plans that
- generate the objectives that
- create demands for resource allocation that
- must be translated into dollars in a proposed budget.

Later, the approved budget becomes an MBO document that:

- permits securing the resources (personnel, equipment, supplies, facilities, education, and training) to
- carry out objectives that
- implement programs (for patients, personnel, the community) that
- fulfill the organizational goals.

Chapter 8 provides a detailed explanation of ABP as a nurse-manager technique.

Securing Involvement

By definition, MBO is a technique that includes the preparation of mutually established objectives. ROPEP, for example, involves preparing agreed-upon standards of performance. Other management techniques also require the participation and involvement of personnel with their own managers in the development of standards and objectives, and in evaluating performance results.

The word "involve" by definition means to include, draw in, embroil, engross. The word "participate" by definition means to take part, join, share. For human beings generally, the foregoing types of action are natural tendencies—until learned behavior seems to indicate otherwise (Maslow, 1970; McGregor, 1960). Yet many nurse managers appear to be uneasy with, or unskilled in, the process of securing meaningful involvement. The reasons often include the fact that they really don't know how to do it; they haven't learned the skills; they have had no model to follow (no boss of their own who has ever been a skilled facilitator); or they see no reason for trying.

A major reason for securing involvement in the processes we have described is that better performance results can be obtained by doing so. At least this has been the experience of many nurse managers. They often discover also that they enjoy their managing more. In addition, employees at every level can meet some of their human needs and achieve greater job satisfaction through meaningful participation and involvement.

You can secure more involvement and participation by your people through use of the following suggestions:

1. Act as though you want your people involved.

    Never be too busy to listen (even though it takes time), or your people will think you really don't want to hear them or involve them.

2. Ask for help. (Invite participation.)

    There once was a nurse manager who, whenever she was asked by an LPN what to do about a patient problem, would tell the LPN what to do. One day when the LPN asked about how to handle another problem, the nurse manager asked, "What do you think?" "Huh?" responded the LPN, in a mild state of shock. "I asked you to tell me how you think you can solve it," said the nurse manager. "That's what I thought you said," answered the LPN, "but I didn't think you really meant it." Then the LPN proceeded to give her own idea and was encouraged to try it. It worked.

3. Use "Tips for Leading Discussions."

    These tips may help you, as they have helped others, to get good results in leading group discussions. They work well also in face-to-face discussions with another person, as in interviews, performance evaluation, and problem solving. (These "tips" can be found in *HELP with Management by Objectives* (Ganong & Ganong, 1975).

Management involves getting meaningful results through and with other people. MBO helps to do it better. Securing successful involvement is a key to MBO.

NURSING BY OBJECTIVES

Managing patient care is different from managing personnel who are members of a patient care unit. The differences are both in kind and degree of activity. Managing unit personnel involves assigning care for the entire group of patients. This is the basic concept, even though it may be modified depending upon the setting and the nurse manager. Managing patient care involves the concept of one nurse and one patient working together to carry out the medical care plan and the nursing care plan for that patient. While this concept can rarely be implemented without modification, application efforts to carry out the concept are being made by nurses with such titles as nurse practitioner, primary nurse, and clinical specialist.

Nursing by Objectives (NBO) is a results-oriented technique using mutually-established patient care objectives, an implementation schedule, and evaluation of results and patient progress. It applies the management-by-objectives approach at the unit level with the focus on the one nurse/one patient relationship. The emphasis is not the performance of tasks for patients. It is upon helping patients achieve their goals. This means establishing a helping relationship between nurses and patients, a relationship in which patients are recognized as being in charge of themselves (insofar as they are able) and nurses are facilitative managers of goal achievement in accordance with the patient care plan. Primary nursing puts to work the elements of NBO better than any other nursing care modality.

The following list summarizes the purpose of NBO and the variety of factors that influence how well the patient and the nurse can work together to achieve their mutual objectives. Very likely you can add additional factors.

INFLUENCING FACTORS

Patient	*Nurse*
Own human needs	Own human needs
Specific health problems	Medical plan of care
Medical care plan	Nursing care plan
Family involvement	Discharge planning
Degree of dependency	Teaching process
Learning process	Organizational environment
Others	Others

By using mutual understanding, trust, cooperation, and skill, the goals of both the nurse and patient can be achieved.

The foregoing introduction to nursing by objectives is intended to help develop an awareness of NBO as a management technique that assists in achieving patient care goals. NBO is specifically and directly related to the nursing process for each individual person. Therefore, it becomes an integral part of assessing, planning, implementing, and evaluating each person's needs and plan of care. Think of it as a series of concentric circles cyclic in nature with NBO at the center as the specific management technique; the nursing process as the outer circle; and the middle circle as the integrating model of the management process.

Some of the similarities and distinctions between nursing management by objectives and nursing by objectives are summarized in Table 5-2. An understanding of this comparison will help all nursing unit personnel participate easily and effectively in the use of management by objectives.

An Example of Interrelated Goals

Dorothea E. Orem has written, "The nurse's special interest is the continuing therapeutic care which the patient requires.... The nursing focus takes into account both the medical point of view and the patient's point of view" (Orem, 1971, p. 49).

The implementation of NBO takes into account the goals and objectives of the patient's doctor, together with three other aspects of nursing goals and objectives: (1) your own, as the patient's nurse; (2) the patient's, as a person; and (3) the family's, as healthcare consumers.

For example, consider again the three short-range goals for a married female patient, age 40 (see page 110), who has successfully undergone surgery and initial recovery for an abdominal hysterectomy. The patient's goal is to move about without pain; the husband's goal is to reassure his wife that she is still loved and needed; and the nurse's goal is to prevent circulatory complications.

Note that each goal is set by the individual involved—the patient, the husband, and the nurse. All are meaningful and need attention. The nurse needs to be aware of all three goals with an understanding that, while each person

Table 5-2 Comparison Summary

Feature	NMBO	NBO
Aim	Goal achievement	Goal achievement
Focus	Personnel management	Patient care management
Method	MBO technique	MBO technique
Objectives	Oriented to nursing management objectives	Oriented to direct patient care objectives
Motivation	Self (nursing personnel)	Self (patient)
Involvement	Nurse managers/personnel	Nursing personnel/patient/family
Process	Problem solving/unit management	Problem solving/nursing process

can set objectives to meet parts of each of the goals, no one person can meet all of the goals. The patient, husband, doctor and nurse must all work together to satisfy all these goals. For patient-care objectives to be practical at the direct care level, it is necessary to determine selectively which of the components of an objective are appropriate and useful in a given situation. Let's follow through with the three separate goals and see what objectives might assist the three parties involved to achieve those goals.

The patient's goal is to move about without pain. One of the patient's objectives might be to learn to support the area of incision with her hands during the first 48-hour postoperative period. A second patient objective is to request a pain medication 20 minutes before attempting to get out of bed (for three postoperative days).

The husband's objectives can be (1) to demonstrate on each visit, through words and attitude, his continuing love, devotion, and need for his wife, and (2) to remind and assist her in her pain-control practices. And the nurse, to meet the goal of preventing circulatory complications, has an objective to schedule and assign staff to help the patient increase the number of occasions for exercise at regular intervals on each successive postoperative day.

Note that the husband's objectives, if carefully set and carried out, help to meet his needs as well as his wife's needs and goals. Similarly the nurse, in setting and carrying out his/her objectives, will help achieve his/her goal while helping both husband and wife meet their objectives—and hence meet their goals. But this kind of mutually satisfying outcome is not likely to be achieved if the several persons involved set their goals and objectives independently of one another.

As we learn more and more to include the patient and family in the patient's care, we need to practice the setting of mutual goals. Setting goals with instead of for people may take place between the doctor and nurse, the doctor and patient, the nurse and the patient, the patient and family—any combination that the patient's needs indicate. This mutual goal setting must be documented in the patient's medical record. The goals that involve the nursing staff with patient and family may be noted on the nursing care plan. The goals are based upon the needs and problems of the patient. Specific nursing orders are then identified on the nursing care plan to meet each need or problem.

NBO and PONS

When a person enters today's healthcare system, that person assumes the role of patient. Similarly, when people work in any healthcare organization, they assume the role designated by their titles. But each of us has many roles in our life and work. And whatever role we assume, we bring ourselves into the situation as persons. Goals and objectives are set by persons. Systems are designed by persons. But a technique or system is only as effective as the person who uses it. This is as true for NBO as it is for any other technique or process. We believe that nurses can make a conscious decision to identify meaningful goals and objectives mutually with doctors, patients, and families—and with other healthcare personnel. Regardless of the pressures brought to bear on nurses by the organization in which they work, only the nurses themselves can ultimately decide to set mutual goals and objectives.

If you are like many nurses you can recall one or more occasions when you've said, "Oh, I can't do that. I can't learn to practice MBO. I just can't be a manager." The next time you say, or are tempted to say, "I can't" change it to "I won't do that; I won't learn to, etc." Nearly always the "I won't" is a more accurate statement than the "I can't." As a nurse you can do almost anything you really want to do—if you are willing to pay the price in time, effort, and the acquisition of newer knowledge and skills. If you can visualize how what you decide you can do will result in better care for your patients and greater work satisfaction for yourself, you are likely to want to pay the price in return for the benefits. In economic and budgetary terminology, this is known as the price/benefit ratio. As Katherine B. Nuckolls has said, "Ultimately, the person who really determines what the nurse can do is the nurse herself. Her perception of her role and her expectations of herself will be the most important determinants of her behavior" (Nuckolls, 1974, p. 630).

NBO and PONS are two techniques or systems that complement one another. Table 5-3 is a summary comparison of the basic components of both, presented in the context of the management functions of plan, do, and control.

HUMAN MODE AND TECHNICAL MODE IN MBO

Clearly we have emphasized the human elements of MBO as much as the technical aspects of the subject. This is necessarily so. MBO is not a new program or system to be superimposed upon an existing organizational way of getting results. MBO provides, however, a possible new outlook, a different way of trying to accomplish the major purposes of the agency and its subdivisions. It also points the way to the need for sharpening the skills of managers who have the responsibility for getting results—through the use of MBO and such additional techniques as the managers use in carrying out their functions.

Nurses are in the fortunate position of being able to accommodate the principles and practices of MBO quite readily. MBO fits a familiar pattern of the nurses' educational preparation. It is consistent with the nursing process.

Table 5-3 Comparison of NBO and PONS

NBO		PONS
	P	
Set a goal	l	Principles of practice
Set objectives	a	The nursing process
	n	
Work toward the objectives and goals	D o	Problem-oriented nursing record
	C o	
Evaluate level of achievement of goals and objectives	n t	Nursing audit
		Nursing inservice and continuing education
	r o l	

It is easily adapted to nurse manager responsibilities via NMBO and to patient care management responsibilities via NBO. The revelation for some nurses that "Why, this is very much like what I have been doing all along!" may come as a surprise. Such a reaction can be helpful or hurtful—helpful, if it leads to more skillful use of MBO to strengthen present practices in personnel and patient care management, but hurtful if it leads to thinking MBO has nothing to offer nurses, the nursing department, or patients. MBO has much to offer because it can become the means to greater agency-wide cooperation and effectiveness.

AGENCY-WIDE USE OF MBO

In many healthcare organizations, the method of introducing MBO and other management techniques has been based upon a business or industrial model. Examples used in MBO orientation and training sessions have in many health agency applications been selected from business or nonpatient-care situations.

We have reversed the customary approach. We have presented MBO as a technique for nurse managers. An obvious reason for this is to increase the likelihood that nurses will understand, accept, and use this valuable method for managing. Another vital reason is the fact that the nursing department in the typical hospital spends upwards of 40 percent of the institution's operating expenses each year. In addition, the day-to-day patient care activities of the nursing department reach out to involve all other departments of the organization. Finally, nursing departments are often led by excellent managers; and often it is the best managers who can see the value of an improved technique or method, will adopt it, and use it in the interest of high-quality, optimum-cost patient care.

Marvin Weisbord has put some of these considerations into sharp focus. He writes:

> ... consider a connection between deteriorating doctor-nurse relationships and rising hospital costs. There are in the main three things hospital patients need: Clinical care, personal attention, and help in getting a complex system to focus on their own case. Doctors provide the first service. Increasingly, aides do the "hands-on" care, clerks the paperwork, allied technicians the clinical tests, and ombudsmen the patient advocacy. Nurses, who might provide a link between clinical and administrative tasks, are being squeezed out. RN's often don't want the narrow jobs, for they are trained to greater responsibility.
>
> They cannot use their knowledge well in the present setup, despite the fact they spend more time with patients, and often understand better than anyone the complex relationship among physical, emotional, social and administrative problems. With clinical and administrative training, they might make excellent hospital integrators—much better, in fact, than doctors or administrators. Instead, they are opting for the Identity game—seeking to become nurse practitioners—because nobody, themselves included, can visualize a more appropriate use for their training (Weisbord, 1976).

It should be clear that we believe that nurse managers sometimes are, and certainly can become, "excellent hospital integrators." This is most likely to happen only when all managers on the healthcare team understand each other's roles and cooperate with those persons—nurse managers or others—who are willing and able to assume the hospital integrator responsibility.

Experience has demonstrated that all hospital department heads are usually willing and able to benefit from management development efforts that focus on management functions, techniques, and skills. Department heads learn to conceptualize and understand their managerial roles better, to enjoy their work more, and to contribute more effectively to the goals of the hospital. MBO is one such technique that deserves agency-wide understanding, strong implementation leadership from the chief executive, and consistent follow-through as part of day-to-day management. MBO serves as a method for integrating personal and departmental objectives. MBO facilitates interdisciplinary efforts to achieve the broad goals of individuals and the healthcare agency. MBO works best when it is used in this manner, rather than being carried out as a separate program apart from the day-to-day use of the management process. Subsequent chapters present additional management techniques—performance evaluation, nursing audit, budgetary planning—from the same point of view. They work best when used within the same framework of concepts and philosophy as MBO. Altogether, these techniques help nurse managers to carry out their management functions.

NOTES

Bakke, E. W. Teamwork in industry. *The Scientific Monthly*, March 1948, *66*, 213-220.

Combs, A. W., Avila, D. L., & Purkey, W. W. *Helping relationships: Basic concepts for the helping professions*. Boston: Allyn and Bacon, 1971.

DiVincenti, M. *Administering nursing service*. (2nd ed.). Boston: Little, Brown, 1977.

Drucker, P. M. *Management: Tasks, responsibilities, practices*. New York: Harper & Row 1974. (Excerpt reprinted with permission.)

Ganong, J., & Ganong, W. *HELP with management by objectives*. Chapel Hill, N.C.: W. L. Ganong Co., 1975.

Johnson, G. V., & Tingey, S. Matrix organization: Blueprint of nursing care organization for the 80s. *Hospital & Health Services Administration*, Winter 1976, *21*(4) 27-39. (Provides a brief explanation of the project management concept.)

Maslow, A. H. *Motivation and personality* (2nd ed.). New York: Harper & Row, 1970.

McGregor, D. Do management control systems achieve their purpose? *AMA Management Review*, February 1967, *56*(2).

McGregor, D. *The human side of enterprise*. New York: McGraw-Hill, 1960.

Myers, M. S. *Every employee a manager*. New York: McGraw-Hill, 1970, pp. 69-70.

Nuckolls, K. B. Who decides what the nurse can do? *Nursing Outlook*, October 1974, *22*.

Orem, D. E. *Nursing: Concepts of practice*. New York: McGraw-Hill, 1971.

Weisbord, M. R. Why organization development hasn't worked (so far) in medical centers. *Health Care Management Review*, Spring 1976, *1*(2). Excerpt reprinted with permission of Aspen Systems Corp.

Reading List

Books

Bakke, E. W. *The bonds of organization: An appraisal of corporate human relations*. Hamden, Conn.: Archon Books, 1966.

Cornuelle, R. *De-managing America—The final revolution*. New York: Random House, 1975.

Deegan, A. X., II. *Management by objectives for hospitals*. Germantown, Md.: Aspen Systems Corp., 1977.

Morrisey, G. *Management by objectives and results*. Reading, Mass.: Addison Wesley, 1970.

Odiorne, G. *Management decision by objectives*. Englewood Cliffs, N. J.: Prentice-Hall, 1969.

Articles

Adams, R. H. Goalstorming. *S.A.M. Advanced Management Journal*, Summer 1979, *44*(3), 55–61.

Cain, C., & Luchsinger, V. Management by objectives: Applications to nursing. *Journal of Nursing Administration*, January 1978, *8*(1), 35–38.

Cannon, J. Using MBO in managing contracts. *Health Care Management Review*, Winter 1978, *3*(1), 41–51.

Gerstenfeld, A. MBO revisited: Focus on health systems. *Health Care Management Review*, Fall 1977, *2*(4), 51–57.

Migliore, R. H. The use of long-range planning/MBO for hospital administrators. *Health Care Management Review*, Summer 1979, *4*(3), 23–28.

Sherwin, D. S. Management *of* objectives. *Harvard Business Review*, May–June 1976, *54*(3), 149–160.

A Results-Oriented Performance Evaluation Program

"HOW AM I DOING?"

All members of a nursing staff need to know how they are doing. You and others have a right to receive answers to the often-voiced questions, "Where do I stand?" and "Is my work OK?" You may get answers from the people you are working for—the patients, the doctors, your own nurse supervisor, someone in administration, or other personnel. When any of these people tell you, "You've done a good job!", you feel great. You like praise because it satisfies your basic need for self-worth, self-respect, status, and ego satisfaction.

You hurt if you are deprived of this kind of need satisfaction. You probably feel this hurt just as much as when you are deprived of other basic biological requirements for remaining healthy—such as the need for air, water, and food. If you are told, "That was a poor job" or "You really made a bad mistake" or "Why can't you do it right?" you are likely to feel bad. You hurt. You hurt because one of your basic human needs has been assaulted. Other employees, given similar messages, respond in much the same way as you. This is a simple fact whether or not the persons involved comprehend the significance of Maslow's hierarchy of human needs and their influence upon motivation as described in Appendix I. But every nurse manager in today's healthcare agencies should understand and be able to use this theory.

Consider the strength of your own emotional reactions when your nurse manager tells you positive or negative things about yourself or your work. Then it really is "for counts." You react to negative criticism with identifiable feelings even when you know that such criticism is justified. You, like other people, have a fairly accurate idea of how well you are doing your job. You feel it inside yourself when you have done a good day's work. And you usually know it, without anyone telling you, when you have blundered. But what is most disheartening is when the boss gives you an evaluation which is at odds with your own honest evaluation of yourself. And other people, under similar circumstances, feel very much as you do.

This is a problem. It is a problem in many hospitals because of the awkward situation in which the department heads and nurse managers find themselves. They know they are required or expected to evaluate the employees they supervise. But they often are frustrated, uncomfortable, even hostile to the whole routine because they know or feel that:

- the existing evaluation procedure is inadequate for its purpose.
- the techniques for evaluation are unsatisfactory for measuring results.
- they are not sufficiently familiar with the performance of the person being evaluated.
- they lack training in the necessary interviewing and counseling skills.
- they have insufficient time to do evaluations.
- their guilt feelings tend to make them angry with the people they must evaluate.

What managers want from a performance appraisal system and what they get from it frequently are two different things. Managers expect and hope that appraisals will perform two primary functions: (1) effectively measure employee competence, and (2) enrich the employee's experience in the job. However, recent research on the subject indicates that the majority of appraisal systems currently in use are neither effective nor valid for either purpose (Olmos, 1979).

In such circumstances it is no wonder that nurse managers often resent the time and effort devoted to personnel evaluations, and that the intended purpose of the evaluation process is served so poorly. In St. Joseph Hospital, St. Paul, we asked a group of twenty head nurses who had already expressed their dissatisfaction with the existing employee appraisal form to respond to these questions: "How would you design a performance evaluation plan? What characteristics should it have? What conditions should such a plan satisfy?"

These head nurses, working in nondirected, simultaneous knee-group (small identity group) discussions, developed a significant number of recommendations and criteria for such a performance evaluation plan in less than one-half hour. They felt that such a plan should provide for self-evaluation, not just an evaluation by one's own nurse manager; that evaluations should be scheduled more often than once a year; that the evaluation conference should address itself to the question, "What are my goals and objectives?"; that evaluation should help answer personal self-development needs; that different plans should be permitted for different departments, rather than insisting upon one hospital-wide evaluation plan; that the evaluation include responsibilities and leadership requirements; that head nurses should maintain on their own units the necessary records for evaluation purposes; that review dates for evaluation sessions should be staggered to avoid having many persons scheduled for review within a few weeks' time once a year; that a simple grading scale should be used; that different types of plans should be permitted for different job levels; that the evaluation sessions should elicit feelings, attitudes, and understandings about the implementation of important nursing programs such as nursing audit, PONS, and MBO; that evaluations should help to identify employees who have aspirations for growth and who intend to remain with the hospital; that evaluations should be carried out only by nurse managers who are intimately familiar with the work results of the person being evaluated; that the evaluation forms should allow space for comments, examples, critical incidents, and follow-through plans; that standards of performance should be established against which actual work performance will be judged.

This list shows that pragmatic head nurses not only have justifiable criticism of existing employee appraisal programs, but also have excellent suggestions for an improved plan which they believe they could use with more enthusiasm and success. In the instance cited, such a plan was instituted and included practically all of the features which the nurses recommended. The performance evaluation plan described herein successfully meets these same criteria.

The JCAH 1980 Standard II for Nursing Services (see Appendix K) reads as follows: "The nursing department/service shall be organized to meet the nursing care needs of patients and to maintain established standards of nursing practice." The interpretation of this standard includes, among other items, the following special attention to performance appraisal:

> A written evaluation of the performance of registered nurses and ancillary nursing personnel shall be made at the end of the probationary period and at a defined interval thereafter. An annual evaluation is recommended. The evaluation must be criteria-based and shall relate to the standards of performance specified in the individual's job description. Job descriptions for each position classification shall also delineate the functions, responsibilities, and specific qualifications of each classification, and shall be made available to nursing personnel at the time they are hired and when requested. Job descriptions shall be reviewed periodically and revised as needed to reflect current job requirements.

This chapter describes a highly effective results-oriented performance evaluation program (ROPEP). It meets and exceeds the JCAH requirements as set forth above. ROPEP is being used by more and more administrators, department heads, nurse managers, and other supervisory personnel to: (1) identify performance responsibilities, (2) develop measurable standards of satisfactory performance, (3) encourage employees to evaluate their own work performance, (4) provide an objective basis for praising a creditable performance, (5) assist employees in identifying their own needs for additional knowledge and skill, (6) help employees achieve maximum satisfaction from their work; and, when they so desire, qualify themselves for jobs of greater responsibility.

INTRODUCTION TO PERFORMANCE EVALUATION

The term "performance evaluation" carries different meanings for different people. This is to be expected, since people's interpretation of a work-related word or phrase is based upon their own individual work experiences and the management techniques or personnel appraisal methods used in their places of employment. Performance evaluation as used in connection with ROPEP is defined as *the measurement of the results of a person's work effort compared with previously agreed-upon standards of performance.* This definition is broad enough to apply to the employee performance evaluation process at all job levels in every type of organization. It is specific enough to differentiate it from the variety of other terms used, sometimes erroneously, as synonyms.

Zollitsch and Langsner, devoting over 92 pages to "Fundamentals of Employee Evaluation" in their book *Wage and Salary Administration,* found over 70 different titles and descriptive terms used in connection with the evaluation of employees (Zollitsch & Langsner, 1970, p. 362). These terms included performance rating, appraisal and development rating, merit rating, efficiency rating, measuring performance, worker appraisal, and performance review. What's in a name? A great deal! Does it make any difference what name is used to describe the technique? Yes! It makes a difference because of the unfavorable experiences of employees who have been subjected to or required to use so many of the poorly designed or ineffectively applied rating systems in the past.

The focus of many rating or appraisal methods has been on characteristics of the employee rather than upon the employee's demonstrated performance results. In fact, too many hospitals and other healthcare agencies still use appraisal forms that require supervisors to "measure" such factors as initiative, loyalty, cooperativeness, creativity, dependability, stamina, appearance, personality, potential, or interpersonal relations. The use of these kinds of characteristics for rating purposes causes unnecessary resentments, diverts attention from more meaningful objective measures of work results, subverts the laudable goals of the evaluation process and often contributes to making the entire program a matter of ridicule and scorn by both hourly paid employees and managers.

An alternative to the attribute-oriented appraisal just described is a results-oriented performance evaluation. "All one can measure is performance. And all one should measure is performance" (Drucker, 1974, p. 479).

Abe Lincoln's oft-quoted statement is relevant here: "I do the very best I know how—the very best I can; and I mean to keep doing so until the end. If the end brings me out all right, what is said against me won't amount to anything. If the end brings me out wrong, ten angels swearing I was right would make no difference."* We believe that these words express succinctly the attitudes of most of the thousands of healthcare employees with whom we have worked. We believe that these workers at all levels deserve evaluation methods that treat them more like adults than children, and that give recognition to their common sense, their worth as individuals, and their human needs.

Some further clarification of terminology will help avoid later confusion and misunderstandings. "Job Evaluation" is the management technique for determining the relative worth of individual jobs in an organization so as to establish a wage classification system for that organization. "Employee Evaluation," sometimes called merit rating, is the subjective process of appraising employees' relative worth to the organization in terms of their abilities, job performance, and potential. Thus while job evaluation measures the relative worth of jobs, employee evaluation measures the relative worth of employees.

Theoretically, therefore, when both techniques are used effectively, the amount of each employee's pay is determined by the worth of his job together with the measure of his own individual worth. Such a method attempts to provide equitable pay for persons doing the same or different jobs.

For example, the pay range for the LPN I classification may be $4.50 to $4.90 per hour (based upon job evaluation). Sue Smith, LPN, may be receiving $4.60 per hour while Alice Atwood, LPN, is paid $4.75 per hour (based upon their individual employee evaluations). Similarly, two persons who work in the LPN II classification of $4.90 to $5.32 per hour (based upon job evaluation) may be receiving the same pay of $5.10 per hour if they have the same relative worth as individuals (determined by employee evaluation). At the same time these LPN IIs may have merit ratings equal to Alice Atwood's, the LPN I, as judged on the employee evaluation scale.

---

*Attributed to President Lincoln in a conversation with his Secretary of State, William H. Seward.

OTHER FACTORS INFLUENCING WAGES

From a practical standpoint, a variety of other factors have a great influence upon the actual wages and salaries paid to individuals. Such factors include length of service, supply and demand, competition, ability to pay (financial conditions), wage and price controls, labor unions, philosophy of the organization as interpreted by management, personal preferences, fringe-benefits package, and current goals and priorities of the organization. In the final analysis, techniques such as job evaluation and employee evaluation are methods for assisting managers in establishing a fair day's pay for a fair day's work. They help to narrow the range of judgment within which a manager has to make decisions affecting each employee's pay. To this extent, these techniques and others like them can be useful.

Some organizations, however, have adopted a policy of disassociating employee evaluation from the process of setting wage rates and salaries for individuals. This is in recognition and acceptance of the influence of the aforementioned factors that dictate what changes occur in wage payments from year to year. Such a policy has the advantage of permitting the employee evaluation process to take place in an atmosphere free of the concerns related to pay adjustments. The major focus of attention can then be the performance of the employees in carrying out their job duties and responsibilities, and how employee and manager together evaluate the performance results.

ROPEP DEFINITION CLARIFIED

ROPEP is an effective method for the evaluation of performance results. The key words in the definition of performance evaluation (as previously stated in this chapter) can now be examined for their meaning in the light of the prior discussion. *Performance evaluation* is the *measurement* (the determination of degree of conformity with criteria of quality and quantity) of the *results* (consequences, outcomes) of a person's *work effort* (on-the-job activities and exertion) *compared* (examined in order to note the similarities or differences) with previously *agreed upon* (jointly developed in advance with accord by the manager and the employee) *standards* (acknowledged measures of comparison for qualitative or quantitative value; criteria; norms).

The following sections of this chapter describe the several phases of introducing and implementing ROPEP so that performance evaluation, as defined and clarified above, may become a reality. The four necessary phases are as follows: Phase 1, Preparing Performance Descriptions; Phase 2, The

Initial Application; Phase 3, The First Evaluation Cycle; and Phase 4, The Work Evaluation Cycle.

PHASE 1: PREPARING PERFORMANCE DESCRIPTIONS

A performance description has some similarities to a job description, but the two are basically different because they are developed for two different purposes. The job description, by its very title, describes a job. It is prepared by a process of job analysis. Its purpose is primarily to provide the necessary descriptive job information for job evaluation. A performance description, by contrast, describes performance responsibilities. It is prepared by a process of performance analysis carried out by employees with their own managers (supervisors, department heads, bosses). Its purpose is to reach agreement and understanding, between employee and manager, regarding the employee's performance responsibilities so that meaningful, ongoing self-evaluation can take place.

A performance description is defined as a statement of the purpose of a person's job functions, the major performance responsibilities (grouped by persons to whom the responsibilities exist), and measures of satisfactory performance. The emphasis in the preparation of a performance description is upon reaching a mutual understanding between employee and manager regarding who is to do what for whom, when, and how well; so that there can be later understanding and agreement regarding what was done for whom, when, and how well. When an organization, a department, or an individual manager decides to use the ROPEP method, the essential first step is to prepare performance descriptions. This is a time-consuming but rewarding process. This section describes how to do it.

ROPEP requires the preparation of performance descriptions, rather than the conventional job descriptions. These performance descriptions, sometimes called *job performance descriptions*, look different from the usual performance descriptions because they *are* different. They are organized differently because their focus is on performance responsibilities to specific persons, and on standards of performance for each key performance responsibility. They were designed this way originally (in the late 1960s) because we recognized the need for a sound management approach to the task of making each person on the nursing staff accountable for the quality of patient care.

Prior discussion has already emphasized that performance descriptions are the outcome of the combined efforts of each manager and the employees who work for that manager. The process of coming together to discuss the performance responsibilities and the measures of satisfactory performance and of reaching mutual understanding and agreement regarding them is even more important than the actual wording of the statements that become the written form of the performance descriptions. Once understanding is achieved, the interpretation of the words and the meanings of the perform-ance descriptions are likely to be uniform. Lacking such mutual understand-ing, agreement upon the other phases of the performance evaluation process becomes much more difficult.

One of the best ways for two persons to reach an understanding is for them to talk together fully and openly. When the two persons involved are a nurse manager and a staff member, it is necessarily the manager who must set the example and create the climate for such open discussion. An essential ele-ment is the manager's ability to draw out the employee's views with suitable questions, then to listen carefully to what the employee says. This is a skill too often poorly developed by some managers. Listening is difficult; listening takes time; listening is hard work; listening is tiring. Listening skill is essen-tial, however, and it can be developed.

Performance Description Worksheet

Another important way to help personnel understand performance re-quirements is the use of a Performance Description Worksheet. A sample of such a worksheet is included in Appendix D. This type of worksheet, to be completed by every employee in every job, provides for valuable input by the people who know the most about their performance responsibilities—namely, the people doing the work. When all of the responses from all of the employees with the same job title are summarized, a wealth of information is available for preparing a meaningful first draft of the major performance responsibilities for that particular job—as described by the employees themselves. Similarly, employees' answers to the question, "How do you know when you are doing a good job?" provide some excellent clues to suitable measures of satisfactory performance.

The Performance Description Worksheets can be distributed by nurse managers at small departmental or unit meetings. The purpose of the worksheets can then be explained, with time for questions and answers. It is helpful to state the purpose of the worksheets, and instructions for com-pleting them, directly on the worksheet forms. This will minimize misunder-standings.

Should these worksheets be signed or should they be completed anony-mously? We believe they should be signed. To do otherwise is to start off on the wrong foot with a program designed to strengthen the most important of all on-the-job relationships—that between employees and managers.

Anonymous questionnaires smack too much of the kind of gameplaying that ROPEP seeks to eliminate. Admittedly there may be some organizational circumstances that dictate unsigned responses when the worksheets are used for the first time. Whenever this is the case, it is symptomatic of significant administrative, supervisory, or labor relations problems that deserve attention before ROPEP is introduced.

As with PONS and MBO, the introduction of an important technique such as ROPEP often is long delayed, awaiting a top-level administrative exploration, decision, and implementation effort. This is unfortunate, because more often than not there is no need for a uniform plan to be used agency-wide. In fact, there may be valid reasons for using varied approaches, different starting dates, and different implementation steps within different departments of a hospital. With this in mind, we provide in Appendix D some guidelines and specific implementation steps which can be used by nurse managers independently within their own areas of responsibility. The steps are remarkably simple. They make sense to nurse managers who have followed them. All that you need in order to do the same thing yourself are some of the characteristics of being a nurse manager previously discussed: motive force, willingness to take some reasonable risks, ability to use the Decision Worksheet, a sense of agreement with McGregor's Theory Y and Myers' enriched job concept, and a desire to follow the simple instructions.

The approach, as you will see in Appendix D, is first of all to prepare your own performance description. The fact that you take the initiative (instead of your boss doing so) makes no difference. The more to your credit! It is important, however, that you seek the involvement of your boss. Both you and your boss need to agree upon what you should be doing for whom, when, and how well. Then when you want an answer to the question, "How am I doing?", both you and your boss will be evaluating the same things by the same standards of satisfactory performance.

The Complete Performance Description

Appendix G provides an example of a performance description for a head nurse. An example of a performance description for a staff nurse position (RN II) as developed by nurse managers in one hospital may be found in Appendix D. The content of this description includes the position title and department name, titles of the employees supervised by the RN, and a brief statement of the purpose (or primary function) of the nurse classified as RN II. Then the performance responsibilities and the standards of satisfactory performance are presented in a two-column format, as follows:

Major Performance Responsibilities	Performance Standards
To patients (or other agency clients) To medical staff To own nurse manager To unit personnel To committees To other department personnel To other organizations To self	(For each item, a statement is made of the measurable conditions that will exist when performance is satisfactory.)

The major performance responsibilities listed are what the RN IIs in this hospital have to do in their work, listed under the person or persons for whom the responsibilities are performed. In the right-hand column, opposite each item of major responsibility, is the statement of measurable conditions that will exist when performance is up to standard. Each of these measures completes the sentence beginning, "Performance is satisfactory when . . . ." The final section of the performance description is a listing of the qualifications necessary to become an RN II as established for this hospital department of nursing service. The qualifications section may or may not be included as part of a performance description, depending upon the total purposes which the description is intended to serve. This section is useful when a wide-track careers program (with clearly defined career ladders) is being instituted to identify promotional opportunities within the organization and tell employees how to qualify for them.

PHASE 2: INITIAL APPLICATION (INTRODUCTION/EDUCATION)

When nurse managers prepare to initiate their first ROPEP evaluations with their departmental employees, they will find that each employee is at a different stage of readiness. Those who have had the opportunity to participate in Phase 1 and have actively contributed to the development of their performance descriptions are likely to be the best prepared. Newer employees and others who for one reason or another were not able to participate directly in Phase 1 will be far less informed and will require the greatest amount of initial orientation to the first use of the performance descriptions for the self-evaluation procedure.

Exhibit 6-1 is a Manager's Guide and Checklist for the Use of Performance Descriptions in Role Clarification and Performance Evaluation—An Employee Self-Evaluation Method. The emphasis is on self-evaluation of

Exhibit 6-1 Manager's Guide and Checklist for the Use of Performance Descriptions in Role Clarification and Performance Evaluation

An Employee Self-Evaluation Method

A. Meet with each employee to discuss and reach a mutual understanding of responsibilities and the standards of satisfactory performance.
_____ 1. Review the performance description.
_____ 2. Ask for comments and questions.
_____ 3. Clarify and amplify the performance description through discussion.
_____ 4. Explain the self-evaluation procedure (including the exception principle).

B. Establish a plan for regular employee self-evaluation.
_____ 1. Set a date for completion of first self-evaluation.
_____ 2. Obtain from employees their own written comments regarding how well they think they are meeting the standards for their performance responsibilities. (The Self-Evaluation of Performance record may be used.)

C. Meet with employees individually to review their self-evaluations.
_____ 1. Set dates for the discussions.
_____ 2. Meet with the employees individually and listen to their comments.
_____ 3. Agree whenever possible with the employees' own performance evaluations of the major performance responsibilities.
_____ 4. When you disagree with the self-evaluation of a responsibility, ask the employees to explain again their reasons for their own evaluation. Then indicate why you feel that the performance results are better than, or not as good as, the employees' own evaluations.
_____ 5. Reach agreement upon those performance results which need strengthening, if any.
_____ 6. Develop suggestions for improvement with the employees, if any are necessary. Help identify available resources or new challenges.
_____ 7. Agree upon specific follow-through action. Identify objectives to be met.

Source: Ganong, J. and Ganong, W. *Help with results-oriented performance evaluation.* Chapel Hill, N.C.: W. L. Ganong Co., 1974, p. 41.

performance results by each employee. This is a necessary step. As Frederick Herzberg says: "A real method of instilling the potential of accountability is to remove the crutch of inspection and instead directly identify the performance of the work with the individual" (Herzberg, 1974, p. 74). To do otherwise is to perpetuate the record of failure, friction, and frustration that has been characteristic of traditional employee appraisal and performance review plans in so many healthcare organizations. Herewith is a detailed explanation of each step included in the guidesheet for the Employee Self-Evaluation Method.

Manager's Guide to Using Performance Descriptions

Here is an elaboration of each step outlined on the manager's guide and checklist (Exhibit 6-1).

A. Meet with each employee to discuss and reach a mutual understanding of performance responsibilities and standards of satisfactory performance.
   1. Review the performance description.
   This step is considerably simplified when the employee helped to prepare the statements in the performance description. When this is the case, there may be a temptation to omit this first step on the assumption that it is not necessary. Resist such a temptation. Circumstances change. Ongoing work experiences can change a person's viewpoints and interpretations. A person's apperceptive mass continues to evolve. So while this first step may take less time with the employee who was involved in the first writing of the performance description, include this step always with each and every employee as part of every periodic evaluation discussion.
   2. Ask for comments and questions.
   The intent in this step is to encourage an open, free, and easy exploration of what the employee's work is all about—its purpose, what has to be done for whom, and so on. How each manager brings about this kind of discussion depends greatly upon the manager's own individual style. What works well for one person may not work so well for another. However, a vital factor that has a great influence upon the level of communication that takes place is the attitude that the manager brings to the discussion. This will be communicated and will influence what happens. Some tips for stimulating productive discussion are included in these pages.
   3. Clarify and amplify the performance descriptions, through discussion.
   This is especially essential for the first meeting with employees who have not previously seen the performance description for their jobs. This can-

not be hurried. Whatever time it takes will be time well spent. (How long does it take and how much does it cost to process a grievance? A labor arbitration case? A lawsuit in court?) Ask repeatedly, "What does this mean to you?" Request, "Tell me in your own words what this means." Reiterate, "The reason we are doing this is so that both you and I have the same understanding about your work and what we can expect of each other." Say, "What I think I heard you say was ... (repeat what employee said). Do you mean that ..." (try to give same message in different words of your own choosing). Give an example to illustrate the meaning; say, "For example, if a patient asks to be helped out of bed, then slips and falls on the floor, do you mean that you would ... (etc.)?"

4. Explain the self-evaluation procedure (including the exception principle).

The self-evaluation aspect of ROPEP is a theme that requires emphasis throughout every step of ROPEP. Explain, "The reason for our having this kind of a self-evaluation program is so that you can feel comfortable doing your work without having me looking over your shoulder. Most people don't like the idea of a manager being a 'snoopervisor.' I don't like it either. The best way for both of us to get along together is for us to understand what both of us (you and I) consider to be satisfactory performance of your responsibilities. So let's take a look at these again."

Explain that:

    (a) The *first* regular performance evaluation discussion will include *all* of the performance responsibilities.

    (b) Subsequent regular evaluations (once or twice per year) will focus on those performance results that are either exceptionally outstanding or exceptional because they do not meet the standard of satisfactory performance. This is the *exception principle*. All other performance results require no attention because they are satisfactory.

    (c) Performance evaluation is really an ongoing day-to-day process. Thus there are likely to be many occasions between regular evaluation review sessions when the performance descriptions will need to be used to clarify questions, remind each other of performance standards, help to plan skill-improvement programs, and for other work-related purposes.

B. Establish a plan for regular employee self-evaluation.

1. Set a date for completion of first self-evaluation.

A date for completing the first self-evaluation may be set during the foregoing discussion in Step A4. Much depends upon the readiness of the individual employees. One person may require more than one discussion to complete steps A1 through A4. Another person may be ready to carry out his own self-evaluation immediately following step A4.

The manager will be able to judge how soon to allow the self-evaluation step to be completed. The manager can say, "How soon will you want to complete your first self-evaluation of performance?" There is usually no need to hurry it. For one person it may be within the month; for another, two or three months.

2. Obtain from employees their own written comments regarding how well they think they are meeting each of their performance responsibilities.

Remind employees to include every performance responsibility in this first self-evaluation. An extra copy of the performance description can be used by the employees on which to record their comments. For subsequent evaluations, the form in Appendix D can be used. Whatever form is used, the employee is expected to submit it to the manager by the set date.

Encourage employees to discuss with you (as manager) their efforts at self-evaluation if they wish to do so. They may need nothing more than to have some time with you to tell you how they are progressing and to have you agree with the kinds of words they are using. This interchange prior to the actual evaluation discussion can be highly valuable in preparing both employee and manager for a productive follow-through.

C. Meet with employees individually to review their self-evaluations.

1. Set dates for the discussions.

Establishing and maintaining a schedule for evaluation discussions is an indication of the importance attached to this activity by the nurse manager. Allow ample flexibility in the time planned for each individual evaluation discussion so that there will be no need to cut short a discussion that is proving to be lengthy but productive. It is good practice to schedule no more than one person for an evaluation session on any one day.

2. Meet with employees individually and listen to their comments.

Even when the manager has the employee's written self-evaluation comments in advance of the discussion, there is merit in permitting the employee to explain the self-evaluation verbally in the evaluation session. It is part of the process of maximizing communications and understanding at a most crucial point in the procedure.

3. Agree whenever possible with the employee's own performance evaluation of the major performance responsibilities.

The purpose of this procedure is to reach a meeting of minds (the manager's and the employee's) regarding the employee's performance results. Seek areas of agreement, not disagreement. The main question to be agreed upon for each performance responsibility is: "Has performance been satisfactory or not satisfactory, as measured against the stated standards in the performance description?"

4. When you disagree with the self-evaluation of a responsibility, ask the employee to explain again the reasons for the evaluation. Then indicate why your evaluation of the performance results are better than or not as good as the employee's own evaluation.

If both the employee and the manager have the same understanding of the responsibilities being evaluated and of the standards of satisfactory performance, then any disagreement in an evaluation would stem from differing knowledge of actual performance results (or differing interpretations of those results). The process of examining each of the three aspects in turn for any performance responsibility on which there appears to be a lack of agreement will minimize the likelihood of unnecessary misunderstandings.

The manager should maintain adequate personnel records to provide factual back-up data for unsatisfactory performance as well as for exceptionally good performance. Such documentation is essential for a number of valid purposes related to accreditation standards, nursing audit, patient care, lawsuits, labor relations when unions are involved, and effective personnel administration. One of the useful documentation methods is the critical incident technique as described in *Nursing Evaluation: The Problem and the Process* (Fivars & Gosnell, 1966).

5. Reach agreement upon those performance results which need strengthening.

This step is not always necessary with all employees for every regular performance evaluation. One of the fallacies connected with employee evaluation practices is the idea that there is always something wrong with employees or with their performance. Rating forms frequently seem to encourage emphasis on weaknesses rather than strengths. No wonder the appraisal procedure has such a bad reputation!

It is not necessary to make a special effort to find evidence of poor performance results that require improvement. Managers need not feel that they are poor evaluators if they cannot always identify weaknesses in employees' performances. On the contrary, managers should take credit when they have provided the kind of training and leadership that minimizes or eliminates unsatisfactory performance results.

But when performance results have been less than satisfactory, they must be faced for what they are. Hopefully, both the manager and the employee will recognize and agree upon the evidence of unsatisfactory performance results. Whenever there is a lack of such agreement, and the manager is convinced that the results for a given major performance responsibility are clearly unsatisfactory, the manager must make his own evaluation known to the employee and proceed in whatever manner is most likely to secure a satisfactory level of performance.

6. Develop suggestions for improvement with the employee. Help identify available resources.

Again, as in item 5, this is not always a necessary part of the self-evaluation process with every employee. Significant numbers of employees are likely to be delivering satisfactory performance for all of their major performance responsibilities. Many of this group of employees are valuable in their present jobs, have no need to improve their performance, and have no desire to qualify for higher-paid positions. They form an important and usually stable portion of the workforce. They are using their assets well and deserve credit for doing so.

When improvement is required on one or more performance responsibilities, ask the employee, "What do you want to do about it?" If improvement is to occur, it has to come about through the efforts of the individual employees. They have to motivate themselves to make improved performance happen. The manager can suggest sources of help and guidance when these are wanted. When necessary, the manager can prescribe the remedy necessary to secure results.

7. Agree upon specific follow-through action.

This is the specific outcome of a regular performance self-evaluation discussion. This step answers the questions, "What happens now? What do we do next?" For some employees the follow-through is signified by a parting comment on the part of the manager, "Keep up the good work." For other employees there will be an understanding of agreed-upon action by the employee (and perhaps the manager also) that will lead to the correction of those performance results that have been unsatisfactory. This agreement should be in writing and should follow the general pattern of the management-by-objectives technique—set a goal; set a date; evaluate. The objectives worksheet (found in Appendix D) provides a simple way to record this information for future follow-through.

The Meaning of Satisfactory Performance

There are some evident similarities between ROPEP and Nursing Audit as management techniques. Both are evaluative processes. Both establish standards of performance for measurement purposes. Both seek to provide criteria that will lead to employee performance results that assure the optimum delivery of patient care services. Both use a "go, no-go" concept of measurement (as discussed in Chapter 7).

The measure of satisfactory performance as used in connection with major performance responsibilities in patient care is a demanding standard. Thus the statement, "Performance is satisfactory when there are no documented errors," means no errors—none at all. There are few jobs in the world of work where such a stringent standard is required. But can any other standard prevail in any aspect of healthcare so vital, for example, as that of giving medications? Drucker makes the point nicely in writing about decision making and the need for compromise in order to balance conflicting objectives, conflicting opinions, and conflicting priorities.

> One has to compromise in the end. But unless one starts out with the closest one can come to the decision that will truly satisfy objective requirements, one ends up with the wrong compromise—the compromise that abandons essentials.

> For there are two different kinds of compromise. One kind is expressed in the old proverb 'Half a loaf is better than no bread.' The other kind is expressed in the story of the Judgment of Solomon, which was clearly based on the realization that "half a baby is worse than no baby at all." In the first instance, objective requirements are still being satisfied. The purpose of bread is to provide food, and half a loaf is still food. Half a baby, however, is not half of a living and growing child. It is a corpse in two pieces (Drucker, 1974, p. 479).

PHASE 3: FIRST EVALUATION CYCLE (IMPLEMENTATION)

ROPEP may appear to be a detailed, time-consuming procedure. It is. But what are the alternatives? Other employee appraisal techniques are time consuming also and often generate results that are far from satisfactory. ROPEP builds upon a combination of the human and technical modes in management that work well at all organizational levels. The focus is upon people doing the work of the organization—the needs, goals, and performance of people as related to the needs, goals, and performance of the organization. Thus ROPEP is an integral part of a management-by-objectives program within an organization.

Figure 6-1, entitled Management by Objectives for Nursing, summarizes in six steps the functioning of an *integrated MBO System* that uses performance descriptions as the basis for employee performance evaluation in relation to individual objectives within the pattern of the broad departmental and organizational goals. In the example, the position used is that of a nurse manager (head nurse, supervisor, patient care coordinator, assistant director of nursing service, etc.). The six steps of the ROPEP/MBO procedure are: (1) identify purpose and performance responsibilities (to whom); (2) list the major job segments (details of performance responsibilities); (3) develop standards of satisfactory performance; (4) set goals, objectives, and target

Figure 6-1 Management by Objectives for Nursing:
A Graphic Outline of the ROPEP/MBO Procedure/
The Nurse Manager's Job Responsibility

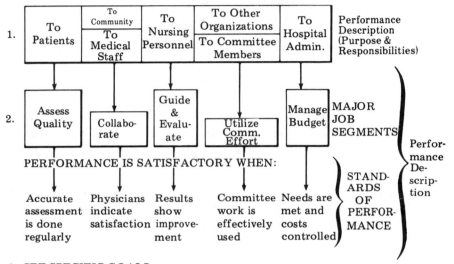

4. SET SPECIFIC GOALS

    Set Objective
    Set Target Dates

5. DO THE TASKS NECESSARY TO MEET THE SET OBJECTIVES

6. REVIEW PERFORMANCE ON SET TARGET DATE

    Set New and Revised Objectives
    Set New Target Dates

---

dates; (5) work toward achievement of objectives; and (6) review performance results; plan new objectives and target dates.

The consistency of relationships between and the similarities of purpose for the various management techniques and the management functions are evident. Management techniques (by whatever name) are action plans, procedures, or programs to assist nurse managers in using their skills to perform one or more management functions. The management techniques of ROPEP and MBO may be carried out in a variety of ways in different agencies and under a variety of names or without any identifying names at all. The merit in having a name to identify a worthwhile method or procedure is that it facilitates communications about it, minimizes misunderstandings, distinguishes it from other less satisfactory versions intended for the same purpose, and helps in the training of newer nurse managers in the art and science of their profession.

Where to Begin

Organizations, like people, must start from where they are when they undertake a new learning or developmental program. Each is at a different state of readiness. Some hospitals have had considerable experience with one or more types of appraisal systems. Others have had little or none. Some organizations will want to adopt ROPEP as part of building a strong personnel program with effective manager-employee relations to minimize the likelihood of a union. Others will begin to use ROPEP *because* they have a union.

But while there may be variations in how to begin to implement ROPEP, it is sound practice to begin with the administrative and management group. No managers at any level should be expected to carry out any of the ROPEP steps with employees under their direction until they have been on the receiving end of the process themselves. Is this dictum idealistic? Yes! Is it too idealistic for most healthcare agencies? No! One of the reasons for the failure of appraisal systems generally is that administrators and chief executives have approved the installation of such systems for use by middle managers with lower-echelon employees without having been willing to implement the plan with the people who work directly for them. Had they done so, many of these appraisal plans would have been abandoned before they were exposed to the justified disdain of managers at lower organizational levels. ROPEP should not be introduced into a hospital whenever the administrator or chief executive is unwilling to use ROPEP first with those persons who report directly to him or her. This admonition should be heeded for a number of reasons:

- Top administrative and middle management personnel require effective evaluation of their own performance for the same reasons as do others in the organization. The use of ROPEP at the higher organizational levels is even more essential than at lower levels because of the great impact that satisfactory or unsatisfactory individual performance of top-level managers has upon organizational goal achievement.
- The critical, analytical use of ROPEP by top administrators will contribute to whatever adaptations may be necessary for its most effective ongoing use within that hospital or agency.
- Managers learn by doing, just the same as other people. Part of the learning process is to carry out all of the steps of ROPEP "for real," in-

cluding developing the measures of satisfactory performance, self-evaluation, and follow-through of the MBO cycle.

- ROPEP gains in credibility, just as does any other technique, when the manager can say to employees with conviction, "This is not just for you. My boss uses it with me, too."
- There isn't any other successful way to do it. Review the ROPEP-MBO cycle as part of your management functions. It will be obvious that the suggested approach for using ROPEP does not add work. It simply helps to organize and systematize the already essential elements of the manager's performance responsibilities—at all levels.

Steps B1 and 2, and steps C1 through 7, of the Manager's Guide and Checklist for ROPEP (as shown in Figure 6-1 and discussed in the accompanying description) present a way to plan and carry out the initial self-evaluation with employees when ROPEP is just beginning. Subsequent self-evaluation discussions follow easily at appropriate intervals, and will require less total time than the first series of evaluations using the two-column performance descriptions as the results-oriented basis for measurement. As the process continues through several evaluation cycles over the first year or two, the exciting benefits of ROPEP will become apparent as an essential basic technique in the nurse manager's repertoire.

PHASE 4: WORK EVALUATION CYCLE (CONTINUATION)

Much emphasis has been placed upon the mutual development of performance descriptions which represent an understanding between employee and manager regarding who is to do what for whom, when, and how well. These same elements of performance were used as the basis for the self-evaluation procedure that has been described.

The early phases of setting up and initiating ROPEP are necessary for a successful performance evaluation program. This is true for any management technique—the preparation and beginning phases are more time consuming than the ongoing use and maintenance of the program. Yet suitable help and guidance can minimize the time requirements for introducing the program and completing the performance descriptions. An additional benefit of such help is the training of the management personnel who will coordinate the program and serve as organizational resource persons.

The six steps of the ROPEP-MBO cycles (Figures 5-5 and 6-1) demonstrate how the performance evaluation concept is broadened to include all aspects of a person's performance goals—the regular job performance responsibilities as well as those periodically assigned performance objectives.

The latter are a natural outgrowth of the ROPEP method since some objectives will relate to necessary action needed to secure a satisfactory level of performance for one or more major performance responsibilities. There is a danger, however, in overemphasizing the identification and attempted correction of deficiencies. Certainly errors and grossly unsatisfactory performance cannot be allowed to continue. But the focus needs to be on identifying the *strengths* of individuals and in building upon these strengths for the benefit of all. To do otherwise is to ignore the findings of motivational research as well as to blind ourselves to the meaning of the life/work experiences of each one of us.

This section considers the ongoing, continuous evaluation process once the initial developmental stages of ROPEP have been completed and the first self-evaluation cycle has occurred. An important reminder is that ROPEP is *not* a once-a-year enforced appraisal routine scheduled to coincide with the "annual merit increase." This phrase is one often used, tongue-in-cheek, by those who recognize the hypocrisy of the term "merit" for a wage adjustment process that is influenced primarily by a variety of other factors described early in this chapter.

More often than not the governing principle that appears to dictate wage adjustments is: "Every employee worth keeping is worth paying as high an across-the-board general increase as we can afford." Such a policy is understandable in these times of major financial stress due to inflation and the increasing restraints imposed by union contracts and consumer- or government-inspired wage and price controls. Such a principle *implies* performance evaluation in the phrase "worth keeping." Some employees may not justify an increase in wages based upon their performance. But they receive the increase nonetheless. Some of them by any objective measure should have been dropped from the hospital payroll years ago. These are the "touchy" cases that require special attention and action. In any event, the sham and cost of an annual formal personnel appraisal in the traditional mode is unnecessary to justify the nickel-and-dime "merit" wage adjustments that have been so typical.

·While ROPEP will assist meaningfully in the annual wage adjustment decisions, this is not its primary purpose. Its principal purpose is to provide a technique and the tools to assist nurse managers in getting people to do well what has to be done because *they* want to do it.

The Day-to-Day Use of ROPEP and MBO

The point has been made previously that an effective performance evaluation procedure is not an "add-on" to a manager's regular workload. More accurately, ROPEP and MBO become an integral part of the manager's three main functions: planning, doing, controlling. Compare the three management functions with the three steps of ROPEP and of MBO. These are summarized as follows:

ROPEP Cycle	Management Functions Cycle	MBO Cycle
Identify performance responsibilities and standards	Plan	Set goals and objectives
Perform job segments	Do	Perform necessary work
Measure performance against standards	Control	Review progress (was objective achieved on time?)

These cyclical processes are going on daily in one form or another for managers and other employees alike. They are neverending. They are mutually dependent and supportive. They are this way because they are based upon proven principles and practices of participation and involvement of people working together toward common objectives. When ROPEP and MBO are seen as month-in and month-out, year-round ways of managing, the occasions for discussing self-evaluations of performance are many. These occur naturally in the course of a day's work and by plan when needed. Effective managers know that evaluation discussions are most worthwhile when they occur soon after the specific performance results that drew attention.

The more formal semiannual or annual general reviews using the complete performance descriptions can be scheduled if desired. But these need not be grouped together in one month of the year. Like the billings for renewals of magazine subscriptions or for automobile drivers' licenses, they can be scheduled to spread the workload throughout the year by using employment anniversary dates, birth dates, or a similar method.

Insofar as individual performance goals and objectives are concerned, they too are always in varying stages of identification, initiation, effecting, and completion. Even when MBO objectives are related to budgetary planning, as is often the case, an effective ABP (annual budgetary planning) program will minimize an excessive concentration of objectives-related effort in any one month.

ROPEP: A Program Performance Plan

Figure 6-2 provides a summary of the four phases of introducing ROPEP. This program performance plan is designed so that it can serve as a worksheet to assist you and others who may wish to introduce the ROPEP concept in your own agency or department. The program worksheet is intended to provide a flexible guide which can be adapted to your own situation with its unique organizational interrelationships, level of receptivity to newer management methods, and timetable requirements.

The Systems Syndrome

Crystal balls went out of style years ago as part of the manager's tool kit. In actuality they never worked much better than Ouija boards. Hunches, sixth sense, and feelings about situations and people have been more reliable when recognized for what they are and checked out accordingly. But managers tend to continue looking for a magic formula to help them do what they have to do—manage.

The trend toward the installation of and reliance upon systems is one manifestation of this understandable desire of managers to simplify their work of planning, doing, and controlling. Systems are necessary. But they are no better than the persons who use them and manage them. Experience has demonstrated that well-motivated personnel using a poorly designed system ("no system at all") can achieve better performance results than poorly motivated personnel with a far more sophisticated system.

Some of the reasons for this phenomenon of motivated performance are set forth clearly in the writings of Douglas McGregor, Abraham Maslow, Peter Drucker, Frank Goble, and similar researchers and observers of people at work. Their message is clear. It is what effective managers have discovered repeatedly for themselves. This is the fact that managers cannot *make* employees give top performance results. Only the employees can *make themselves* give their best performance. If there is any kind of crystal ball insight, a magic formula for managers, it lies in the awareness of this simple truth and how to create the motivational climate that permits employees to do their best. Some clues are provided herein, and in a later chapter.

Satisfactory versus Top Performance

Why does ROPEP use standards of *satisfactory* performance instead of some higher goal of excellence? Perhaps the reasons are already evident. They include:

Figure 6-2 Program Performance Plan and Worksheet

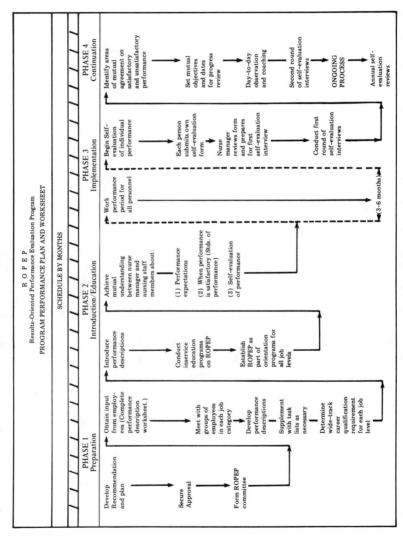

Source: Ganong, J. & Ganong, W. *HELP with results-oriented performance evaluation.* Chapel Hill, N.C.: 1974, p. 105.

- ROPEP intends to be realistic in regard to what level of performance should be expected as a "fair day's work for a fair day's pay."
- The "satisfactory" standard is a demanding one, especially when the measure is "no errors" in the critical tasks of patient care.
- Managers and supervisors have learned through hard, frustrating experience the fallacies and hazards of more complicated appraisal methods.
- The *satisfactory* evaluation principle is consistent with labor-union philosophy and practice, as well as with sound personnel-administration policy.
- Excellence in performance often occurs in spite of, not because of, an appraisal program. Excellence is achieved by people with pride in their work, by people who get satisfaction from their work.

This last reason is most significant. Healthcare organizations need to strive for top performance and excellence today more than ever before. Competition, always a motivational factor in general-business organizations, is affecting hospitals and the healthcare industry too. Healthcare organizations must attract and hold as many people as possible who will do the work that has to be done—satisfactorily. ROPEP will help and contribute to creating a climate for top performance.

Creating a Top-Performance Climate

Every organization, every department, tends to reflect the person at the head of it. That person's character, values, and management concepts inevitably have a profound influence on creating the climate for performance. Recognizing this, there is much that all nurse managers can do to affect the climate within which their people work. Tools, techniques, and skills are necessary. Among these are communications skills that will help with the success of a program such as ROPEP.

It remains our conviction, however, that the character, values and attitudes of the nurse manager are paramount to successful performance. The nurse manager is the role model who trains, leads, and evaluates the unit team workers who provide the level of care received by the patients. The challenge and responsibility are great. The rewards for satisfactory performance are highly personal and gratifying.

Later chapters include a variety of items that can be of assistance to managers who are attempting to implement ROPEP, MBO, and other management techniques. The emphasis in these aids is not on systems and techniques in the traditional framework of management control. They stress a way of thinking about management and a set of value concepts that give balance to both the human mode and the technical mode. They are implicit in the following ROPEP Precepts:

1. Criticism has a negative effect on achievement of goals.
2. Honest appreciation has a positive effect on motivation.
3. Performance improves most when specific achievable goals are established.
4. Defensiveness resulting from a negative appraisal produces inferior performance.
5. Coaching should be a day-to-day, not a once-a-year, activity.
6. Mutual goal setting, not criticism, improves performance.
7. Interviews designed primarily for the purpose of performance review should not unduly influence a person's potential for salary increase or promotion.
8. Participation by employees in the objective-setting procedure helps produce favorable results.
9. In summary, compare the old review methods with the new results-oriented review procedure:

Focus of Old Review Methods	Focus of New Results-Oriented Review Methods
1. Personality	Specific goals and objectives
2. Weaknesses	Strengths (limited criticism)
3. Unilateral goal setting	Mutual goal setting
4. Annual review	Day-to-day coaching
5. Looking back	Looking to future

SUMMARY

Figure 5-5 in Chapter 5 shows how ROPEP and MBO work together as closely related techniques to help managers do their jobs. The mutual goal-setting (MGS) method described by Olmos is a participative appraisal technique that shows how ROPEP and MBO can be adapted and individualized in a specific hospital setting. The benefits speak for themselves: improved morale, clarified job responsibilities, mutually-set measurable performance standards for tasks ("objectives" in the MGS plan), and better orientation for new employees. "The bottom line on mutual goal-setting is improved job performance, which carries with it higher levels of employee motivation and efficiency—the very things managers want from an appraisal system" (Olmos, 1979).

Another writer makes a similar point, but with a different emphasis. "Management by objectives and performance appraisals are inextricably bound together. There should be a subtle linkage but not necessarily a direct relationship" (Gerstenfeld, 1977). Figures 5–5 and 6–1 show how these two management techniques are linked together. See also "MBO and performance appraisal" (Golightly, 1979). Other chapters—especially Chapters 7, 8, 9, and 13—demonstrate how the use of MBO and ROPEP are fundamental to quality assurance, budgetary planning and control, staffing and scheduling, and successful use of career ladders.

Now ask yourself, "How satisfied am I with the performance appraisal system in my nursing department? How well does it meet the criteria for a results-oriented performance evaluation program?" Exhibit 6–2 lists such criteria. Your answers are vitally important. If your appraisal/evaluation methods are not in tune with the times—from a nursing management point of view—you must take action to improve them. You owe this to your nursing personnel, to your patients, and to yourself.

Be careful how you go about improving your system. Don't feel you are locked in to a hospital-wide or government-mandated plan that doesn't work well. (If you must, you can still use such plans on a pro forma basis while developing and using a real results-oriented performance evaluation program for your own purposes within the nursing department.) Some *real professionals* in nursing management are doing this already. So can you. You can't afford to wait for someone else to do it for you. Too much hangs in the balance.

We say these things with due deliberation. Consider!

- *Item:* The JCAH requires regular performance appraisals.
- *Item:* The American Hospital Association's (AHA) most recent guide to performance appraisal is nearly ten years old and is attribute-oriented rather than results-oriented or objective-oriented.
- *Item:* The AHA booklet concludes, "The failure rate of employee appraisal systems is alarmingly high" (AHA, 1971).
- *Item:* Olmos, quoted on the second page of this chapter, writes, "The majority of appraisal systems currently in use are neither effective nor valid ..." (Olmos, 1979).

The foregoing is a shocking state of affairs. Remember, what is being discussed is a management technique that goes to the very heart of the manager/employee relationship. Even when nurse managers do not recog-

Exhibit 6-2 Criteria for an Effective Performance Evaluation Process

1. builds upon the findings of the behavioral sciences—what we know about people and organizations
2. helps to satisfy, rather than assault, basic human needs
3. adapts to individual differences
4. focuses on strengths of individuals, not their weaknesses
5. relates individual performance results with work unit goals and objectives
6. measures performance results, not personal traits
7. utilizes mutually-developed (understood and agreed-upon) standards of performance
8. provides opportunity for accurate self-evaluation
9. is independent of wage and salary considerations
10. facilitates agreement upon evaluation outcomes between boss and subordinate
11. is economical to use
12. adheres to organizational philosophy and to pertinent governmental or contractual regulations from a legal standpoint
13. uses a simple OK/NOT OK (satisfactory/not satisfactory) rating of results for each key performance responsibility
14. emphasizes the process of achieving mutual understanding and agreement, rather than the trained use of particular evaluation instruments and forms

Source: Ganong, J., and Ganong, W. *Help with results-oriented performance evaluation.* Chapel Hill, N.C.: W. L. Ganong Co. 1974, p. 12. For full elaboration see *Nursing job performance appraisal* by same authors, Aspen Systems Corp., to be published.

nize an ineffective appraisal system, the nurses and other personnel know how it feels. And the *new breed* of nursing staff are likely to be aware of their rights in connection with a poorly designed or poorly implemented appraisal plan. (See *Legal Aspects* in Chapter 2.)

We recognize that a better management technique per se doesn't assure salvation; yet the better-designed system can be a great help to nurse managers. This is especially true for those who agree with the comments of a noted manager, researcher, and author.

Workers are more perceptive than most managers realize. Whether their formal education is high or low, workers quickly see through managers who try to exploit and deceive them. It is essential that people within an organization receive fair treatment. When justice prevails, it is important that workers know it. ... Hand in hand with the need for justice is the need for a climate of trust. Unless this exists, all motivational attempts will fall far short of their full potential" (Goble, 1972).

NOTES

American Hospital Association. *Employee performance appraisal programs: Guidelines for their development and implementation.* Chicago: Author, 1971. Reprinted with permission.

Drucker, P. F. *Management: Tasks, responsibilities, practices.* New York: Harper & Row, 1974, p. 479. Excerpts reprinted with permission.

Fivars, G., & Gosnell, D. *Nursing evaluation: The problem and the process.* New York: Macmillan, 1966, pp. 9-25.

Ganong, J., & Ganong, W. *HELP with results-oriented performance evaluation.* Chapel Hill, N.C.: W. L. Ganong, Co., 1974.

Gerstenfeld, A. MBO revisited: Focus on health systems. *Health Care Management Review,* Fall 1977, *2*(4), 51-57.

Goble, F. *Excellence in leadership.* New York: American Management Association, 1972.

Herzberg, F. The wise old turk. *Harvard Business Review,* September-October 1974, *52*(5).

Olmos, S. Employees help to define their jobs. *Hospitals,* June 16, 1979, pp. 79-81.

Zollitsch, H. G., & Langsner, A. *Wage and salary administration.* Cincinnati: South-Western Publishing, 1970.

Reading List

Books

Carter, J. H., Hilliard, M., Castles, M. R., Stoll, L. D., & Cowan, A. *Standards of nursing care: A guide for evaluation* (2nd ed.). New York: Springer, 1976.

Drucker, P. F. *The effective executive.* New York: Harper & Row, 1966.

Drucker, P. F. *Management: Tasks, responsibilities, practices.* New York: Harper & Row, 1974.

Ganong, J., & Ganong, W. *HELP with management by objectives.* Chapel Hill, N.C.: W. L. Ganong Co., 1975.

Ganong, J., & Ganong, W. *HELP with results-oriented performance evaluation.* Chapel Hill, N.C.: W. L. Ganong Co., 1975.

Ganong, J., & Ganong, W. Evaluating staff performance. In A. Marriner (Ed.), *Current perspectives in nursing management.* St. Louis: C. V. Mosby, 1979, Chapter 6.

Ganong, J., & Ganong, W. *Nursing job performance appraisal.* Germantown, Md.: Aspen Systems Corp., to be published.

Mager, R. F. *Analyzing performance problems.* Belmont, Ca.: Fearon, 1970.

Mager, R. F. *Goal analysis.* Belmont, Ca.: Fearon, 1972.

Maslow, A. *Eupsychian management.* Homewood, Ill.: Dorsey Press, 1965.

Maslow, A. *Toward a psychology of being.* Princeton: Van Nostrand, 1968.

Maslow, A. *Motivation and personality.* New York: Harper & Row, 1970.

McGregor, D. *The human side of enterprise.* New York: McGraw-Hill, 1960.

Myers, M. S. *Every employee a manager: More meaningful work through job enrichment.* New York: McGraw-Hill, 1970.

Odiorne, G. *Management decision by objectives.* Englewood Cliffs, N.J.: Prentice-Hall, 1969.

Articles

Bennett, A. Executives work hard to evaluate. *Modern Healthcare,* June 1979, *9*(6), 53-54.

Brady, R. MBO goes to work in the public sector. *Journal of Nursing Administration,* July-August 1973, *3*(4), 44.

Crowder, D., & Bennett, A. Total commitment to goals is secret of hospital's success. *Hospitals,* July 1, 1976, *50*(13), 104-109.

del Bueno, D. Implementing a performance evaluation system. *Supervisor Nurse,* February 1979, *10*(2), 48-52.

Douglas, J., Grimes, A. J., Ivancevich, J. M., & Klein, S. M. A progression training approach to management by objectives. *Training and Development Journal,* September 1973, *27*(9), 24-30.

Dracup, K. Improving clinical evaluation. *Supervisor Nurse,* June 1979, *10*(6), 24-27.

Engle, J., & Barkauskas, V. The evaluation of a public health nursing performance evaluation tool. *Journal of Nursing Administration,* April 1979, *9*(4), 8-16.

Golightly, C. "MBO and performance appraisal." *Journal of Nursing Administration,* September 1979, *9*(9), 11-20.

Hayes, J. L. How am I doing? Standards tell. *Modern Healthcare,* August 1975, *4*(2), 61.

Herzberg, F. The wise old turk. *Harvard Business Review,* September-October 1974, *52*(5), 70-80.

McConkey, D. D. Applying management by objectives to non-profit organization. *S.A.M. Advanced Management Journal,* January 1973, *38*(1), 10-20.

McGregor, D. An uneasy look at performance appraisal. *Harvard Business Review,* May-June 1957, *35*(3), 89-94.

Moore, M. A. Philosophy, purpose, and objectives: Why do we have them? *Journal of Nursing Administration.* May-June 1971, *1*(3), 9-14.

Nuckolls, K. B. Who decides what the nurse can do? *Nursing Outlook,* October 1974, *22*, 626-631.

Palmer, J. Management by objectives. *Journal of Nursing Administration,* January 1971, *1*(1), 17-23.

Samaras, J. T., Stewart, S. H., Gerould, M. T., Bebee, L. G., & Boatright, D. T. Wage evaluation methods: A model for nurse administrators. *Journal of Nursing Administration,* June 1978, *8*(6), 13-21.

Chapter 7

Quality Assurance

QUALITY THROUGH ACCOUNTABILITY

Every healthcare agency needs to evaluate the quality of care patients receive and the quality of nursing staff performance. The entire concept of accountability in nursing rests on the ability to demonstrate the nature and quality of performance delivered by nursing personnel. The need for such accountability is dramatized by the rising cost of care—without an equivalent rise in quality or proof of that quality. Caring and quality are intimately intertwined. Pirsig addresses this issue:

> I talked about caring ... and then realized I couldn't say anything meaningful about caring until its inverse side, Quality, is understood. I think it's important now to tie care to Quality by pointing out that care and Quality are internal and external aspects of the same thing. A person who sees Quality and feels it as he works is a person who cares. A person who cares about what he sees and does is a person who's bound to have some characteristics of Quality (Pirsig, 1974, p. 269).

Nurses are developing ways to identify and use meaningful quality assurance components. As a result of this effort, definitions of quality assurance abound. One comprehensive definition can serve the nurse manager well:

> Quality assurance involves assuring the consumer of a specified degree of excellence through continuous measurement and evaluation of structural components, goal-directed nursing process, and/or consumer outcome, using pre-established criteria and standards and available norms, and followed by appropriate alteration with the purpose of improvement (Schmadl, 1979, p. 465).

Quality nursing care is dependent on the accountability of the individual nurse for the nursing process used in delivering care and the outcomes to the individual patient as a result of that care. We must face up to accountability if nursing is to come into its own as an autonomous member of the helping professions. As nurses achieve more autonomy and freedom (coupled with higher levels of formal education, more status, and pay), nurses can expect increased responsibility and accountability and the legal consequences of each. Froebe and Bain (1976) conceive of accountability as acknowledging definitive delegated function as one's right and duty within a system of interrelated functions. These same authors define accountability as "a measure of individual, group, or institutional efficiency and productivity that is judged against a predetermined guide or standard by both the agent and the client." Accountability means one is *answerable* for one's actions to a person or a group. In nursing, then, the individual nurse (i.e., the primary nurse) is answerable for the actions he/she takes based on predetermined standards of nursing practice. The nurse manager is similarly accountable.

Building Accountability

The nurse manager can help the nursing staff assume more accountability by using the following guidelines:

- Clarify responsibilities and standards of performance.
- Make responsibilities realistic and progressive.
- Evaluate progress frequently.
- Realize that only the *person* can make accountability really work.
- Use the motivators: Achievement, Recognition, Work Itself, Responsibility, Advancement, Growth. (See Chapter 10.)
- Help nurses meet their own needs in the process of achieving agency and department goals.
- Be sure the nurses can handle the responsibility and then hold them accountable.

Many of the nurses giving care in the wide variety of hospitals and related care facilities are new professional nurses right out of nursing programs. The nurse manager can help these new professionals build accountability by taking the following behavioral factors into account:

- treating the new nurses as professionals
- accepting their newness
- accepting the young nurses as persons
- using the problem-solving approach rather than the workload concept
- asking for their new knowledge

- identifying professional needs in both technical and human modes of behavior
- having dialogues, not monologues
- being clear about expectations and standards
- identifying strengths and recognizing them
- focusing on the mutual goals of the new nurse and the organization
- keeping their end of the bargain
- being alert to costs and quality
- focusing on standards rather than personalities
- focusing on policy as guides to action
- rewarding professional behavior by word and deed
- being role models
- responding favorably to change
- using the human and technical modes of behavior themselves
- using quality assurance programs (Ganong & Ganong, 1978, p. 142).

Nursing and nurses are continuing to build an accountable posture in the healthcare field. McClure points out that in spite of many problems,

> some progress has been made in moving the nursing profession toward a more accountable posture. In practice settings, such developments as primary nursing and nursing audits offer evidence of a willingness to achieve a more responsible attitude toward the quality of care rendered to patients. Among nursing faculty, the continuing critical examination of curriculum, combined with a greater willingness to accept input from nursing service, also indicates a new regard for accountability (McClure, 1978, p. 48).

Documenting Accountability

The nursing process requires both doing and documenting. Quality in nursing care can be enhanced if nurses master the *use* of the nursing process in a caring way and *document* it so outcomes and process are retrievable. Each step of the nursing process requires documentation. This is an essential part of being accountable. Figure 7-1 details the flow of that accountability.

Documentation is the process of recording in the patient's medical record pertinent information about the patient gathered by the nurse through assessment and evaluation.

Ainsworth puts it very well:

> Forms permit a uniformity in the documentation of patient care. Since several nurses and other health professionals will provide care for an individual patient, uniformity makes the medical record a

Figure 7-1 The Nursing Process: Doing and Documenting

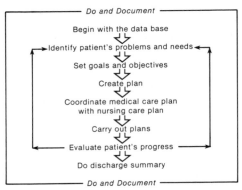

Source: Ganong, J., and Ganong, W. *HELP with nursing audit and quality assurance* (3rd Ed.). Chapel Hill, N.C.: W. L. Ganong Co., 1978, p. 84.

more easily used document which serves as a means of communication among the members of the health care team providing care to an individual patient. If data are recorded in a uniform way, they can be more easily compiled for statistical reporting and evaluation.

Forms are used in the quality assurance program to promote an orderly and rational application for the nursing process in its implementation. At first glance, the forms may appear to be complicated and cumbersome and to require too much time to complete. However, each form is designed to identify a specific essential step in the application of the nursing process. The discipline required in completing each form will lead to the development of an orderly thinking process as the nurse assesses, plans, implements, and evaluates the nursing care plan for each patient. Repetitive use of these forms will, therefore, reinforce this mental process and result in the desired goal for this entire program, namely, a change to a goal- and problem-oriented approach to nursing care (Ainsworth, 1977, p. 51).

The problem-oriented record, through the use of the following forms, can provide a simplified way to document the use of the nursing process with individual patients:

- a data base that provides base line information gathered during the initial assessment at the time of person's admission as a patient

- a numbered problem list that describes each of the patient's identified problems
- a nursing care plan that is based on continual nursing assessment and the nursing diagnosis. This plan incorporates the nursing orders.
- progress notes that spell out in factual form the patient's actual progress, using subjective and objective notations and the assessment and plan that result from those notations
- flow sheets that permit the orderly recording of repetitive information. These supplement and *do not* replace the progress notes.
- discharge summary that records the status of the person at time of discharge as a patient.

Whatever forms are used, the principles of a problem-oriented record can be used. The documentation by the nurse must in all instances be succinct, legible, factual, meaningful, and accurate. The nurse is responsible for *documenting* and accountable for what is *documented*. The quality of care is reflected in the quality of documentation. The recording of the date, time, signature, and title of the nurse attests to that accountability.

STANDARDS AND CRITERIA

A standard is an acknowledged measure of comparison for quantitative or qualitative value, criterion, or norm. A criterion is a standard rule or test on which a judgment or decision can be based. It is essential to establish clinical nursing criteria against which to measure patient outcomes and the nursing process.

Careful choice of words and accurate use of terminology can ensure the understanding and acceptance for a quality assurance program. The following definitions will help clarify key terms used in connection with nursing quality assurance.

Retrospective: Referring to a review or contemplation of things in the past.

Closed Chart: The completed patient record for a discharged patient, in the custody of the medical records department.

Open Chart: The patient record for a patient still receiving care within the hospital or agency.

Retrospective (Closed Chart) Audit: An inspection of a closed chart to evaluate its documentary reliability, completeness, and compliance with the standards for nursing care as established by the agency, the nursing department, and the professional, governmental, and accrediting groups.

Process Audit: The inspection of the nursing process as carried out and documented by nursing staff to evaluate compliance with established standards of nursing practice.

Outcome Audit: Identifies patient outcomes (satisfactory and unsatisfactory) and the patterns of nursing care that appear to be responsible.

Structure Audit: The inspection of the management process as carried out and documented by nurse managers.

Marion E. Nicholls provides a helpful explanation of outcome (ends) standards and process (means) standards:

> Nursing care standards can be divided into ends and means standards. The ends standards are patient oriented; they describe the changes desired in a patient's physical status or behavior. The means standards are nurse oriented; they describe the activities and behavior designed to achieve the ends standards. Properly stated, nursing care objectives are the ends standards and the plan of care (or nursing orders) is the means standard. Although the ends and means standards are interrelated, different information about each is required to determine if they are being met. An ends standard requires information about the patient. A means standard calls for information about the nurse's performance. To be effective as standards, objectives and plans must meet three criteria. The statements must be understandable. They must be achievable in terms of the resources of the patient, the nurses, and the agency. And, if control is to be achieved, they must be measurable (Nicholls, 1974, p. 456).

Standards are established by and received from a variety of sources including federal, state, and local units of government, licensing agencies, accrediting organizations (JCAH, NLN), professional organizations (ANA), trade associations (AHA), institutions (hospital, mental health center), departments (nursing, medicine), patient care units (CCU, OR, psychiatric), and individuals (one's own personal standards). Standards, from whatever source and however developed, must be readily available to all members of the nursing staff on the patient care units. Only when they are understood and used can they be documented and audited.

Standards are intended to provide a basis for measurement which is objective, achievable, practical, flexible, and acceptable. One type of standard is broad in nature and serves a particular purpose by providing guidelines. These are structure standards, such as those set forth by ANA and JCAH.

Another more specific type of standard is needed for the nursing audit. It identifies what element of care is being evaluated by an inspection of a patient's chart. An element of care that is of major consequence to the patient includes the expectation of this element's presence in a chart (i.e., yes or no; or 100 percent, always; and 0 percent, never). Exceptions must be clearly defined, as acceptable within the range of normal professional expectations.

Standards need to be broken down to elements of care or *criteria* that can be used to measure nursing performance and patient outcomes. A comprehensive mechanism for measuring the quality of nursing care was developed by investigators from the Division of Nursing at Rush-Presbyterian-St. Luke's Medical Center and the Medicus Systems Corporation. Three hundred criteria were designed to measure quality and were tested for validity in 19 hospitals around the country. These criteria are the basis for the Medical Center's Quality Assurance Program in Nursing, a national model instituted in 1974 (Promise, 1976).

Nursing staff performance evaluation based on predetermined standards is a part of a Total Quality Assurance program. Evaluation of performance relates to the process audit and peer review. This is the purpose of the Results-Oriented Performance Evaluation Program (ROPEP), which goes beyond the conventional performance appraisal based on personality traits. (See Chapter 6.)

A Quality Assurance Program

A quality assurance program takes into account the *structure* within which care is given, the *outcomes* to the patient, and the *process* of giving the care.

The essential components of a quality assurance program include that it will:

- establish standards for *structure*
- establish criteria for *process* and *outcomes*
- audit against standards and criteria and evaluate results
- identify strengths and deficiencies in *process* and *outcomes*
- evaluate nursing staff and personnel performance. Peer review can be used.
- make recommendations for improvement of nursing *process* and patient *outcomes*
- implement recommendations
- re-audit for results

Froebe and Bain (1976) describe a sample package of tools that are intended for use in a quality assurance program for nursing service. Included are:

- history
- problem-oriented record
- audit
- client evaluation
- care plan
- rounds

A quality assurance program of any magnitude needs to be well coordinated, and a program coordinator may be needed. The coordinator plans, organizes, develops, implements, and evaluates the Quality Assurance Program (QAP) for Nursing in cooperation with the nursing and medical staffs and other hospital departments, and submits regular progress reports and QAP recommendations to nursing administration. In addition, a coordinator:

- works closely with medical staff, patient care evaluation committee, and medical records department on quality assurance, PSRO, and related matters
- serves on hospital and nursing committees that deal with patient care matters. Cooperates with peer review committee
- coordinates the development of nursing standards and criteria for use in measuring the quality of care through process and outcome audits
- recommends to nursing administration changes necessary to improve the quality of care
- provides feedback to nursing unit staff about the results of nursing audits
- complies with nursing division standards for all nursing audits (ANA, JCAH, Medicare)
- chairs regular nursing audit committee and takes responsibility for minutes and their distribution to hospital and nursing administration and medical staff chairperson.

THE NURSING AUDIT

The nurse manager has available a variety of management techniques to assist in delivering and evaluating quality patient care. One of these techniques is the nursing audit. Nursing audit is, first of all, a method for assuring documentation in keeping with the standards established by the agency, the nursing department, and professional, governmental, and accrediting groups. Nursing audit is, therefore, part of the nurse manager's function of *controlling*, the third element in the three-phase management process.

As with other techniques, auditing works best when it is used as part of an integrated system—such as a Problem-Oriented Nursing System (PONS).

One of the strengths of this system is its emphasis on assuring that patient needs and problems are identified and met with an appropriate level of care that is reflected accurately in the nursing audit results.

Nursing audit provides the inspection method that compares results with the predetermined standards and criteria. As the audit is refined and improved, it measures more accurately than earlier methods the quality of the documentation of nursing care. Experience in every field of human endeavor indicates that when quality and performance standards are established, with results being measured against such standards, the results improve. There is increasing evidence that nursing audit helps improve nursing results.

The guidelines for nursing audit take into account the variables among healthcare agencies and their relative performance capabilities. Every agency is expected to adapt to its own uses the fundamental philosophy and basic steps of nursing audit so that demonstrable progress and improvement can be achieved. It should be noted, however, that nursing audit is no cure-all. Documenting the level of quality that is delivered will not, in and of itself, improve the quality of care. You cannot inspect quality into a service; quality must be built into the service. In healthcare agencies the level of quality is determined at the point of service during all four phases of the nursing process. But audit certainly makes personnel more aware of the need for accurate and concise documentation in order to "prove" the care that has been given and the progress of the patient as the result of that care. Nurses must document, in the patient record, their contribution to helping resolve the identified needs and problems of patients and their families.

Management techniques alone cannot improve the quality of care. People improve quality through their use of techniques and skills, and no technique is ever any better than the skills of the person using that technique. This is as true for nursing audit as it is for other management and clinical techniques. Nurses are among the people who provide services to, for, and with patients and their families. Therefore nurses determine the quality level of the care being provided. But the patient is the one who experiences (feels, knows) the quality of care being received. And whatever the level of care may be, as experienced by the patient and his family, it deserves to be reflected as accurately as possible in the audit results. The purposes and benefits of the nursing audit were discussed in Chapter 3 as a vital component of PONS. Our purpose now is to present sufficient details of the nursing audit procedure so that it can be understood as a useful nursing management technique.

ORGANIZING FOR NURSING AUDIT

Nursing audit has become mandatory for three basic reasons: the increasing cost of care; the need to improve quality of care; and the need for proof of the quality of care actually delivered—for yourself, your agency, third-party payers, and interested others. Costs, quality, and accountability are all inextricably woven together in the minds of consumers. With little or no choice or control over these factors, consumers—frustrated and apprehensive—seek ways to relieve their concerns.

Nursing staff members also seek to relieve the causes of their own frustrations. There is ample evidence of individual motivation, as well as departmental and institutional motivation, to improve the auditing process. Now there is available a tested and refined audit technique; and there are urgent reasons to put it to work. Some of the reasons for an audit are implicit in the definition of the term. "Audit," as a noun, means an examination, adjustment, or correction of records or accounts; as a verb, "audit" means to examine, verify, or correct (accounts, records, or claims). The implications for nursing personnel are clear; it is not adequate simply to provide satisfactory patient care. Such care must be fully documented as part of the patient's record.

The Joint Commission on Accreditation of Hospitals (JCAH) has summarized the basic requirements for audit. The hospital governing body has ultimate responsibility for the quality of care. The governing body delegates the evaluation of patient care provided by physicians to the medical staff and delegates the evaluation of patient care provided by others—nurses and allied health professionals—to administration. The medical and nursing staffs can use any organizational method they choose to accomplish audit. The audit procedure should include the following six steps:

1. standards and criteria established
2. measurement of actual practice against criteria
3. evaluation of results
4. action taken to correct deficiencies
5. follow-up and reassessment
6. report to nursing service, administration, and medical staff.

The nursing administrator, as the delegate of the hospital administrator, has the responsibility to: (1) initiate and maintain a nursing audit program, (2) organize for audit using a method decided upon within nursing, (3) include the six basic steps in the audit procedure, and (4) evaluate all patient care services under the direction of the nursing department.

The first step in organizing a nursing quality assurance program is establishing a nursing audit committee. The nursing administrator, in consultation with key personnel, establishes the committee with representation from the units and departments responsible for providing nursing care, maintaining records, and unit management. The nursing audit committee may replace one or more existing committees or it may become a responsibility of an existing committee (such as the patient care committee). To make such a determination, the purposes and functions of existing committees must be compared with the purposes and functions of the audit committee.

This committee is charged with the initial task of developing guidelines for an audit program, setting clinical standards and criteria for measurement of results, deciding on forms, and performing the pilot audits to gain experience and test the instruments to be used. Following this preparatory work, the committee continues the ongoing process of guiding the planning, evaluating, recommending, teaching, communicating, and corrective activities essential to the audit process.

Nursing audit, as part of a quality assurance program, requires a considerable degree of cooperation between the medical records administrator, the nursing administrator, and the audit committee. The responsibility of the medical records administrator does not include evaluating the adequacy of the nursing records nor their value in assisting the physician in his/her management of patient care. This responsibility lies with the audit committee and the nursing department. But the medical records administrator (or designee) is a valuable member of the audit committee. Once standards and criteria have been established, the medical records department can do the retrieval of data needed for the nursing audit committee to evaluate the findings.

The nursing audit committee should be a standing committee of the department of nursing and should submit monthly and annual reports to the nursing administrator. Actual audits may be performed by personnel within specialty areas (i.e., medicine, surgery, obstetrics, pediatrics, psychiatry, cardiac care, emergency care, etc.) or by representatives from these specialties serving on the standing committee. Larger agencies may decentralize the auditing to subcommittees.

Membership of the audit committee should include representatives of all levels of professional nursing including patient care coordinators, supervisors, head nurses, staff nurses, clinical specialists, and nurse clinicians. The chairperson may be the quality assurance coordinator, or may be appointed, selected by the group, or designated based upon performance responsibilities and job title. Where applicable, licensed practical nurses, nursing assistants, and other types of patient care personnel may be members of the audit committee. The medical records administrator (or designee) should be a regular member of the committee.

The functions of the audit committee may be summarized in two phases. During the first phase, the committee meets regularly to develop purposes and objectives; establish standards and criteria; establish guidelines for conducting audits; decide upon the necessary forms (using JCAH forms or adapting other forms to your needs); initiate the auditing process; practice auditing to become proficient; keep brief, pertinent minutes of all audit committee meetings including date, place, time, names of members (and guests) present, topics discussed, action agreed upon, recommendations, and progress on previous recommendations. The second phase begins the actual implementation and maintenance of the audit procedure. The ongoing responsibilities of the committee include:

1. Plan audit sessions and schedule on a monthly basis (or periodically as required) to accomplish goals and objectives.
2. Arrange for Medical Records to pull charts for retrospective (closed chart) audits and retrieve data.
3. Evaluate audit results in committee.
4. Conduct process audits by observing direct nursing care; interviewing patients and personnel; auditing closed and open patient records, and other nursing records.
5. Prepare summaries of all audits for use by the nursing department and patient care units, and to serve as a report to hospital administration. JCAH requires that copies of such summaries be sent to the director of nursing, chief of the medical staff, and to the board of trustees via the hospital administrator.
6. Teach professional nursing personnel the auditing process so they can become involved and share audit results with all nursing personnel.
7. Assist nursing staff in using audit results to improve care and the documentation of care.
8. Make recommendations to appropriate hospital and nursing committees for policies, procedures, systems, services, and materials or equipment that can improve care.
9. Keep brief, pertinent minutes of audit committee meetings (as in the first phase).

When the nursing staff and the medical staff combine to form a single audit committee, the above functions can be incorporated into that committee's activities. In any case, cooperation between the medical and nursing staffs in auditing is important and needs to be encouraged.

WORKING COMMITTEES:

A Nursing Audit Committee on Every Unit

One example of a committee plan with many benefits provides for decentralizing the audit function to the patient care units. Table 7-1 shows the structure, membership, and relationships of the committees. On the patient

Table 7-1 Summary of Working Committees Membership

Personnel Titles (Other comparable titles may be substituted)	Coordinating	Systems and Procedures	Employee Needs	Staff Development	Audit/Nursing Care	Nursing Care Teams
Dir. of Nsg. Serv./PCA	Ch.					
Assoc. Dir. of Nsg. Serv.	*				Ch.	
Asst. Dir. Nsg. Serv. Days	*	Ch.				
Asst. Dir. Nsg. Serv. Eve.	*		Ch.	*		
Asst. Dir. Nsg. Serv. Nite	*	*				
Coord. Inserv. Ed./Staff Development	*	*		Ch.		
Supervisor, Evenings		*	*			
Supervisor, Nights		*	*			
Hd. Nurse/Pt. Care Coord.		Rep.	Rep.	Rep.	*	Mgr.
Charge Nurse		Rep.	Rep.	Rep.	*	Mgr.
Staff/Primary Nurse		Rep.	Rep.	Rep.	*	*
Licensed Pract. Nurse		Rep.	Rep.	Rep.		*
Nurse Aide		Rep.	Rep.	Rep.	Rep.	*
Orderly		Rep.	Rep.	Rep.		*
Ward Clerk/Unit Sec.		Rep.	Rep.	Rep.		*

KEY: * = Regular member.   Rep. = Selected representative of group.
      Ch. = Chairman.   Mgr. = Unit manager (add team leader as necessary).

Source: Ganong, J., and Ganong, W. Reducing Organizational Conflict Through Working Committees. *Journal of Nursing Administration,* January–February 1972, 2, p. 12. Reprinted with permission of Nursing Resources, Inc.

care units the audit activity is carried out by the Unit Nursing Care Committees. The purpose of each nursing care committee is to plan, coordinate, measure, and improve the 24-hour nursing care activities for each nursing unit and specialty department so that the delivery of patient care will be consistent with the objectives of the nursing unit, the department, and the hospital for quality care. Members include, for each nursing unit and specialty department, the head nurse, days, as chairman; the head nurse (charge nurse), evenings; and the head nurse (charge nurse), nights. (For the specialty departments such as OR and ER, membership will be modified to fit the existing situation.)

The purpose of each nursing care team is to involve nursing unit shift personnel in the effective delivery of patient care, through the use of the nursing process for each patient. Members include for each nursing unit and specialty department the shift head nurse as chairman and all other unit personnel on the shift: staff nurses, licensed practical nurses, nurse aides, orderlies, and unit secretaries. Where regular nursing care teams have already been used effectively, they may be continued as the basis for this link in the committee network.

This type of committee structure provides for the meaningful involvement of nursing personnel in committee work. It facilitates the job enrichment concepts of Frederick Herzberg, M. Scott Myers, and others. Skillfully used, these concepts greatly enhance the likelihood of success with a nursing audit program and its contributions to optimum patient care.

THE NURSING AUDIT TECHNIQUE

Retrospective audit, as defined, attempts to determine the degree to which the patient's chart accurately reflects the quality of nursing care received by the patient and whether or not the care given is clinically sound and meets a standard of optimal care achievable by the healthcare agency. The retrospective audit procedure may focus on either an outcome audit or a process audit—or both. The outcome audit identifies patient outcomes that are satisfactory or unsatisfactory and is intended to identify also the patterns of nursing care that appear to be responsible. The process audit is a deeper probe of already recognized or suspected problems in the nursing care process.

Outcome audits focus on two factors—Discharge Status and Complications. The three components of discharge status are health, activity, and knowledge. In order to determine discharge status and complications, it is necessary to establish a base-line assessment. For this reason the audit committee may need to refer to the initial assessment (data base) to compare the patient's status at the time of discharge with the status at the time of admission.

A quantitative standard should be established for each component. The standard identifies the expected status of the patient in respect to each component at the time of discharge. The quantitative standard is always 100 percent for all assessment and discharge elements and 0 percent for complications. Exceptions, when stated, indicate the circumstances under which a nonstandard condition is justified.

Here are the audit steps.

1. The first step in the audit procedure is to establish standards and criteria. Standards are designed to provide measurement criteria and must be objective, achievable, practical, flexible, and acceptable.
2. The second basic step is measurement. This means to secure the charts from Medical Records (possibly by random selection), excerpt the necessary data from the charts, then on a quantifiable basis demonstrate how well—by actual measurement—the results conform to the established criteria. Once the procedure is established, this can be done by trained clerks.
3. The third basic step is to evaluate the observable variations and decide which are justifiable in terms of the criteria and acceptable nursing practice, and which are unjustifiable and represent actual deficiencies. Probable reasons for such deficiencies need to be established. This must be done by nurses.
4. Step 4 is to take suitable corrective actions to prevent recurrence of such deficiencies. This is a most important part of the audit cycle, and one that is perhaps most difficult to handle. The efforts of a variety of personnel are required to carry out the action steps which may include direct one-to-one counseling, longer-range inservice education programs, or modification of staffing in particular situations. In other cases the deficiency analysis may suggest clarification of or revisions in existing policies and procedures, or the development of new policies, forms, or procedures.
5. Step 5 is the follow-through. This is the clincher, and answers the questions, "Did the action occur, and was it helpful in securing improvements?"
6. The last of the six basic audit steps required by JCAH is to prepare and distribute suitable summary reports to nursing service, hospital administration, and to the executive committee of the medical staff.

As a management technique, then, nursing audit can be viewed as part of the evaluating and planning phases of the management process. It is ongoing rather than sporadic. Monthly and quarterly comparisons of results provide a way to determine the efficacy of the audit program.

AN APPLICATION IN PUBLIC HEALTH NURSING

Nursing audit is helpful in a variety of settings, not just in hospitals. The nurse manager in a public health agency needs to apply nursing audit as a facet of quality control. Applications in public health pose special kinds of challenges and opportunities. Public health nurses need to identify and set outcome standards for particular population groupings, such as the high risk mother and the postpartum mother and infant, rather than for disease entities and surgical procedures. Infant and child immunization programs and adult screening programs present another challenge and opportunity for the audit committee. Fortunately, nurses are developing innovative ways to meet the challenge while finding new job satisfaction in the process.

A pertinent example is the Cumberland County Health Department in Fayetteville, North Carolina. (Exhibits can be found in Appendix H.) The nursing director designated a nursing audit committee comprised of nine nursing staff members who had participated in a nursing audit workshop. Together they surveyed the literature, explored a variety of resources, and with the encouragement of their director used their ingenuity to initiate the audit program. The committee established the following goals and plan of action:

Short-Range: Improve documentation of Maternal/Child Health records (initiated by MCH Program nurses) through setting nursing standards for MCH Records.

Long-Range: Improve documentation of public health records through the establishment of nursing standards for all areas of public health nursing and, through improved documentation, show proof of the quality of nursing care being delivered.

Steps to Achieving Goals:

1. Establish nursing standards for all areas of public health nursing.
2. Audit records for which standards have been established to determine quality of documentation.
3. Examine the results of the nursing audit and make recommendations regarding gaps in documentation (and possibly education) to supervisory personnel and nursing staff.
4. Execute follow-up and reassessment three to six months later.

Results of the public health agency retrospective audit and quality control check are shared with the maternal/child health nurse based at the hospital and with the district public health nurses so that they can act on recommendations to improve the quality of care and the documentation of that care.

SECURING ACTION ON AUDIT REPORTS

One result of nursing audit analysis and problem identification is a recommendation for action to the person or department head who can make a decision and implement it. Thus it is a committee responsibility to summarize a recommendation succinctly and to provide justification and support for the recommendation.

An effective tool to use for presenting recommendations is the Committee Follow-Through Memorandum (Exhibit 7-1). It requires reducing the recommendation to a relatively few words and limiting the supporting justification to major items only, such as cost, benefits, and suggestions for implementation. Thus for some recommendations that are rather extensive in their complexity and implications, the memorandum serves as a cover sheet for

Exhibit 7-1 Committee Follow-Through Memorandum

TO:_____ DATE: _____

FROM: _____, Chairman of _____ Committee

SUBJECT:_____

Recommendation:

Justification (*Cost, benefits, suggestions for implementation*):

(*Attach supporting documents as necessary.*)

- -

FOLLOW-THROUGH ACTION:

____ Approved as recommended
____ Approved with modification
____ Disapproved for reasons as stated
____ Referred back to committee

Comment:

Signed _____ Date_____

additional pages of audit findings, analysis results, estimates of cost and savings (if any), suggestions for implementation, and so on.

The principle that applies here is that of the doctrine of completed staff work. This means that the committee should be sure to do its homework. It should present the recommendation in such a way that the decision-making process becomes as easy as possible for the person to whom the memorandum is addressed. This can happen when the recommendation is stated simply and clearly and the justification is objective, incisive, and persuasive.

In a very real sense the task of securing approval for a recommendation is a selling job. The following are guidelines for selling a desired course of action:

Make Ready: Know your prospect (needs, wants, goals).

Approach with Benefits: Answer the prospect's unspoken question, "What will this do for me?"

Stimulate Desire: Appeal to self-motivation. (Sell the sizzle, not the steak.)

Tell Facts: After the foregoing steps.

Eliminate Retardants: Foresee objections; remove them as obstacles.

Request Action: Ask for what you want done.

Then secure reactions and feedback, and follow through appropriately to assure action. Obviously the audit analysis and findings provide important facts, but they alone may not secure approval of the recommendations. So do your homework; complete your staff work by thinking through the implementation process that may be necessary; provide answers for the possible objections that may enter the decision-maker's mind (costs, complications, interdepartmental problems, legal or policy concerns, etc.). Make it as easy as possible to secure the answer you seek.

REPORTING AUDIT RESULTS

The sixth basic step in the audit procedure is to report the results of the auditing process periodically. This provides a record of the committee's work, a summary of audit activity, an organized presentation of general findings, the recommendations for action that have been presented, the follow-through action that has taken place, and what has been the impact of such follow-through on the problem conditions.

One type of periodic report form is shown in Exhibit 7–2, the Audit Summary for a specific patient care unit. When this is used effectively by the nurse managers with personnel on the units through the Working Committees Plan, the audit program becomes a vital part of every employee's job. A

Exhibit 7-2 Audit Summary

TO: Ward or Unit _____ Date_____
FROM: Audit Committee   Signed_____, Chairman
RE: Audit Topic: _____

QUALITY CONTROL CHECK OF NURSING PROCESS
____ Number of Open Charts Audited
____ Number of Patients Observed/Interviewed
____ Number of Personnel Observed/Interviewed

RETROSPECTIVE AUDIT OF PATIENT OUTCOMES
____ Number of Closed Charts Audited

FINDINGS AND RECOMMENDATIONS
1. Indications of quality care:

2. Outstanding problems:

3. Indications of improvement:

4. Recommendations for improvements:

5. Special comments:

main concern of most patient care personnel is the quality of care; and given the opportunity and leadership, they will contribute creatively to improving patient care practices.

The reporting function is a vital one in the auditing process. It provides a necessary communications link for feedback and evaluation purposes to the patient care units, nursing administration, hospital administration, and the medical staff. Feedback of nursing audit results to the nursing staff on the patient care units is also essential. Audit committees must use a variety of methods for providing informative, useful feedback. An Audit Summary and the Committee Follow-Through Memorandum are written communications. Face-to-face verbal feedback is highly desirable, too. Each audit committee member can become a personal ambassador to serve as a liaison between the committee and the head nurse or coordinator for one or more patient care units. Tactful, personal follow-through can add greatly to the effectiveness of the entire audit program.

A follow-up audit of the same audit topic should be carried out within a few months after recommendations and feedback have been given. The follow-up audit provides solid evidence of whether or not improved documentation and/or patient care quality has been achieved.

The feedback process is intended to be more than one-directional. The audit committee itself needs regular feedback and evaluation if it is to perform effectively and meet its responsibilities. When the committee seeks and encourages such feedback it is most likely to receive it. The evaluation of the audit committee's performance can be achieved through a variety of measures. These include a regular reporting of the quantity of audits performed, the quality of audits completed, a statistical comparison of findings and follow-through action, and subjective evaluation of how well each of the stated committee purposes and objectives is being met.

NURSING AUDIT AND THE NURSE MANAGER

Auditing is an inspection process. It compares results with standards and criteria. Thus it is a most useful tool for the nurse manager. Every organization requires its own relevant inspection procedures. In general manufacturing where the measurement of size and dimensions is critical, "go, no-go" gauges are used. The item is either satisfactory (within standard) or it isn't. In the auditing of patient care and patient records there is a similar identification of those elements of care which represent "go" or "no-go" quality. Elements are either present (100 percent STD) or not present (0 percent STD) for acceptable clinical performance. Audit necessarily provides for acceptable variations for identifiable reasons. These too must be defined and documented as described earlier.

The guidelines for nursing audit take into account the variables among healthcare agencies and their relative performance capabilities. The thrust is for every agency to adapt to its own uses the fundamental philosophy and basic steps of nursing audit so that there can be demonstrable progress and improvements. Nurse managers welcome such programs for improving patient care through professional, businesslike methods. Nurse managers make them work well for their intended purposes.

Nursing audit is only one part of the growing trend toward a system of nursing that has as its focus the prevention of illness and care of patients based upon their identified problems and needs. In such a problem-oriented system it is essential to establish outcome and process standards of care as a basis for nursing practice, nursing documentation of that practice, and the auditing of both the practice and the documentation. The success of such a system rests largely upon the ability of nurse managers to assure that nurses use the nursing process effectively—that they assess, plan, implement, and evaluate on a continuous basis in all patient situations.

Goals and objectives need to be mutually set and agreed upon by nurses and patients (along with other health professionals) so that everyone is working toward the same ends. MBO and Nursing Management by Objectives blend well with the problem-oriented system and its audit component. After all, standards and objectives have much in common, even by definition. It is timely to begin involving the patient and the patient's family more directly in establishing objectives. Nurses must plan and carry out patient care with the patient whenever possible, rather than at or for the patient.

Job satisfaction is essential for the nurse. Results-oriented performance evaluation, based on the philosophy and principles of MBO, adds another personally satisfying dimension and provides for feedback and self-evaluation of performance with patients. ROPEP rests solidly on the establishment of standards of personnel performance. Coupled with standards of nursing care for use on the patient care units and for nursing audit purposes, there is the promise of being able to maintain a consistently satisfactory level of quality in nursing staff performance and patient care. Nursing audit, as one means of measuring quality of care, is a healthy indicator for the future direction of nursing and patient care under the leadership of professional nurse managers.

NOTES

Ainsworth, T. H., Jr. *Quality assurance in long term care.* Germantown, Md.: Aspen Systems Corp., 1977.

Froebe, D. J., & Bain, R. J. *Quality assurance programs and controls in nursing.* St. Louis: C. V. Mosby, 1976, pp. 9, 10.

Ganong, J., & Ganong, W. *HELP with nursing audit and quality assurance* (3rd ed.). Chapel Hill, N.C.: W. L. Ganong Co., 1978.

Ganong, J., & Ganong, W. *101 tremendous trifles.* Chapel Hill, N.C.: W. L. Ganong Co., 1978.

McClure, M. L. The long road to accountability. *Nursing Outlook,* January 1978, 26(1), 48.

Nicholls, M. E. Quality control in patient care. *American Journal of Nursing,* March 1974, pp. 456–459.

Pirsig, R. M. *Zen and the art of motorcycle maintenance.* New York: Bantam, 1974.

Rush-Presbyterian-St. Luke's Medical Center. Measuring the quality of nursing care. *Promise,* May 16, 1976. Chicago: Author, 1976.

Schmadl, J. C. Quality assurance: Examination of the concept. *Nursing Outlook,* July 1979, 27, pp. 462–465.

Reading List

Books

Brunner, L. S., & Suddarth, D. S. *The Lippincott manual of nursing practice.* Philadelphia: J. B. Lippincott, 1974.

Cantor, M. M. *Achieving nursing care standards: Internal and external.* Wakefield, Mass.: Nursing Resources, 1978.

Carter, J. H., Hilliard, M., Castles, M. R., Stoll, L. D., & Cowan, A. *Standards of nursing care: A guide for evaluation* (2nd ed.). New York: Springer, 1976.

Cazalas, M. W. (Ed.). *Nursing and the law* (3rd ed.). Germantown, Md.: Aspen Systems Corp., 1978.

Davidson, S., Burleson, B. C., Crawford, J. E. S., & Christofferson, S. *Nursing care evaluation: Concurrent and retrospective review criteria.* St. Louis: C. V. Mosby, 1977.

Ganong, J., & Ganong, W. *HELP with nursing audit & quality assurance* (3rd ed.). Chapel Hill, N.C.: W. L. Ganong Co., 1978.

Jacobs, C. M., & Jacobs, N. D. *The PEP primer.* Chicago: Joint Commission on Accreditation of Hospitals (JCAH), 1975.

Mayers, M. *A systematic approach to the nursing care plan.* New York: Appleton-Century-Crofts, 1972.

Mayers, M. *Standard nursing care plans.* Palo Alto, Ca.: R/P Co., Medical Systems, 1974, 1975.

Mazur, W. P. *The problem-oriented system in the psychiatric hospital.* Garden Grove, Ca.: Trainex Press, 1974.

Neelon, R. A., & Ellis, G. J. *A syllabus of problem-oriented patient care.* Boston: Little, Brown, 1974.

Phaneuf, M. C. *The nursing audit: Profile for excellence.* New York: Appleton-Century-Crofts, 1972.

Vasey, E., & Riley, M. *Quality assurance: Peer review for nursing.* Pittsburgh: Western Pennsylvania Regional Medical Program, 1975.

Weed, L. L. *Medical records, medical education, and patient care.* New York: Appleton-Century-Crofts, 1972.

Woolley, F. R., Warnick, M. W., Kane, R. L., & Dyer, E. D. *Problem-oriented nursing.* New York: Springer, 1974.

Yura, H., & Walsh, M. *The nursing process.* Washington, D.C.: Catholic University of America Press, 1967.

Articles

Brown, B. (Ed.). Quality assurance and peer review. *Nursing Administration Quarterly,* Spring 1977, *1*(3), entire issue.

Cook, G. Rx for the maladies of health care: A medical revolution in the making. *The Futurist.* June 1979, pp. 179–183.

Danbert, E. A. Patient classification system and outcome criteria. *Nursing Outlook,* July 1979, *27*(7), 450–454.

Kerr, A. H. Nurses' notes: That's where the goodies are. *Nursing '75,* February 1975, pp. 34–41.

Moore, K. What nurses learn from nursing audit. *Nursing Outlook,* April 1979, *27*(4), 254–258.

Nursing Clinics of North America. I. The problem-oriented record. II. Quality assurance. June 1974, *9*(2), 213–379.

Trussell, P. M., & Strand, N. A comparison of concurrent and retrospective audits on the same patients. *Journal of Nursing Administration,* May 1978, *8*(5), 33–38.

Chapter 8

Cost Containment through Annual Budgetary Planning

THE NURSE MANAGER'S ROLE IN COST CONTAINMENT

Professional nurse managers are acutely aware that money is the least common denominator of the 5M management formula (see Chapter 11). All of the other elements of the formula—manpower, material, machines and equipment, even the Big M for Manager—translate into money. Money is the ultimate unit of measure. Budgeting has to do with the flow and utilization of money. Thus the skill with which managers plan and control the budget becomes a key measure of managerial performance. And this means cost containment, now and for the foreseeable future.

> In the hospital industry, nursing costs are considered to be the largest challenge. Nursing, the largest employee unit, utilizes the greatest volume of supplies, has the greatest fluctuations in activity levels, and thus has the crushing opportunity either to improve or to justify its use of "manhours."
>
> To meet these challenges, nursing administrators keenly feel the need for sophisticated, understandable, valid, and reliable budgeting, forecasting, cost-accounting, and cost-saving tools and technologies (Mayers, 1979, p. xviii).

Most nurse administrators and managers are accustomed to managing in an environment of cost containment. Over the years their requests have been met—all too typically—by "It's not in the budget," "We can't afford it," or "Not this year." Yet today's cost-containment crunch is new and different. As discussed in Chapter 2, the environmental pressures have changed. Hospital administration has changed. And nursing management has changed. More than ever before, nurse managers are expected to be *professional*—not just as nurses, but also as managers.

Thus the modern nurse manager must be able to contribute to the hospital's or agency's budgetary planning and control process and integrate with it the other operational management techniques presented in this book. It has been our experience that nurse managers, given the information and the tools to use, learn to become highly effective in discharging their budgetary responsibilities—because they learn how to manage well those factors affecting costs. One case example is included as Appendix L.

This chapter is devoted to budgeting as related to operating expenses because this is the portion of the total budget over which nurse managers have major influence. They can *do* something about operating expenses. They have little or no control over the capital budget—the planned expenditures for major projects, items of equipment, or facilities that will be amortized rather than being paid for as part of the current year's expenses. Yet nurse managers need to be sufficiently familiar with the budgeting procedure for capital items so that they can submit budgetary requests for equipment or facilities when they believe these can be justified on the basis of cost/benefit or on the basis of their expected contribution to patient care programs.

CASH FLOW

Cash flow refers to the rate at which monies are received and spent. Every household manager experiences a cash flow problem when the rate of money coming in for a period of time is less than the rate of spending for the same period. The problem is acute when no reserves are available to be drawn upon for that portion of current expenses not covered by current income. Hospitals experience the same difficulty. A front page story entitled "Providers Clamor for Stalled Medicaid Checks" in a Raleigh, North Carolina newspaper read in part,

> Anxious nursing home and hospital administrators called Thursday for quick resolution of a Medicaid contract dispute that is tying up more than $3.3 million they are due for treating low-income patients. . . . Switchboards at the state office were swamped Thursday with calls from concerned hospitals and other healthcare providers—some complaining that they urgently needed their checks in order to meet their payrolls.

Similar examples abound.

Nursing administrators and managers in the typical hospital have not, until recently, been able to influence the rate of income received by the hospital. That situation has begun to change. For example, note the corporate goals for Nebraska Methodist Hospital (NMH) in Appendix F. Item IIA reads, "Expand and develop sources of revenue other than normal hospital services." During the mid-1970s, NMH's dynamic nursing administrator, Edna Fagan, was helping to meet this objective by serving as a consultant and conducting fee-for-service nursing management workshops in various parts of the country. The nursing administrator and the president of Bayfront Medical Center, St. Petersburg, Florida, have conducted primary nursing workshops and consulted on a fee basis. This income goes into an educational fund for members of the nursing department.

Another trend is to charge separately for nursing services. Nurse managers need to be deeply involved in the process of making this happen. A pertinent example is St. Luke's Hospital Medical Center in Phoenix. As reported in *A Patient Classification System for Staffing and Charging for Nursing Services,*

> One of the original intents for developing this system was to establish cost-related patient charges. At St. Luke's the patient is charged separately for room, dietary, and nursing care. The nursing care charge is a variable charge based on patient acuity and staffing requirements (Cisarik, Higgerson, & Van Slyck, 1978).

The patient charge system is outlined in this brief but worthwhile report. It is available at modest cost from St. Luke's Hospital.

The medical staff, of all hospital-related groups, has the greatest influence on the volume of hospital income and the rate at which it is received. It is the physicians and surgeons who provide the patients and who influence when the patients enter the hospital and how long they stay there. And it is the patients, whose hospitalization initiates the payment process, who provide (through whatever payment channel) the greatest portion of the hospital's income. But even though the doctors largely control the income-producing process by writing the orders for their patients, they play little or no direct role in spending or controlling the operating expenses of the hospital—except insofar as they use the hospital facility and personnel in the pursuit of their hospital-related medical practice. They do, of course, have a significant indirect influence on some aspects of the expense budget and on many aspects of the capital budget. Witness the attempts to initiate control mechanisms on burgeoning capital expenditures, ranging from the Health Systems Agencies to the National Center for Healthcare Technology (Cherry, 1979).

Possibly in the coming decade or two we will see some nurses influencing hospital income in the same manner as doctors do now. This will happen as private nurse practitioners earn the right to admit their own patients to hospitals. There are sharply contrasting views about this possibility. Dean

Dorothy Novello believes that nurses can function autonomously, practice independent of the physician in any setting, and accept responsibility and accountability. Economist Eli Ginzberg, however, predicts a substantial increase in physicians in the years ahead and thinks nursing lost its chance to assume a greater role in physician care by not getting into the nurse practitioner movement sooner. He challenges the idea of nurses practicing independently. "Nursing is tied to medicine. Nursing has a role to assist and intervene but not alone. Nurses can't do surgery or prescribe for pain" (NLN Convention, 1979).

CONTROL OF EXPENSES

Operating expenses, the day-to-day costs of maintaining and running a hospital or other healthcare agency, are considered to be controlled by hospital administration and the department heads. In point of fact, however, it is the people who work in the hospital, all of the employees at every level, who spend the money that makes up the greatest portion of the operating expense budget. This is a stark and simple fact. The employees use up the minutes and hours of each working day that are translated into payroll dollars, the largest single item of operating expense. And employees are the ones who spend the money paid for materials and supplies, since they actually use those supplies and materials in their daily work. Employees, therefore, individually and as an entire group, control a major portion of hospital expenses. A payroll clerk or an accounts payable clerk may write the checks but have no control over the actual expenditure of money.

Any observant manager recognizes the truth in the statement, "Your people can pull the rug out from under you any time they want to." Staff members can help or prevent the achievement of objectives and cost containment efforts, because they can control what happens to every expense dollar. In his hard-hitting article, "Do Management Control Systems Achieve Their Purpose?" McGregor (1967) concluded that traditional management control systems often fail because of noncompliance by employees who perceive in such systems the threat of punishment, a lack of trust, and a negative impact on their own human needs. They retaliate simply by not complying with demands for change, using their own imagination to beat the system, and sometimes fudging the data to distort the control reports. McGregor's recommendations for a managerial strategy that encourages employee involvement and commitment are summarized in Chapter 5. The theme of this book and our reasons for including so much of the humanistically-oriented philosophy, techniques, and principles of managerial leadership are related directly to McGregor's message. These techniques and principles reflect also the findings of other realistic researchers, as well as our own work experiences and observations of organizational behavior.

THE FINANCIAL ORGANIZATION CHART

The nurse manager's fiscal responsibility is dramatized through a Financial Organization Chart for the operating expense budget of a department of nursing. The first example, Figure 8-1, is a university hospital of approximately 350 beds. The total annual operating budget of $5.7 million, for which the director of nursing has responsibility, is approximately 40 percent of the total operating budget for the entire hospital—a percentage quite typical for general hospitals in the 300- to 500-bed size category. Variations from this figure are usually due to the inclusion or exclusion of certain departments (OR or Central Supply, for example) in the nursing service budget.

Note in the example that the patient care units are grouped in eight clusters, each group having its own nurse manager reporting to the director of nursing. These eight nurse managers have individual responsibility for operating budgets ranging from $321,000 to $798,000, depending on the number, size, and nature of the patient services offered in each group of units. Payroll expenses alone make up over 90 percent of the operating expenses for this department of nursing. Here again, the percentage is typical for comparable hospitals. No wonder, then, that escalating wages over the past decade have had such an impact on the costs of hospitalization. And no wonder that nurse managers have been exhorted to operate with minimal staff, use the lowest salary classification of personnel who can do the work, avoid scheduling staff for overtime work, and take advantage of every other means possible to contain payroll expenses. Many nurse managers feel, with considerable justification, that they have been fighting a losing battle because of the wage/price spiral, the state of the economy, and the difficulty (in many areas) of recruiting the kind and quantity of personnel they need to build stable, competent patient care teams.

In the second organization chart example, Figure 8-2, the arrangement of the unit clusters and the reporting relationships as shown were developed by nurse managers to meet existing needs and opportunities and to serve as the basis for a longer-range developmental plan. The chart indicates that responsibility for day-to-day operations is shared by two associate directors reporting to the director of nursing service. The head nurses report either to a supervisor or directly to one of the two associate directors. The clinical specialists also report to one of the two associate directors and serve in a staff capacity for their respective unit clusters. As clinical specialists, they are

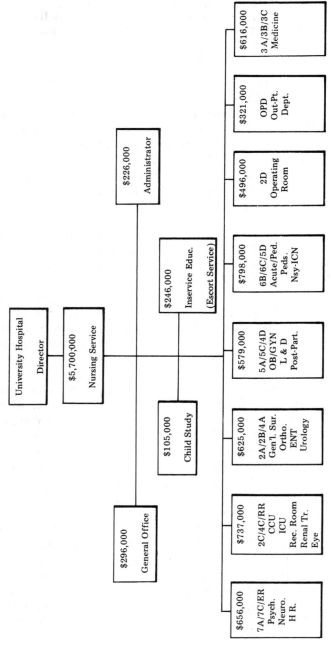

Figure 8-1 A Financial Organization Chart for Nursing Service Operating Expense Budget, 1975–1976 (All Figures to Nearest Thousand Dollars)

available also to the entire department when their individual clinical skills are required. The projected operating expenses for the fiscal year have been added to the chart. The recommendation and rationale for adopting the organizational plan as shown was as follows:

Recommendation: Adopt the organizational structure depicted on the attached chart, effective July 1.

   Rationale: This organizational plan—

1. provides maximum capability to support cost-containment goals of administration
2. continues our hospital's tradition of providing the best in patient care
3. builds upon the assets and demonstrated potential of nursing personnel
4. provides for flexibility and rapid response to changing demands and conditions
5. has the built-in mechanism for effective budgetary control
6. vests authority and accountability in those key nursing personnel who have responsibility for day-to-day operations and patient care
7. provides adequate and competent staff support to the nurse managers
8. strengthens the department's ability to achieve interdepartmental, hospital-wide communications and cooperation.

Chapter 10, in the section on organizing for motivational management, as well as Chapter 2, presents additional concepts and considerations relating to organizational structure.

Budgeting and cost containment will continue to be vital areas of concern for nurse managers. To cope with these matters, nurse managers deserve the best available practical staff support and service. Some nursing departments are providing such help within the department of nursing by establishing a position of Coordinator of Systems and Planning, or comparable title. A performance description is included in Appendix G. Persons in such a position, suitably qualified, earn their salaries many times over each year through savings and improvements in staffing, methods, and procedures; work simplification; new product analysis; and so on. They are nursing management engineers, with or without portfolio. They provide vital supporting services on demand to the nurse managers who have the direct fiscal responsibility on each unit, unit cluster, section, and division of the nursing department. Working together, they can demonstrate laudable results in operational management.

Nurse managers can set up simple graphs and charts (e.g., person hours/patient day, operating expenses/month) to help control expenses on a

Figure 8-2 Budgetary Control Responsibility within the Department of Nursing

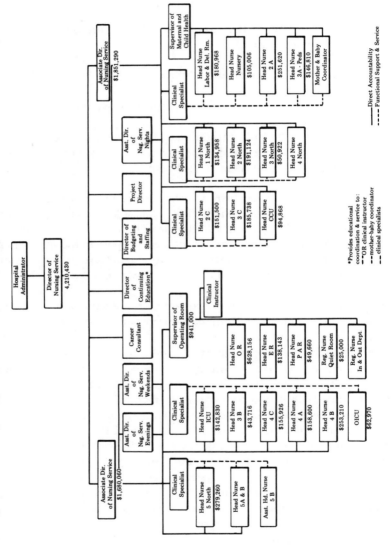

day-to-day basis and contribute to real cost-containment results. *In our experience an organizational approach works better than a more limited systems, technically-oriented approach.* The organizational approach is one which places responsibility for fiscal management in the nurse managers at every level and provides them with the resources they need to carry out that responsibility. Under such circumstances the nurse managers deliver commendable and often unexpected results in money management and patient care.

> Cost effectiveness and management responsibility for nursing service administrators begin with the budget process. This budgetary responsibility and accountability should be extended to each staff nurse so that all nurses understand individual responsibility in the financial aspect of patient care. If staff nurses are involved in determining the budget for their unit, they can better understand the need to monitor patient care hours, supplies and other indicators of budget control (Brown, 1978, p. vi).

The remainder of this chapter is devoted to annual budgetary planning and control as part of each nurse manager's responsibilities for patient care programs and human resources management. Budgetary planning and control (in the sense of feedback, measurement, and evaluation) provide the management technique which, fully utilized, serves as the bottom-line indicator of the caliber of managerial leadership and performance.

INTRODUCTION TO ANNUAL BUDGETARY PLANNING (ABP)

When we first wrote about "ABP for Nursing Administration" (Ganong & Ganong, 1973), we used ABP as the abbreviation for Annual Business Plan, a deliberate carryover of a term used in general business situations for the type of comprehensive planning process described. Our reason for using "business" in the title was twofold: (1) the healthcare industry is usually cited as the first or second largest in the country, and the time is long overdue for coming to grips with the business issues involved, using the appropriate terminology for doing so; and (2) nurse managers recognize that the business of healthcare organizations is patient care and that businesslike plans of care and businesslike methods for the delivery of such care lead to best results for patients and consumers generally.* We find no one to dispute that position with any serious conviction.

---

*For a scholarly, documented analysis supporting this view, see The Industrialization of Service. *Harvard Business Review.* September–October, 1976, *54*, 69–70.

The pace of change being what it is, however, we take no umbrage at those nurse managers who are not yet ready to adopt the Annual Business Plan terminology for use within their own nursing department. This is in recognition of the fact that in many hospitals the nurse managers are just beginning to play a significant role in budgetary planning and control. In such hospitals the use of an ABP program for annual budgetary planning with realistic involvement of the nurse managers is a major progressive step toward improved hospital-wide management.

In other hospitals we find situations in which an administrator, controller, or business manager is far too ready to pass over to the nursing administrator a disproportionate share of the burden for budgetary matters. In view of the fact, therefore, that annual business planning is necessarily a hospital-wide function, this chapter presents ABP in that context, but with the focus on the nurse manager's role in budgetary planning and control. As stated in the first sentences of AHA's 1961 publication *Budgeting Procedures for Hospitals*, "Planning future operations through budgeting is an integral part of successful businesses today. Similar planning is equally important to successful operation of our hospitals" (Cappleman, 1961, p. 1).

Just a few years ago the nursing administrator's role in budgetary planning was concentrated into a relatively few weeks or months prior to the end of the fiscal year (Ganong & Ganong, 1976). Times have changed, as reflected in so much of the current literature.

> In contrast to the generally accepted belief in nursing that preparing next year's budget is an annual event, budgeting really begins with the premise that its planning and control is an ongoing activity. Too often our attention is directed to this end, usually accompanied by frenetic activity in the few weeks or months prior to the beginning of a new fiscal year. However, understanding the ongoing nature of the budgetary process is essential if the director of nursing service is to maintain the necessary control (Porter-O'Grady, 1979, p. 35).

Figure 8-3 presents a program performance plan for a nursing department's annual budget considered as part of the hospital's annual business plan. The time span shown is the twelve-month period preceding the beginning of a new fiscal year on July 1. The July through June fiscal year is the one most commonly used in hospitals. The sequence of steps in the ABP process is listed from top to bottom in the Activities column, while the scheduled time for carrying out each step is shown in the horizontal block spanning the number of weeks required to complete the activity. The titles in the "Who Will Do or Help" column indicate the persons who will assume primary

Figure 8-3 Annual Budget Plan (ABP) for Department of Nursing*
Fiscal Year July, 1, 1977–June 30, 1978

SCHEDULE ACTIVITIES	JUL	AUG	SEP	OCT	NOV	DEC	JAN	FEB	MAR	APR	MAY	JUN	WHO WILL DO/HELP
1. Establish Objectives for the Fiscal Year 1977–1978	■												Dir. of Nursing Assoc. Director
2. Identify Key Issues	■	■											Dir. of Nursing Assoc. Director Pt. Care Coords.
3. Analyze Performance and Resources		■	■										Dir. of Nursing Controller Pt. Care Coords.
4. State Basic Assumptions				■									Pt. Care Coords. Dir. of Nursing
5. Set Unit Objectives					■	■							Pt. Care Coords. Unit Staff
6. Develop Program Strategies and Action Plans						■	■						Pt. Care Coords. Unit Staff
7. Forecast Income						■	■						Controller
8. Develop Operational Plans								■	■				Pt. Care Coords. Unit Staff
9. Prepare Budget Recommendations									■				Pt. Care Coords. Dir. of Nursing Assoc. Director
10. Submit Budget; Review, Revise, and Secure Approval											■	■	Dir. of Nursing Assoc. Director Pt. Care Coords.

* Adapted from Ganong, J., and Ganong, W. ABP for Nursing Administration. *Journal of Nursing Administration*, May–June 1973, *3*, 6. Reprinted by permission of Nursing Resources, Inc.

responsibility for completing the particular planning activity by the scheduled date. Specific titles for personnel will vary with the size and nature of the agency. For example, a nurse with the title of Coordinator for Systems and Planning, reporting to the director, can become a key person in the ABP process. This title would be substituted for associate director and/or others when such a person is part of the staff. The director of nursing has responsibility for maintaining the schedule whether or not the persons with the titles indicated are members of the nursing department. Missed due dates will seriously impair the orderly progression of the entire planning sequence. The numbered paragraphs that follow relate to the numbered activities in Figure 8–3.

1. Establish the departmental objectives for the fiscal year. These objectives stem from the goals of the nursing department. The annual objectives are the specific operational results which the nursing department intends to accomplish, and are related to the long-range planning for the entire hospital as enunciated by the administrator or other chief operating executive. Such objectives are more quantitative and measurable than those usually included in the typical statement of philosophy and objectives drawn from existing nursing department manuals. When a management-by-objectives program is in effect, the annual objectives are part of the MBO plan. Such objectives are the stepping stones of progress leading to the achievement of the broad departmental goals for the fiscal year.

> *Example:* One nursing objective is to select a patient care coordinator for each of two pilot groupings of related units (maternal and child care, and three medical-surgical units) as a step toward better utilization of all personnel while maintaining or improving the quality of patient care. The related hospital objective, part of the administrator's annual business plan, is to move toward more decentralized management of hospital departments having similar operational characteristics and similar problems for the purpose of cost containment and more effective performance.

2. Identify key issues. Key issues are factors that need identification because of their likely impact upon the operation of the patient care units during the year. The following key issues have obvious implications for the entire hospital's annual business plan.

> *Examples:* (A) The planned retirement of a well-liked neurosurgeon with a large practice, with no replacement in sight, will affect the OR schedule and the surgical floor census.
>
> (B) The imminent merger of this hospital with another will affect the nursing department's organizational relationships; formal completion of incorporation is expected early next year.
>
> (C) Organizing attempts by two different labor unions that seek to represent nurses will likely result in an election before the end of this year.

3. Analyze past performance, available resources, expected demands, and known constraints. This involves three major aspects. The first is the review of past performance results, existing organizational assets and resources, and a realistic assessment of limitations and constraints affecting the scope of realistically obtainable objectives. This first step is an inward look at your own organization. It is a kind of intraorganizational audit.

Example: Assume an objective of adding four beds to an existing 10-bed ICU, to be effected by August 1. In order to estimate the effect of the four additional beds on the operating expenses per bed, an examination must be made of current operating expenses per bed in the existing 10-bed ICU as related to occupancy rate, trend of supply costs, and physician attitudes toward the use of the unit for their patients. The 40 percent increase in bed capacity may result in an increase of operating expenses per bed by an amount significantly less than or greater than the 40 percent increase in the number of beds. The accuracy of the forecast and its influence on the nursing budget depend largely on how well this analysis is carried out.

The second aspect is an outward-looking step. It is a type of community-oriented survey to update your knowledge of your market, to use a respectable business term. It answers such questions as: Who are your consumers of patient care? What are their characteristics—age, sex, culture, socioeconomic status, health status, etc.? What services have they been using and in what volume? What community changes may affect the mix of such services that should be available in the year ahead?

Example: A large influx of younger families into new real estate developments in the hospital area is causing an increasing use of the OB, GYN, PEDS, and ER departments. This will influence space, equipment, and staffing requirements for the year ahead.

The third aspect is competition analysis, also an outward-looking step. It provides information about other healthcare agencies in your market area and what their plans are so that your hospital and nursing department can relate such information to your own planning.

Example: The recent opening of a private nursing home in your area last summer is expected to reduce the pressures to expand your extended care facility. The new nursing home, together with the plans of other community agencies and the opening of a retirement village in another town, may dictate maintaining the present size of your own extended care facility or even a planned reduction in such service.

4. State basic assumptions. These are expectations which must be stated in writing, to avoid embarrassing and costly misunderstandings, communication breakdowns, and failure to attain an objective. The basic assumptions in this plan should be prepared by the end of November by each patient care coordinator.

> *Examples:* (A) Mrs. Acey will be available to become the patient care coordinator of units 7, 8, and 10 to replace the supervisor who is moving to Florida in the fall of this year.
>
> (B) The supply of trained LPNs being supplied by local sources can be increased by 15 percent per month beginning September 1.
>
> (C) Some form of mandatory rate control will be instituted in this state by the springtime two years from now.

5. Set unit objectives. The unit objectives are the specific operational results which each unit plans to accomplish during the fiscal year. Such objectives reflect objectives of the department of nursing as set forth in Step 1, but are translated into detailed terms specific to each unit. These objectives are prepared by the patient care coordinator of each unit, to be completed no later than December 31.

> *Examples:* (A) Install additional autoclave in CSR. (Expected delivery date is early September.)
>
> (B) Prepare LPNs to assume an increasing share of technical duties. (Program plans and dates to be supplied by inservice director and head nurses.)
>
> (C) Provide inservice programs for RNs on the problem-oriented nursing system (September through March).
>
> (D) Revise current cyclical schedule to provide for every other weekend off (effective date October 1).
>
> (E) Establish nursing audit standards and criteria for eight additional disease entities.

6. Develop program strategies and action plans. This step considers the strategies and tactics to be used in each unit's "marketing" program (service offerings and how to interest potential users in them). The input of prior steps provides the necessary data for the formulation of the action plans and strategies. The unit profile (described in Chapter 10) can be helpful also. This step is necessarily a coordinated effort by the patient care coordinator of each unit, with the help of the director of nursing service and pertinent members of the medical staff working closely within the policies and objectives of the institution. The completion date is the end of February two years hence.

> *Example:* The OB department will initiate a planned program beginning October next year to better compete with the "loss-leader" (services below cost) services of a local proprietary hospital that has affected the census in OB and related income. Possible activities include closer contacts by the admitting department with the appointment secretaries in the offices of OB/GYN physicians, a stepped-up teaching program for expectant mothers, and a follow-through service to involve the visiting nurse association—together with an information program to publicize these services.

7. Forecast income. The income forecast is an essential ingredient of the budgetary plan in order to predict: (a) how achievement of stated objectives may increase or decrease the amount of income for the year; and (b) where the money is coming from to pay for the costs of approved programs related to specific objectives. The nursing department usually has little or no responsibility for direct input to this step. The income forecast is to be developed by the controller during January and February.

> *Example:* The planned program for OB services (see example in Step 6 above) is expected to make little impact on the OB census during the coming fiscal year and will cost approximately $3,000. The expectation for the following year will be increased utilization and income of about 10 percent.

8. Develop operational plans. These plans set forth in as much detail as possible the full annual plan prepared by each unit to achieve the approved objectives. Completed by March 31st, this plan permits budget preparation in time for board approval prior to the beginning of the new fiscal year.

> *Example:* An operational plan includes a 12-month timetable of activities, staffing requirements and schedules, recruitment efforts, utilization of agency resources, services required from other internal or external sources, rate of expenditure of funds, and so on.

9. Prepare budget recommendations. The budget summarizes in dollars what the ABP means in terms of income and expenditures. It projects the rate of expenditure of funds allocated to permit progress toward established objectives and provides a measure of performance results on a monthly basis.

Example: If none of the $3,000 allocated for the OB program (see examples in Steps 6 and 7) has been spent by the February date, then performance progress on this objective will be behind schedule and will re-quire review and possible rescheduling.

10. Submit budget; review, revise, and secure approval. This is the last step in the ABP process. In far too many hospitals, Steps 9 and 10 are considered to be the sum and substance of annual budgetary planning. Note that with ABP, the budget is simply the outcome of the foregoing steps that provide the basis for the budget itself.

THE MEANING OF ABP FOR NURSE MANAGERS

It should now be clear why the term Annual Budget Plan is so meaningful for nurse managers. ABP really refers to your annual management plan for the nursing department. The budgeting process, carried out as described by the ten-step program performance plan, brings together all of the elements of the nursing management process—the unifying theme throughout this book.

ABP is a technique which, like the other management techniques, helps nurse managers carry out their management functions of planning, doing, and controlling. Each management technique provides particular help with one or more functions. And each technique in itself contains all three elements of planning, doing, and controlling.

Here is a summary of how the ABP technique relates to and involves a balanced use of other nursing management techniques:

- Management by Objectives: ABP is the essence of MBO. Every objective has a price tag. The budget adds up the prices and helps decide upon the priority and scheduling of objectives. (See also *goalstorming* in Chapter 5 reading list article by Adams, 1979.)
- Problem-Oriented Nursing System: PONS (Chapter 3) has its focus on the patients and their care programs. The objectives for patient care programs are at the heart of all other hospital and nursing objectives, and become high-priority considerations in the ABP Steps 1 through 8.
- Results-Oriented Performance Evaluation Program: ROPEP (Chapter 6) is vital to Step 3 of ABP and to the nature and likelihood of achievement of the objectives, strategies, and operational plans developed in Steps 5, 6, and 8.

- Nursing Audit: Auditing (Chapter 7) is critical to the control aspects of MBO, PONS, ROPEP, and ABP.
- Motivational Management: Creating a motivational climate and a "motivating gap" (Chapter 10) are parts of a technique for nurse managers that influence especially the implementation and evaluation phases of ABP.
- Wide-Track Careers: The WTC program (Chapter 13), as part of human resources management, is an ongoing part of every ABP. The success of WTC has a direct influence upon the nurse manager's success in using the other techniques.

"Learning by doing," an age-old, valid principle of education, has special meaning for those nurse managers who would learn budgeting. You will learn how to prepare and control budgets if you do it within your own agency, preferably with expert guidance. You may benefit from courses of instruction or from reading about the budgeting process if the content is specifically designed to meet your needs. In our experience, however, a far better investment of time is that spent in direct on-the-job training in preparing and controlling that portion of your agency budget for which you are responsible as a nurse manager. In so doing you will discover the substance and implications of all the other parts of this book dealing with your functions, techniques, and skills as a nurse manager.

In summary, ABP as a year-round process brings together the techniques and functions of managing in a way seldom achieved previously, so that nurse managers can comprehend, integrate, and carry out with professional confidence their responsibilities for patient care management, operational management, and human resources management.

Nursing administrators can and must develop more refined systems of cost control and financial management in all areas of nursing service. To do this, we must improve our knowledge base by developing population-based data systems, implementing institutional financial reporting systems, working closely with third party payers and being responsive in rate-review mechanisms at both local and state levels. We need to broaden nursing participation in the utilizational review structure. We must work toward an effective health education and prevention program for the consumer in order to assure a high-quality, cost-effective health care delivery system. We must also design new patient care programs to add to institutional financial revenue gain (Brown, 1978, pp. vii–viii).

NOTES

Brown, B. (Ed.) From the editor. . . . *Nursing Administration Quarterly,* Fall 1978, *3*(1). Reprinted with permission of Aspen Systems Corp.

Cappleman, E. N. *Budgeting procedures for hospitals.* Chicago: American Hospital Association, 1961, p. 1.

Cherry, L. Medical technology: The new revolution. *The New York Times Magazine,* August 5, 1979, p. 22.

Cisarik, J. M., Higgerson, N. J., & Van Slyck, A. *A patient classification system for staffing and charging for nursing services.* Phoenix, Ariz.: St. Luke's Hospital Medical Center, 1978, p. 17.

Ganong, J., & Ganong, W. ABP for nursing administration. *Journal of Nursing Administration,* May–June 1973, *3*(3), 6.

Ganong, J., & Ganong, W. *HELP with annual budgetary planning and control.* Chapel Hill, N.C.: W. L. Ganong Co., 1976, p. 7.

Mayers, M. (Series Ed.). Foreword. In E. Schmied (Ed.), *Maintaining cost effectiveness.* Wakefield, Mass.: Nursing Resources, 1979.

McGregor, D. Do management control systems achieve their purpose? *AMA Management Review,* February 1967, p. 6.

NLN Convention: 1979. *Nursing Outlook,* June 1979, *27*(6), 400, 401.

Porter-O'Grady, T. Financial planning: Budgeting for nursing, Part I. *Supervisor Nurse,* August 1979, *10*(8). Reprinted by permission of *Supervisor Nurse Magazine.*

Providers Clamor for Stalled Medical Checks. *The News and Observer,* Raleigh, N.C., May 28, 1976.

Reading List

Books

Cappleman, E. N. *Budgeting procedures for hospitals.* Chicago: American Hospital Association, 1971.

Cleverley, W. O. *Essentials of hospital finance.* Germantown, Md.: Aspen Systems Corp., 1978.

Cunningham, R. N., Jr. *Improving work methods in small hospitals.* Chicago: American Hospital Association, 1975.

Groner, P. N. *Cost containment through employee incentives program.* Germantown, Md.: Aspen Systems Corp., 1977.

Herkimer, J., & Allen, G. *Understanding hospital financial management.* Germantown, Md.: Aspen Systems Corp., 1978.

Hospital Financial Management Educational Foundation. *The budgeting process: Student packet.* Chicago: Author, 1970.

Hospital Financial Management Association. *Planning the hospital's financial operations: Readings in hospital budgeting.* Chicago: Author, 1972.

Marram, G., Flynn, K., Abaravich, W., & Carey, S. *Cost-effectiveness of primary and team nursing.* Wakefield, Mass.: Contemporary Publishing, 1976.

Schmied, E. (Ed.). *Maintaining cost effectiveness.* Wakefield, Mass.: Nursing Resources, 1979.

Trivedi, V. M. *Hospital management systems demonstration: Optimum allocation of float nurses using head nurses' perceptions.* Ann Arbor: University of Michigan, Bureau of Hospital Administration, 1974.

Zollitsch, H. G., & Langsner, A. *Wage and salary administration.* Cincinnati: South-Western Publishing, 1970.

Articles

Boer, G., & Parris, W. Flexible budgeting—A cost control tool. *Hospital Financial Management.* December 1970, *24*(11), 12-14.

Boyarski, R. P. Nursing workweek equalizes shifts, time off. *Hospital Progress,* July 1976, *57*(7), 36.

Bruton, P., & Berkowitz, S. Financial management by objectives in hospitals. *Health Care Management Review.* Spring 1978, *3*(2), 25-32.

Deason, J. M. (Ed.). Flexible budgeting. *Topics in Health Care Financing,* Summer 1979, *5*(4), entire issue.

Ganong, W. L., Ganong, J. M., & Harrison, E. T. The 12-hour shift: Better quality, lower cost. *Journal of Nursing Administration,* February 1976, *6*(2), 17-29.

Herzlinger, R. Fiscal management in health organizations. *Health Care Management Review,* Summer 1977, *2*(3), 37-42.

Houser, R. How to build and use flexible budgeting. *Hospital Financial Management,* August 1974, pp. 12-20.

Levitt, T. The industrialization of service. *Harvard Business Review,* September-October 1976, *54*(5), 63-74.

Munch, J. Let's involve nurses in budget planning. *Hospitals,* February 16, 1974, *48*(4), 75-78.

Wymelenberg, S. New accounting system helps control costs. *Hospitals,* July 1, 1979, *53*(13), 68-70.

Chapter 9

Staffing and Scheduling

THE REALITY OF DELIVERING PATIENT CARE

Nursing in the hospital or long-term-care facility is a 24-hour, every-day-of-every-month-of-every-year reality. While most, if not all, of the other professional and technical personnel shut down daily and weekly operations to go home and be "on call," the nursing staff and personnel continue to integrate patient care and services. This creates a special problem for the department or division of nursing. It requires the continual planning and monitoring of enough nurses and nursing personnel on site around the clock for every patient unit. Often it means not only delivering nursing care but also providing the technical services of other departments such as physical therapy, respiratory therapy, and pharmacy—to name a few.

As soon as, or even before, the doors of a new inpatient facility open for business, the struggle of staffing and scheduling begins—and never ceases. No other profession, not even medicine, is faced with such a demand for relentless, continuous service. DiVincenti cites staffing as one of the most persistent and critical concerns facing nursing service administration and indicates that there is not very much evidence of whether the problem is quantity, quality, or utilization (DiVincenti, 1977). It is likely to be all three.

In a book written for healthcare consumers, there is a chapter on understanding the nursing staff and how it can benefit the patient. The authors point out that it is helpful to understand who's who on the nursing staff. They remind us that it was simpler 50 years ago when there were hospitals with just doctors who examined patients, planned treatment, and wrote orders; and there were nurses who did everything else. There were no other workers. Today, they note, is a different matter. Times have changed and so have nurses. There is a hierarchy of nurses who are specialized and whose duties are stratified (Gots & Kaufman, 1978).

Hospitals and medicine have become more complex in structure, organization, technology, competition, and cost in an effort to keep abreast of the rapid changes in health and illness care. All of this impacts on the nurse manager who has to staff the patient units to meet ever-increasing and shifting demands for the delivery of care. The reality of providing that delivery involves nonstop effort by the nurse manager.

STAFFING AND SCHEDULING DEFINED

Staff is defined as a group of assistants who aid an executive or other person of authority; the personnel who carry out a specific enterprise, as *the nursing staff of a hospital* (American Heritage Dictionary, 1976, p. 1254). *Staffing* means to provide with a staff of employees.

A *schedule* is a timetable or a production plan; in nursing management it usually refers to the time sheets showing planned work days and shifts for nurses and other nursing personnel. *Scheduling* means to plan or appoint for a certain time or date; to make up and enter on a schedule (time sheet). Another way of looking at staffing and scheduling is to view *staffing* as a complex process and *scheduling* as a *task* (West, 1979). The author compares the *staffing process* to the *nursing process* and identifies six essential elements: staffing study, master staffing plan, scheduling plan, position control, budgeting plan, and management information system. In addition, high priority must be given to patients' identified needs which are categorized and summarized by a patient classification system. The JCAH states the requirement for identifying the nursing care needs of patients and the qualifications of nursing personnel to meet those needs as follows:

> STANDARD III   Nursing department/service assignments in the provision of nursing care shall be commensurate with the qualifications of nursing personnel and shall be assigned to meet the nursing care needs of patients. (See Appendix K for interpretation.)

Nurse managers at every level of the nursing organization must understand current thinking on both the process of staffing and the task of scheduling.

STAFFING AND THE MANAGEMENT FUNCTIONS

Staffing is an integral part of all three management functions: planning, doing, and controlling. The following staffing presentation is organized under each of the three functions.

PLANNING

Factors that affect staffing, in order of their priority, include (1) needs of patients, (2) nursing modality, (3) organizational structure, (4) scheduling of staff, (5) mix of personnel, and (6) budget. All six factors are important in the planning of staffing.

1. *Needs of patients.* How many of what kinds of patients require what kinds of care on each shift, 24 hours a day, seven days a week? With suitable guidance, nurse managers can develop a simple form of patient classification. Key nursing staff members must be involved in this development effort if the patient-categorization plan is to be usable and acceptable, fully effective for its purpose, understood, cost-effective, and one to which the nursing staff can be committed. This plan, together with a suitable ongoing analysis of census data (actual and projected, day by day), provides a firm basis for summarizing anticipated patient needs. Periodic review and updating of such a plan will assure its ongoing efficacy.

If the purpose of a patient classification plan is limited, such a plan may be developed in-house quite quickly and at low cost. If a sophisticated plan is needed, with the ultimate purpose of individual charges to patients for the nursing care they receive, the plan may have to be developed with the help of management engineers or consultants. Examples of both types follow. Exhibit 9–1 provides guidelines for the simpler, do-it-yourself approach.

A patient classification plan permits categorization of patients by levels of nursing care required. The resultant totals for each classification provide the basis for defining the nursing workload, the number of nursing care hours required on each shift. Simply said; but not so simply done. It is a complex task to determine the optimum number of nursing hours to be scheduled for how many of what categories of nursing personnel on each shift so that adequate patient care can be provided. The task is far more than an exercise in applying time standards, however these are developed. Nurse managers must be familiar with, and proficient in using, the human mode as well as the technical mode skills.

A useful sourcebook on a patient information and workload management system is *GRASP* by Diane Meyer (1978). It describes a successful application at Grace Hospital, a 160-bed Friesen-designed acute care facility in a North Carolina community of approximately 40,000 population. The design of the units has a direct influence on the staffing requirements. Nursing stations are eliminated; an administrative control center is staffed by an administrative aide; patients' rooms have pneumatic tube stations, work space alcoves, and pass-through cabinets for supplies and medications. Other influencing factors are described in detail.

Exhibit 9-1 Guidelines for Creating a Patient Classification Plan

Introduction: This is an outline for the in-house development by nurses of a simple, limited-purpose patient classification plan to assist with staffing and scheduling. The plan may be for a single unit, a unit cluster, or the entire nursing department.

Step 1: Form a task force composed of nurse managers and staff nurses from the unit (or group of units) concerned. . . . Bring the group together under the leadership of a person (not necessarily a member of the task force itself) who has recognized ability as a discussion group leader (see Ganong, W., & Ganong, J. "Tips for Leading Discussions," 1978, pp. 29–32). Ask the group to identify the factors that influence the level of care required by patients on their units. . . . List these, as offered, on the blackboard (e.g., ambulation, procedures, treatments, medications, activities of daily living, medical care, visitors—whatever is suggested). . . . Include all suggestions.

Step 2: Review the factors. . . . Combine similar ones, add or subtract others. . . . Then list the agreed-upon factors across the top of the blackboard so as to permit adding individual evaluative words (descriptors) under each of them.

Step 3: Work with the group to identify the descriptors which best indicate the range of conditions which can be observed or readily measured (from *minimum* to *maximum*, from *none* to *all*, or whatever terminology is most appropriate). . . . This process helps to refine the number of factors to be used and helps in considering how many levels of patient care you will use.

Step 4: Decide how many patient care categories will be most appropriate. . . . The number may range from as few as three to as many as six. . . . The number should be a suitable balance among various attributes: simplicity for understanding and use, costs involved, and how your plan will facilitate its total purposes. . . . Avoid the temptation to make the plan overly detailed if it is just a means of better organizing and utilizing the nurses' judgments regarding patients' conditions and their effects upon staffing considerations. . . . Set up the form with descriptors arranged hierarchically. . . . Write short guidelines for using the plan.

Step 5: Task force members make a trial use of the typed first draft of the patient classification form to test the descriptors and the number of patient classification categories. . . . Then refine the plan as necessary and introduce it for continuing use.

This classification plan is not intended to be a rigid guide to the allocation of nursing hours. Rather, it is an aid to the professional nurse manager's judgment regarding staffing requirements, considering all factors that influence patient care. Later—through experience, observation, and suitable measurement techniques—time standards can be developed for each patient care category.

Source: Ganong, J. and Ganong, W. *101 tremendous trifles: A collection of management mini-guides,* 2nd Ed. Chapel Hill, N.C.: W. L. Ganong Co., 1979, p. 76c.

Exhibits 9-2 and 9-3 are examples of two components of a well-developed, sophisticated plan that includes patient acuity classification, nurse staffing, patient charges for nursing service, and a validation and audit procedure. It was developed and implemented over a period of years at St. Luke's Hospital Medical Center in Phoenix under the leadership of Ann Van Slyck, Director of Nursing. The authors of a brief manual describing the project admit that,

> The project has been frustrating, discouraging and a source of worry; but more important, it has been challenging, rewarding and worthwhile. . . . The intent of this manual was to share the development process and current products of a sophisticated system that includes patient classification or acuity, nurse staffing and individual charges for nursing care. We have committed thousands of man-hours and dollars to its development. By much trial and error, we have accomplished a system that meets the requirements of our hospital. Although not totally perfect, we believe, with pride, that this is the most comprehensive, yet functional, system in operation in this country (Cisarik, Higgerson, & Van Slyck, 1978, p. 25).

A copy of this worthwhile report is available from the hospital for a modest charge.

2. *Nursing modality.* What is your nursing-care modality—functional, team, case, modular, total care, or primary nursing? Your answer to this question is vitally important for staffing and scheduling since it reflects the philosophical and pragmatic realities of your facility, your department of nursing, and your patient care unit. (See also Chapter 2.)

Planning of staffing must be based on your choice of modality or modalities. Within one hospital it may be possible to use total care in intensive units, primary nursing on some medical or surgical units, and modular nursing on still other units. Staffing needs will depend upon such choices.

3. *Organizational structure.* As a nurse manager, are you committed to a centralized or decentralized structure—in theory and in practice? Having considered your patient/client population and your choice of nursing care modality or modalities, what plan of organization is most appropriate? Once again, the philosophical/pragmatic realities have a great influence. The choice is between a traditional, authoritarian style of management and a participative style that stresses the individual responsibility and accountability of every employee. Your choice has considerable influence on staffing, ranging from numbers and grouping of nursing leadership positions to the numbers and mix of nurses and other nursing personnel.

A decentralized organization permits decision making about staffing and scheduling at the lowest levels of organization consistent with performance

Exhibit 9-2 A Patient Classification Plan

ST. LUKE'S HOSPITAL MEDICAL CENTER
Phoenix, Arizona

PATIENT CARE RECORD · MEDICAL/SURGICAL

ABBREVIATIONS				
N = Nite B = Breakfast				
D = Day L = Lunch				
E = Evening D = Dinner				

			N	D	E
•DISCH TIME	CODE				
POINTS LEVEL		SUB-TOTAL ACUITY 'A'			
26- 37 1					
38- 55 2		SUB-TOTAL ACUITY 'B'			
56- 70 3		SUB-TOTAL ACUITY 'C'			
71- 83 4		TOTAL POINTS			
84-103 5		ACUITY LEVEL			

DATE	•☐ON PASS ☐PRIV. DUTY				DATA PROCESSING COPY

DIET	Refused None	B	L	D
NOURISHMENT	Partial Total			

ACUITY 'A'		N	D	E
DIET	DIET CHECK	2	2	2
	NPO	2	2	2
	SELF	2	2	2
	ASSIST & TRAY	5	5	5
	SIPS/CHIPS	5	5	5
	INTAKE/OUTPUT (FORCE/LIMIT)	5	5	5
	ASSIST FEED	8	8	8
	TOTAL FEED	8	8	8
	GAVAGE FEED	8	8	8
	•TEACHING FEED	8	8	8
	•COMPLEX TOTAL FEED	8	8	8
BATH/LINENS	ENVIRONMENTAL CHECK	1	1	1
	TUB c̄ HELP	1	1	1
	BATH c̄ HELP	1	1	1
	SHOWER c̄ HELP	1	1	1
	SELF-HELP (BEDSIDE)	2	2	2
	HS CARE	2	2	2
	TUB c̄ OCCASIONAL CHECK	2	2	2
	SHOWER c̄ OCCASIONAL CHECK	2	2	2
	COMPLEX HS CARE	4	4	4
	PARTIAL BATH	4	4	4
	COMPLETE BATH	4	4	4
	•COMPLEX BATH	5	5	5
	•TEACHING BATH	5	5	5
	•MULTIPLE BATHS	5	5	5
MOBILITY	Q _____ H.CHECK	2	2	2
	UP AD LIB	2	2	2
	CHAIR	2	2	2
	BRP	2	2	2
	•AMBULATE c̄ HELP	5	5	5
	•BRP c̄ HELP	5	5	5
	•CHAIR & HELP	5	5	5
	BEDREST c̄ BRP/COMMODE	5	5	5
	BEDREST	5	5	5
	COMPLETE BEDREST	8	8	8
	•COMPLEX ACTIVITY	8	8	8
	•TEACHING ACTIVITY	8	8	8
	TURN Q _____ H	8	8	8
	TOTAL LIFT Q _____ H	10	10	10
	STRYKER/CIRCLE BED TURN Q ____ H	10	10	10
	•SOFT/LEATHER RESTRAINTS	10	10	10
	SUB-TOTAL ACUITY 'A'			

ACUITY 'B'		N	D	E
MEDICATIONS	MEDICATION KARDEX CHECK	5	5	5
	ROUTINE c̄ IV's	8	8	8
	ROUTINE c̄ IV's	15	15	15
	MULTIPLE MEDS	15	15	15
	HEPARIN LOCK	15	15	15
	•TEACHING MEDICATIONS	15	15	15
	•ASSESSMENT MEDS	15	15	15
	ROUTINE c̄ MULTIPLE PIGGYBACKS	25	25	25
	•BLOOD TRANSFUSIONS/OBSERVATION	25	25	25
	•ADMINISTRATIVE/FREQUENT INTERVENTION	25	25	25
BEHAVIOR	RESPONSIVE TO CARE	5	5	5
	•DEPENDENT PSYCHOLOGICALLY	10	10	10
	•BARRIERS TO CARE	10	10	10
	•CONFUSED	10	10	10
	•DISORIENTED	10	10	10
	•REPETITIVE REQUESTS	10	10	10
	•LETHARGIC	10	10	10
	•COMATOSE	10	10	10
	•DISRUPTIVE	15	15	15
	•HALLUCINATIONS/DELUSIONS	15	15	15
	•CONFLICT OF EMOTIONS	15	15	15
	•THREATENING PHYSICAL HARM	15	15	15
STATE	SELF RELIANT	4	4	4
	ROUTINE ADMISSION	7	7	7
	•SHORT TERM TEACHING & COUNSELING	7	7	7
	ASSISTANCE c̄ ADL	7	7	7
	•RESTRICTIONS	7	7	7
	PRE-OP PREPARATION	11	11	11
	•COMPLEX ADMISSION/TRANSFER	11	11	11
	POST -OP/POST-ACU (24 HOURS)	11	11	11
	•PHYSIOLOGICALLY UNSTABLE	11	11	11
	•DISCHARGE PLANNING/TEACHING	11	11	11
	•COMMUNICATIONS BARRIER	15	15	15
	•EXTENSIVE NURSING CARE	20	20	20
	SUB-TOTAL ACUITY 'B'			

ACUITY 'C'	(7 · 14 · 20) SUB-TOTAL		
TREATMENT/PROCEDURE	ITEMS—FREQUENCY	TIMES	

SIGNATURES										
NITE		LPN/ NA	SIDE RAILS↑	DAY		LPN/ NA	SIDE RAILS↑	EVE		LPN/ N A	SIDE RAILS↑
		RN	BED↓			RN	B E D↓			RN	BED↓

• REQUIRES DOCUMENTATION

MEDICAL RECORD

Source: Form 302, © 1977 St. Luke's Hospital Medical Center. Used with permission.

Exhibit 9-3 Staffing Matrix—*Registered Nurses*

Full-time equivalent personnel required per patient day = 0.267 (I) + 0.319 (II) + 0.400 (III) + 0.533 (IV) + 0.800 (V)*

Number of Patients	Patient Acuity Classification				
	1	2	3	4	5
1	.267	.319	.400	.533	.800
2	.534	.638	.800	1.066	1.600
3	.801	.957	1.200	1.599	2.400
4	1.068	1.276	1.600	2.132	3.200
5	1.335	1.595	2.000	2.665	4.000
6	1.602	1.914	2.400	3.198	4.800
7	1.859	2.233	2.800	3.731	5.600
8	2.136	2.552	3.200	4.264	6.400
9	2.403	2.871	3.600	4.797	7.200
10	2.670	3.190	4.000	5.330	8.000

*Note (I) (II) (III) (IV) (V) = Number of patients in respective acuity classification

Source: St. Luke's Hospital Medical Center, Phoenix, Arizona. Used with permission.

responsibilities and accountability. A decentralized plan permits and requires maximum involvement on the part of unit nurse managers, staff, and personnel in planning, problem-solving, doing and controlling matters of staffing and scheduling. Experience indicates that decentralization (in the context described here) not only provides for more effective staffing and scheduling but also contributes to a greater economy of operation.

The three broad categories of patient/client groupings (primary, secondary, and tertiary care) influence the ways in which nursing staff and personnel are assigned for patient care purposes. A program caseload is most characteristic of community (public) health agencies. Centralized staffing and/or unit cluster staffing are more characteristic in secondary and tertiary care facilities (hospitals, nursing homes, and skilled care facilities).

Unit cluster staffing is most applicable in medium to large-size hospitals and other agencies where like kinds of patient care units can be grouped together into clusters. The surgical intensive care unit (SICU), coronary care unit (CCU), and medical intensive care unit (MICU) may make up an intensive nursing cluster. Or the obstetrical care units of delivery, postpartum, nursery, and pediatrics may form a family-centered care cluster.

Each unit cluster is responsible for its own staffing. Staff are not floated off the cluster, nor is extra help provided from outside the cluster—unless a true emergency or disaster occurs. This means that the clusters take care of their own needs and problems and are responsible and accountable to one another for the smooth operation of the unit. Peer pressure is most effective in coping with the occasional "problem staff member" who calls in sick frequently and without just cause. This arrangement also takes care of unplanned personal leave time by permitting personnel to swap time with peers.

Unit cluster staffing can be effective from the standpoint of patient care, employee satisfaction, recruiting, and cost containment. Staff members are recruited for specific job openings in a specific cluster. Staff and personnel are oriented to the few patient care units in the cluster, and therefore work in familiar areas where they are knowledgeable. This assures a safer level of patient care. New nursing personnel are assured at the time of employment that they will be expected to float only within the cluster, except in extreme emergencies. Thus the cluster becomes a satisfying workworld.

4. *Scheduling of staff.* How flexible and innovative are you in using scheduling options—flextime; 12-hour shifts; minishifts; four-day, ten-hour shifts; part-time scheduling; or seasonal arrangements? As with the first three factors, nurse managers first must be convinced that they have some options—that choice among these options does make a difference in patient outcome, cost per unit of service, and employee job satisfaction—and that they have an opportunity and responsibility to influence such fundamental decisions. These options are described in readings included in the Reading List at the end of this chapter. See also the section on scheduling later in this chapter.

5. *Mix of personnel.* What kinds and levels of nursing staff and personnel are required and available? How many of each kind are needed? Clearly, the choices exercised in the first four factors affect the answer to this question. One version of the numbers game is to treat staffing problems as though they were determined by Factors 1 and 5 only and can be solved by exercises in addition, multiplication, and division. However, such a view is simplistic and unrealistic.

Admittedly, even with the right mix of personnel, there may be problems of absenteeism, excessive use of sick time, and high turnover. Such evidence of employee disaffection may stem from (and lead to) ill-advised floating of personnel, lack of job satisfaction, and a failure to consider employee needs—thereby continuing a vicious cycle. These problems tend to be symptomatic of significant weaknesses in the nursing-care system, the organizational structure, or the caliber of managerial leadership. Hence, the nursing administration must work to permit a blending of organizational goals with the needs and desires of individuals. Staffing issues can then be dealt with in a balanced managerial perspective.

6. *Budget.* Are available funds well utilized? This is a sound starting point, different from "How much more money do we need in order to give the kind of nursing care we believe our patients/clients need?" Budgetary planning and control is an ongoing, year-round process. An adequate budget is the result of appropriate planning of patient-care programs in the context of Factors 1 through 5 as they apply in your healthcare setting.

Certainly the management of staffing and budgeting is one of *logistics*—defined as "the procurement, distribution, maintenance, and replacement of material and personnel." That takes money; it's a matter of getting it and spending it—wisely.

In summary, staffing the nursing department continues to be a major concern of nursing administrators. Quality of patient care, labor costs and job satisfaction are the factors that must be balanced. Approaches to staffing range from maintaining the status quo (when quality of care is not jeopardized) to treating staffing as a problem of supply and demand (availability of nursing staff versus patient-care workload). Such approaches, by themselves, can be useful in particular circumstances. And nurse managers, like other managers, learn to "play the numbers game" when that becomes the accepted way to adapt to change.

In the long run, however, the resolution of staffing problems requires a more sophisticated managerial analysis and follow-through by nursing administration. Today's nurse manager recognizes that optimum staffing is achieved in any patient-care unit (or group of units) only when there is an appropriate balance among a variety of influencing factors. Wages and number of patients are only two elements in this scheme.

An organizational approach to staffing is different from a purely mechanistic approach. Adequate numbers of staff are important in relation to your nursing system and patient needs. Sufficient money in the budget *is* essential—but only in relation to effective utilization of all resources in a modern management context. More RNs may *be* vital—but only if total numbers of staff are not increased (depending upon the other factors involved) unrealistically.

The workworld of today's professional nurse manager is a dynamic, changing one. Nurse managers should no longer be locked into a conventional fixed budget with control by line items based on simplistic work measurement. The nurse manager who understands how the six factors interact to influence staffing can provide better patient care at lower cost. This approach is characterized by a truly flexible budget, a commitment to a maximum (not-to-exceed) cost per unit of service, and the ability to make shift-by-shift daily adjustments in staffing and scheduling as circumstances dictate.

The nurse manager, therefore, should ask, "How can I best meet the 24-hour needs of the patients in my unit(s)?"

The first step in answering this question may be to encourage change in the habits and attitudes of those who now decide staffing and scheduling matters. The time is coming when the professional nurse manager for a patient-care unit or unit cluster will contract with the director of nursing or hospital administrator for an agreed-upon nursing cost per patient day. This becomes the budget of that unit or unit cluster. Such a budget is realistic and recognizes the nurse manager as a professional decision maker. Such a manager is able to evaluate the six factors discussed above and take the appropriate short- and long-range actions to provide for patient-care needs.

DOING

The implementation of staffing plans initially involves the recruiting, hiring, and orientation of new nursing staff and other nursing personnel at all levels within the nursing department or division. Many RNs are recruited into their first jobs directly upon graduation from nursing school. Many of these nurses experience what Kramer has identified as "reality shock" as they move from an educational to a work environment. Kramer defines reality shock as "the phenomenon and the specific shocklike reactions of new workers when they find themselves in a work situation for which they have spent several years preparing, and for which they thought they were prepared, and then suddenly find that they are not" (Kramer, 1974, pp. vii, viii). The author summarizes the impact of reality shock by noting,

> It will not go away by ignoring it. It will continue to take its toll, both in terms of personal loss and in the loss that nurses who leave might have made toward achievement of our common goal. Reality shock has not been extensively studied before nor studied in an organized manner. Second-culture learning is not something that can be accomplished in school, although the school can do much to begin the role transformation and to motivate the student to develop the tools useful in adapting to and learning new subcultures (Kramer, 1974, p. 233).

Of course, it is extremely important to the nurse manager that the RNs successfully bridge the gap between school and the workworld. Failure to understand and help the new graduate may contribute to two very real problems—turnover and burnout.

Turnover is a fact of life for the majority of nurse managers. Here are some statistics to consider:

> In the metropolitan areas, where job change is easier due to proximity and number of choices, the turnover rate sometimes reaches 150 to 200 percent. It would seem that many nurses change jobs, hoping to find a difference, but generally find the new position quite like the previous one—and quite as frustrating.

> - The National Commission on Nursing and Nursing Education (1970) estimated that the staff R.N. turnover rate was 70% per year.
> - An HEW study ("The Geographic Distribution of Nurses," 1973) found that the mean number of workdays a new, inexperienced R.N. spent on the job before assuming full responsibilities was 39.1, or about eight work-weeks.

> Therefore, if the actual turnover rate is 70%, the average position is filled each 68 weeks, and the new, inexperienced employee is not fully productive 12% of the average tenure (Rowland, 1978, p. 103).

Turnover analysis and control are surprisingly unsophisticated in many organizations. Sometimes the statistics themselves are meaningless or misleading. A most useful guide is *The study of turnover* (Price, 1977). This book presents codifications of the literature about organizational turnover, defines types of turnover measures, and includes research findings. It deserves careful reading by nurse managers considering turnover in the context of the Framework for Nursing Management.

Nurse managers seek ways to keep turnover to a minimum. Some turnover is inevitable. The distinction has been made between *unavoidable* turnover due to family responsibilities (such as marriage, beginning a family, transfer of spouse) and *avoidable* turnover due to unrecognized or unmet needs of nurses by the hospital organization (Tirney, 1976). Avoidable turnover is wasteful, time consuming, and costly. It involves the all-too-familiar labors of recruiting, hiring, orienting, training, and paperwork—as well as the less obvious costs of disruption of patient unit group work and lowered morale of remaining staff and personnel. Zander, writing about primary nursing, refers to *burnover* as follows:

> BURNOVER is another legacy which can either add weight to the rationale for primary nursing or work against it. Burnover is a com-

bination of the professional hazard of "Burnout" (Shubin, 1978) and the institutional problem of turnover. When nurses cannot find within themselves (or in the resources available to them) the strength to balance their ideals with reality, they burn out and become one of an astounding percentage of nurses who leave positions every year. If a nursing department has a firm commitment to primary nursing, including the use of specific built-in resources, primary nursing has the potential of decreasing burnover (Zander, 1980).

It isn't surprising that a syndrome like *burnout* should arise in today's fast-paced, demanding, everchanging healthcare climate. It is a destructive mode of behavior in which the nurse becomes disillusioned, turns conflict inward, and becomes burned out. According to Kramer and Schmalenberg (1977) the nurse who is burned out may appear calm while inwardly frustrated, sometimes becoming a chronic complainer who never really resolves conflict—an unhealthy person.

The nurse manager needs to be aware of burnout before it progresses too far. Like reality shock, it is a real phenomenon and will not just fade away of its own accord. During the role transformation from student to working graduate, the nurse must go through occupational socialization. According to Kramer (1974), this is the process by which people learn to perform the various roles required of them. The socialization process can be facilitated by good judgment on the part of socialization agents in the workplace.

Recruitment

Recruiting professional nurses is an essential part of staffing within the management function of *doing*. Recruitment in the broadest sense includes the hiring, training, and retaining of a competent nursing staff. It is a major challenge to the nurse manager.

Today's competitive healthcare marketplace dictates a comprehensive recruitment program that will *assess* what you have to offer and what is available, *plan* a recruitment strategy, *implement* that strategy, and *evaluate* the results of the entire recruitment effort. A sophisticated, hard-selling, and knowledgeable professional nurse recruiter can help the nurse manager stay ahead of—or just keep up with—the competition. Professionally designed, highly attractive employment packages can help the recruiter in this effort.

In small community hospitals where hiring a full-time recruiter is not viewed as practical, a part-time person is sometimes used. In any event, the following guidelines (adapted from *101 Tremendous Trifles*, Ganong & Ganong, 1979, p. 90a) can be helpful to the nurse manager.

1. *ASSESS.* Take a critical/analytical look at yourself, your department, your healthcare agency, and your community. Prepare a *balance sheet*: list the assets (all of them) and liabilities (all of them) as viewed by your present staff. Involve your RNs in preparing the lists. An organized approach involves using the two audit forms shown as Exhibit 4-1 (Chapter 4) and as Exhibit 13-1 (Chapter 13).

Ask yourself:

Knowing all the plus and minus items, would you want to live and work here?

What kind of nurse-persons do you want to join you?

What will be your *selling pitch* to potential nurse applicants?

What will you emphasize? Play down? Hide? (What risks will you take?)

How will you answer the following questions from applicants?

- "Will I be able to work on the service of my choice?"
- "Will I have to float? Rotate shifts?"
- "What kind of nursing do you have?"
- "What nursing modality do you use? Is it the same on all units?"
- "Do you have a problem-oriented nursing care plan?"
- "Will I be able to manage the nursing care of my patients?"
- "Is your nursing department centralized? Decentralized?"
- "What kind of nurse/doctor relations exist?"
- "Is nursing leadership strong or weak?"
- "What continuing education and inservice opportunities exist?"
- "Do you have optional career ladders (clinical, management, education, and research tracks)?"
- (Add other questions asked by applicants.)

2. *PLAN.* Review your recruiting methods. List each of the different ways you recruit. Tally (for the past three years) how many RNs were obtained by each method—including word of mouth, walk-ins, and so forth. Arrange the list in order of success, from best to worst. Then figure the total costs involved for each recruitment method, including direct expenses and labor costs (estimating, as necessary, if your three-year records are incomplete). Then divide *costs* by *number hired* to get the *cost-per-hire* for each method.

What do you learn from this? How does this compare with the method of recruiting other professionals (medical residents and interns, pharmacists, social workers, etc.)? List ways of recruiting you have not exploited: nursing job fairs (regional, national), career days at your own agency, referrals by own staff nurses, job-specific advertising (*not* "Nurses Wanted"), use of your best nursing professionals (who project the right appeal for specific nurses) for selected recruiting activities, directly approaching the nurse you want, teaching contacts at schools and colleges, teaching and speaking by yourself and by staff, and a planned schedule of news releases featuring nurses and professional nursing.

How well do your past, present, and possible future recruitment efforts reflect the realities of your situation? Is your approach one of "hiring someone to come work for you," or are you "attracting someone to come practice their profession with you?" Develop a theme, a brief statement of the image your agency/department has or is building toward. Some examples are *Excellence in Nursing; Tops in Patient Care; The Hospital That Cares:* and *People Caring for People.* Use this theme in all your literature, advertising, letterheads, new releases, and other printed materials.

Prepare your sales kit with all the foregoing in mind. Prepare your nurse recruiter to know your short- and long-range goals and what kinds of persons you need when for specific RN positions. Prepare your RN staff members who will assist in the total effort; and especially challenge your nurse managers to compete for the nurse applicants whom *they* need.

Use role-playing sessions to help test your materials and approaches and to help develop recruiting/interviewing/selling skills. Practice the professional approach—MASTER salesmanship—to achieve your recruitment sales goals.

M—Make ready (know the needs of your RN prospects)
A—Approach with benefits (for your prospect)
S—Stimulate desire (help the RN prospect *want* to buy)
T—Tell facts (so that assets outweigh negatives)
E—Eliminate retardants (foresee obstacles to action)
R—Request action ("May I take your application now?")

Clearly you need a good product to offer to good prospects. This means you may have to review your total nursing program in terms of what today's graduate nurse seeks in terms of professional practice opportunities. Our *Framework for Nursing Management* (Chapter 2) summarizes the pertinent components of such a review. See also our *Nursing Organization Inventory Checklist* (Figure 13-1). You may need to spend time, effort, and money to update your department and program, but the long-term results will provide a most favorable cost/benefit ratio in terms of *recruiting, training,* and *retaining* a qualified staff to practice professional nursing.

A *Program Performance Plan* will help plan the necessary steps including, as pertinent: revisions affecting nursing modalities appropriate for individual units; staffing and scheduling practices (unit cluster staffing, bidding system for permanent shifts); decentralization of responsibility and authority; specific development of nurse managers; career ladder options, staff development; job and salary evaluation; performance evaluation; and much else. This is because successful recruitment is directly related to all other aspects of human resources management and patient care management. See Chapter 5 on MBO and "Administrator must share authority" (Bennett, 1980).

3. *IMPLEMENT the recruitment program.* The Program Performance Plan becomes your *recruiting implementation guide*, just as a nursing care plan (based upon skillful patient assessment) is your *nursing implementation guide* for individual patients. Instructions for and examples of program performance plans are included elsewhere. Once your plan is developed, *use* it. Update, adjust, and revise it periodically—just as you would a nursing care plan.

4. *EVALUATE your recruitment effort.* Keep a complete running record of all recruitment-related time, expenses, actions (visits, presentations, interviews, follow-through, on-site visits by applicants, applications submitted), offers made/accepted/rejected, hires, employment records, employee care plans developed, length of service after hire—in short, all the details that permit a meaningful evaluation of your recruitment program.

An article published in 1979 provides strong support for the marketing approach to recruiting which we had built into the foregoing guidelines in 1978. The author describes a study he conducted with a hospital to determine if marketing can help recruit and retain nurses. He reports as follows:

The discussions indicated clearly that recruiting was only 25 percent of the problem, so that most of the effort should be on the problem of retention. In marketing terms this is the problem of brand *loyalty*. Keeping customers once they have been attracted may be cheaper than attracting new ones. Similarly, it may be cheaper to retain nurses than to recruit and train new nurses continuously.

To illustrate how the marketing process may be translated into the dual problems of recruiting and retaining nurses, the critical questions were stated in terms of nursing problems, with the marketing counterpart noted in parentheses. Four critical questions were identified as follows:

1. What personal needs do nurses (customers) wish to fulfill in choosing among hospitals (brands)? How important are these needs to nurses?

2. What sources of information do nurses use when choosing a hospital (brand) as a place to work?
3. Do the attitudes of present nurses (customers) within the several nursing services (market segments) indicate problems that may produce a high turnover rate (low brand loyalty)?
4. What job (brand) benefits should be added to attract new nurses (customers) and retain the present ones? . . .

Six months and then several years after the research report was submitted the author conducted follow-up interviews to see if the findings had been applied. The feedback was heartening. A team approach was being used to staff the services. Inservice training was decentralized to the level of specific nursing services. The monetized utility data had been used to support budget requests. Turnover had been reduced. While marketing research cannot take all of the credit, it did provide important information for the decisions that produced the results.

In conclusion, the success of this application of marketing research techniques was in seeing the parallels between the critical questions in marketing and those in the recruiting and retention of nurses. These parallels made it possible to apply or adapt research techniques with known properties. Using known techniques lowers the costs and increases the probability that research will improve decision making (Hughes, 1979, pp. 61-62; 65).

Clearly recruitment efforts must pay off in terms of retention if they are to be cost effective.

Staffing for nursing services aimed toward recruitment without due consideration for retention is meaningless. The director of nursing is cognizant of the many critical considerations that are required to implement and sustain a responsive staffing program. These dimensions require astute attention if nursing is to achieve its mission well in advance of the sophisticated and often ritualistic mechanisms associated with staffing for nursing care (Ferguson, 1977, p. 49).

Consultation and workshop programs help some nursing departments become more professional and successful with their recruiting/retention efforts. One such program is that of Dolores Ziff and Tina Filoromo of the Institute of Pennsylvania Hospital in Philadelphia, "Fundamentals of Developing a Professional Nurse Recruitment Program." See also Ziff and Filoromo, 1980 in Notes.

Temporary Nurse Personnel

Nurse managers face new problems caused by the increasing use of nurse registries for temporary nurses. The changed life styles of a new breed of people are partly responsible. But nursing department policies and hospital employment practices have encouraged the growth of the registries so that today they are big business.

> Hospitals' concern about registries is rising as their use increases. A recent American Hospital Assn. survey of 47 state hospital associations showed that hospitals in 32 states were increasing their use of registry nurses. In some hospitals, registry personnel make up an estimated 50% of nursing staff. One hospital chain spokesman said use of registry nurses has increased the chain's nursing costs by $750,000 (LaViolette, 1979, p. 38).

In response to this concern, some hospitals and hospital associations are forming their own registries. The Joint Commission on the Accreditation of Hospitals includes a section in Standard II on evaluation of temporary nurses from outside sources. (See Appendix K.) Hospitals around the country are trying to cut back on the use of outside registries because of increased costs.

Beyond the immediate problem of what to do about the registries themselves is the larger problem of meeting growing demands for higher salaries, more flexible hours of work, and greater job satisfaction. Rak, the Director of Illinois Hospital Association registry, pinpoints this issue:

> The ultimate solution to hospitals' loss of nurses to registries is to raise nursing wages, make hours more flexible, and offer nurses more meaningful rewards, IHA's Ms. Rak believes. Hospital nursing is "long hours and it's crazy hours and it's low pay," she said. Hospitals are "going to have to do something to make it very attractive" (LaViolette, 1979, p. 39).

Where temporary help is used, nurse managers must integrate the part-time workers with full-time staff and personnel to meet staffing demands and patient care requirements. In the long run, the problems of staffing and scheduling will be resolved most effectively by those nursing departments which implement the concepts of patient care management, operational management, and human resources management set forth in this book. There are no shortcuts.

Helen Hoesing, formerly Patient Care Administrator of Memorial Hospital of Dodge County, Fremont, Nebraska (245 beds), used some innovative approaches to staffing and scheduling. One of these is Cycle Bidding. This and other staffing methods are described in Ms. Hoesing's policies and procedures:

> *Cycle Bidding*—Full-time and part-time employees, following the three-month probationary period, are eligible to bid and receive a posted four-week repeating cycle. Their cycle will not be changed and they will not be required to float to other units or rotate to other shifts. During low census periods they are given the choice of taking an extra "zero plus" day or moving to another unit.
>
> *Float Pool*—Full-time and part-time employees that are not eligible or do not wish to take advantage of cycle bidding are automatically a member of the float pool. To maintain sufficient coverage for each shift, float pool employees are assigned a staffing cycle and following appropriate orientation may be floated to other units and/or scheduled to rotate to a two- or four-week cycle on other shifts. Rotation scheduling will begin with employees having the most recent date of hire (the least number of hours worked if dates of hire are the same) and the need for a full-time or part-time replacement.
>
> *Available Staffing*—To provide additional staffing on a short notice basis, employees may be needed on an "available" basis in certain highly flexible patient census areas such as Labor and Delivery, ICU, Pediatrics, and East Wing. Employees are scheduled as "available" and report for duty within thirty minutes of receiving notice. Minimum compensation is four hours for an eight hour shift paid at the employee's normal rate of pay. Cycle bidding, float pool, and labor pool employees are eligible for available staffing.
>
> *Labor Pool Staffing*—Employees submit the dates and shifts they are able to work and are scheduled or called for duty based on patient staffing needs. Labor pool employees are classified as "standby" employees, do not have a staffing cycle, are not guaranteed any amount of working hours and are ineligible for benefits (Memorial Hospital of Dodge County, 1978, p. 1).

Approximately 70 percent of the nursing department employees use the bid basis. The percentage has grown steadily since it was adopted two and one-half years ago. This, and other progressive policies, have kept Hoesing's department well supplied with nurses and other personnel.

Orientation

To orient means to familiarize with or adjust to a situation. It follows that orientation in nursing is a process of becoming acquainted with and adjusting to your new workworld. Because hospitals are the largest employer of nurses (approximately two-thirds of employed RNs work in hospitals), there is a never-ending need for orientation as nurses are recruited and hired into the hospital system. Orientation in its broadest sense, however, is a very real part of any person's workworld in any healthcare setting including hospital, nursing home, clinic, community/public health agency, school, industrial plant, or private office. A new job, a new situation, and new responsibilities all require some orientation. For the majority of nurses, the first position to which they must become oriented is that of staff nurse. In addition to adequate orientation, a staff nurse also needs wise placement with a suitable nurse manager.

> The management of newly employed nurses' early experiences with their immediate supervisors is crucial to efficient, cost-effective staffing. In order to create a sound psychological contract between new staff nurses and their head nurses, both must clarify their expectations and explicitly communicate them to each other. Mismanagement of mismatched core expectations could lead to overconformity to the hospital's rule—"invisible employees" or "dead wood." Or it could lead to rebellion—individuals expending a great deal of energy rebelling against the hospital's expectations (Frohman, 1977, p. 41).

The author notes that in a hospital setting, the most critical period is the first six months. A part of that time is devoted to formal orientation—the orientation program.

The Orientation Program

The newly appointed nurse needs a formal orientation program. The following guidelines are adapted from Kathleen Bower's (1980) outline for developing such a program.

1. Reasons for Orientation
   - Philosophy
   - Purposes and objectives of an orientation program

- The relationship of the orientation program to Department of Nursing philosophy, goals and objectives, standards of nursing
- Nursing administration commitment to orientation

2. Development of the Orientation Program
   - Involvement of nursing staff
   - Development tasks
   - Relating classroom to clinical orientation
   - Transition problems of the new graduate and the experienced nurse
   - Focus on the adult learner and identified needs

3. Orientation Objectives
   - Purpose of objectives
   - Core and clinical objectives
   - Developing orientation objectives
   - Involvement in developing objectives
   - Revision of objectives and orientation program
   - Orientation manuals and reference resources
   - Evaluating the orientee using orientation objectives

4. Roles in the Orientation Process
   - The nurse administrator and associates
   - Clinical coordinators
   - Head nurses
   - Staff education department
   - The orientee
   - Other staff members

5. Discussion of Common Problems in Orientation
   - Departmental level
   - Unit level

6. Materials for Orientation
   - Needs identification form
   - Orientation packet/manual
   - Core orientation schedule
   - Clinical orientation schedule
   - Evaluation tools

The Orientation Time Frame

Length of time for orientation varies from two to six weeks or longer, according to the beliefs and demands of the organization. Planned time usually includes classroom and clinical activities that provide opportunities for information-sharing and practical skill application. Some time is devoted to the patient unit where the orientee will be assigned. The attitudes of present staff members can make the difference between a productive experience and a disastrous one. The nurse manager and staff members can do much to create a welcoming environment for their newest colleagues.

Remember—never again will nurses be in such a receptive frame of mind as when they first come to work for you. They are eager, ready, and willing to learn. They are highly motivated and want to make a good impression. How you treat each one—as a *child*, or as an *adult* professional *peer*—makes a great difference. You can "win them" or "lose them" immediately.

Organizing Daily Patient Care: An Orientation Challenge

Regardless of the modality of nursing care (functional, team, modular, total care, or primary), most new nurses have to learn how to organize themselves and put the nursing process into action. These skills should be reviewed, taught, and practiced during the orientation process. The problem is most acute when the new nurse is responsible for a specified caseload of patients.

The new nurse can use the nursing process as a guide to the patient care management process. Both are built on the same scientific model (Ganong and Ganong, 1978).

Nursing Process	*Everyday Language*	*Management Process*	
• Assess	• Size up the situation	• Get facts, consider options	*(Plan)*
		• Make a decision	
• Plan	• Decide what to do	• Take action	*(Do)*
• Implement	• Do it	• Measure results, replan	*(Control)*
• Evaluate	• Determine how well it worked		

Here are some organizational guidelines to help the new nurse plan/give/evaluate each patient's care. *First,* size up the situation by *assessing* each patient's problems, needs, and goals. Focus on what the patient requires rather than on tasks and procedures as such. One nurse may have responsibility for ten or more patients (in functional or team nursing). This demands as much organizing ability as is required of a primary nurse with 24-hour responsibility for only four to eight patients.

Second, having considered the options, decide what to do by *planning* to take care of patient needs within the time available and with the assigned assisting personnel. This means establishing priorities and making decisions based on these priorities. Accept the fact that it is not possible to accomplish everything desired for each patient during any one shift, or even during a 24-hour period. Assign and utilize available resources (time, personnel, equipment, facilities, money) for the benefit of the patients.

Third, implement these plans. Implementation is a series of ongoing activities and may require more innovative thinking than any other phase. The never-attainable ideal is for one nurse to have full responsibility for each individually-assigned patient. This means the RN, when on duty, may carry out most direct patient care. This helps assure effective use of the four main aspects of work simplification—eliminate, combine, change sequence, simplify—and requires constant assessment of what is *essential* for each patient as opposed to what is *desirable* or *nice-to-do.* In any event, principles of delegation must be used for all those actions, based on the care plans, which are to be carried out by someone other than the nurse.

The *fourth* step is *evaluation.* Evaluation has to be both specific and constant. It occurs naturally, as part of each day's activities, and by plan, as each identified patient problem receives attention.

The major tools available to the nurse in organizing a workday are: a systematic way of thinking; standards of nursing practice; the nursing care plan; the components of a problem-oriented nursing system; and skills in identifying problems, establishing priorities, sequencing events, making decisions, delegating, and coordinating. (See Exhibit 9-4 for a schematic summary of organizational tools.)

The nurse manager can help the new nurse by being a role model/teacher/counselor. The inexperienced nurse can become an effective organizer of a patient caseload most easily when the nurse manager structures the environment to facilitate the nurse's planning/doing efforts.

- Geographic patient care areas are set up as districts (modules, pods).
- RN stays in assigned district with his/her patients.
- Aides, by whatever title, service the rooms with needed supplies and equipment.
- Instead of leaving the district, the RN uses existing patient call system to contact centrally-located unit clerk for needs.
- Nursing flow sheets, progress notes (and medical records when possible), are located at the patient's room.
- Other features of Nurserver (Friesen concept; Friesen & Silvin, 1975) are adopted as feasible (Blome, 1978).

Scheduling

"The success of a scheduling effort is contingent upon achieving balanced staffing each day of the week to meet the patient care needs" (West, 1979). In order to carry out a carefully devised staffing program, the schedules must provide for the right people in the right places at the right times. Staff and personnel are assigned to patient care units by hourly patterns. Each unit has a written schedule that is maintained on a daily basis.

Exhibit 9-4 A Schematic Summary for New RNs in How to Organize Daily Patient Care

RN Action	Nursing/Management Process			
	Assess	Plan	Implement	Evaluate
Upon arrival, the RN·				
1. reviews patient charts quickly for events, actions on nursing care plans, patient outcomes, changes in medical care plan.	•			•
2. visits each patient for observation and question/answer update; verifies/changes assessment of problems and needs.	•		•	•
3. revises/confirms nursing orders or care plans.		•		
4. reviews patient status, medical and nursing orders with nursing staff who will be assisting.		•		
Then the RN:				
1. implements plans, including diagnostic and therapeutic procedures, medication, IVs.			•	
2. incorporates ADLs as appropriate and necessary.			•	
3. teaches patients and documents patient learning.	•	•	•	•
4. takes time for breaks and meals for self and assistants.			•	
5. observes patients, reviews progress, makes progress notes—factually and briefly (SOAP format helps).	•	•	•	•
6. makes rounds with doctors; has them write their own orders, just as RN does.	•	•	•	•
7. involves family in patient care, teaching/learning. Makes every contact, however brief, count.	•	•	•	•
8. cooperates with others in friendly, professional, helpful way.			•	

Source: Ganong, J., and Ganong, W. *101 tremendous trifles: A collection of management mini-guides.* 2nd ed. Chapel Hill, N.C.: W. L. Ganong Co., 1979, p. 76a.

It is essential that the decisions about changes in schedules be made by the nurse manager (head nurse, coordinator). The clerical aspects of scheduling can and should be performed by clerical personnel. Staffing secretaries perform an invaluable service in carrying out the decisions of the nurse manager by keeping careful records and making appropriate telephone calls when adjustments are necessary. But the staffing secretary should not be expected to carry the responsibility and authority for making scheduling decisions that will affect patient care.

Some guidelines are available to the nurse manager. Price (1970, p. 24) lists the following:

1. A core of personnel on duty at all times with a distribution between shifts and days of the week that is as consistent as possible in relation to patients' needs for care.
2. A pattern of shifts to be worked and days off duty that an employee is sure will not be changed by his employer except in extreme emergencies.
3. A means of temporarily changing an employee's work pattern, if he finds that necessary.
4. Fair and just treatment of all employees in regard to hours.
5. A method that takes the least possible amount of a nurse's time and that can easily be taught to others.

These guidelines indicate the importance of once again keeping a balance between the technical and human modes. This means realizing that scheduling is not just a "numbers game." Decisions about scheduling affect not only the patients but also the lives of nursing staff and personnel.

In 1979 Dr. E. M. Price introduced the new Price Plan for staffing and scheduling. It is the culmination of ongoing work during the 70s to develop a means of coping with changing trends in patient care, the workforce, and economic pressures. The Price Plan incorporates features of the 10-hour day, two 12-hour shifts, part-time scheduling, weekend-only work teams, and seasonal staffing/scheduling arrangements. Yet in its simplicity it goes beyond the mere combining or adaptation of these concepts and practices. It provides for four regularly assigned work groups, two for a day shift of $11\frac{1}{2}$ hours and two for a night shift of $11\frac{1}{2}$ hours, with a repetitive two-week schedule of 7 days of work and 7 days off every two weeks. No more than three successive work days are scheduled during the two-week period. The scheduling plan is shown in Exhibit 9-5.

Clearly such a plan has a great many advantages, and few disadvantages compared with other scheduling plans. It will provide great benefit for those nurse managers and administrators who have the initiative and motive force to introduce it and make it work.

Exhibit 9-5 *Total Unit Schedule:* (All groups repeat own schedule every two weeks)

		Week 1	Week 2
Days	Group A	T W S	S M T F
	Group B	S M T F	T W S
Nights	Group C	M T F S	S W T
	Group D	S W T	M T F S

Source: Price, E. M. *The Price Plan,* 1979. Privately printed and distributed by the author, 500 Evergreen, Inglewood, CA 90302. Used with permission.

Centralized Versus Decentralized Staffing and Scheduling

The decision to use a centralized or a decentralized staffing and scheduling program depends on many elements in the framework of nursing management (Chapter 2). The highly centralized organizational structure, for example, may call for staffing and scheduling decisions controlled at the administrative level. If decision making is decentralized to the unit clusters on individual patient care units, then decentralized staffing is more appropriate and economical. There are programs designed and in use for computerized scheduling with centralized staffing (Ballantyne, 1979). The authors of that system conclude that its success can be attributed to well-defined and well-implemented policies, and to a flexibility of programming that permits nursing to meet all the variables of staffing and scheduling for a large hospital. DiVincenti remarks that "even if scheduling is established by a computer, someone must check to see that the schedule is truly equitable and that it is compatible with actual needs" (1977, p. 131).

With decentralized staffing, each unit or cluster within the overall organization is an individual cost center, with the nurse manager (head nurse or coordinator) responsible for decisions about staffing and scheduling. It is possible and sometimes advisable to combine decentralized and centralized functions within a well planned staffing and scheduling program. Consideration has to be given to the size of the facility and the number and size of patient care units and clusters.

We have already indicated that the Unit Cluster staffing model is a highly effective way to decentralize both responsibility and authority to the patient unit level. Each cluster takes care of its own staffing and scheduling within the framework of overall organizational policies and procedures.

Shift Options

There is nothing magical about the eight-hour shift and the five-day work week. While it is necessary to stay within legal specifications, there are alternative scheduling possibilities. None is perfect. Some will work in one place with some people and will not work in other situations with other people. As a nurse manager, you have to determine what is best and possible in your given situation. The possibilities for variations in the work schedule are limited only by the constraints of technology, employee interest, and the imagination of the schedule designer (Cohen and Gadon, 1978). Some of the options are the 10-hour shift, the 12-hour shift, flextime, full-time weekends only, temporary help, and seasonal scheduling. Both full-time and part-time options are worthy of consideration. Hospital departments of nursing are making schedules more flexible in an attempt to keep their own nurses and establish part-time positions for nurses who are available with some notice prior to assignment (LaViolette, 1979, p. 51).

The Price Plan just described provides a unique example of a truly innovative shift arrangement. Another shift variation is the use of a weekend-only staff with two 2-day, 12-hour (or 12½ hour) shifts. The staff for these two Saturday/Sunday shifts are hired (or assigned) for this time period only and are considered as full-time employees. Each such employee works 24 hours per week, and is paid for 36 hours (4 hours at time-and-one-half overtime pay each shift) in the case cited—plus nearly full benefits of regular 40-hour per week employees ("A Full-time Job," 1979). With such a plan, imagine how much easier is the scheduling of the regular Monday-through-Friday shifts.

Another arrangement is covering one full-time position with two "regular part-time" employees who accept the responsibility for covering the total shift hours. Such staffing and scheduling options as those described have great potential for meeting staff requirements economically, especially when used within a policy structure which permits each patient care unit, or unit cluster, to develop a plan that best meets the needs of its patients and staff.

Staffing and Scheduling for Primary Nursing

Primary nursing dictates that each nurse be assigned a reasonable caseload of patients (see Chapter 4). For example, in staffing for a unit of 24 patients, the schedule may require four primary nurses to carry six patients each. This will necessitate enough associate nurses to accommodate the time-off and shift assignments of the primary nurses.

The primary nurse may be scheduled to work any shift. It is neither necessary nor advisable to have the primary nurse see and care for his/her patients only on the day shift. A better assessment of patient problems and needs can be made when the primary nurse sees the patient at different times during the 24-hour period of accountability. Support staff such as LPNs and nurse aides may also be scheduled to assist the primary or associate nurse to carry out the plan of care.

CONTROLLING

Staffing and scheduling, as part of the controlling function of the nurse manager, is an ongoing process of monitoring, evaluating, and adjusting the use of people and money in the interest of patient care. This requires an accurate, timely, and pertinent information system. According to West (1979), "A management information system is a group of periodic, retrospective monitoring tools designed to measure past performance and project future needs."

Using the Computer

The use of computers for staffing and scheduling is a reality for many hospital departments of nursing. Computer miniaturization, the result of dramatic changes in electronic technology, has opened the door to more extensive use. "The concept of employing dedicated computer systems distributed throughout an institution has only recently become economically and technologically feasible. In the past, hospital departments seeking computer support were faced with a limited number of options and oftentimes prohibitive costs" (Medicus Microsystems, Inc., 1979).

Computerized information systems are rapidly growing more sophisticated. Nurse managers must keep abreast of such developments.

> A minicomputer has been added to Medicus Microsystems, Inc.'s 5-year-old nurse staffing and quality monitoring system. ... The information system generates long-range and variable (day-to-day, shift-to-shift) staffing recommendations by assessing patient needs and staff capabilities. The system also accommodates a hospital's staffing pattern and quality standards. ...
>
> The Medicus system generates staffing recommendations by assigning values to nursing workloads and personnel capabilities based on the difficulty of handling various assignments. This analytical method was chosen over more widely used time studies because nursing workload is affected by many complex factors not related to time, according to developers of the Medicus system. The

system also incorporates a hospital's staffing pattern goals and adjusts staffing recommendations to accommodate a hospital's quality goals.

The system's quality monitoring index was developed by Medicus and Rush-Presbyterian-St. Luke's Medical Center under a two-year HEW grant awarded in 1972. The computer system scores the quality of care delivered by individual nursing units, providing feedback on the effect of staffing decisions (*Modern Healthcare*, May 1979, p. 85).

Control of staffing and scheduling goes hand in hand with cost containment and annual budgetary planning (see Chapter 8).

Another aspect of the controlling function is evaluation. Criteria for the evaluation of the total staffing program are delineated by the ANA Commission on Nursing Services as follows:

1. The quality assurance program (nursing audit) demonstrates that the objectives of care are met. If they are not met, analysis of the audit findings indicates that factors other than staffing were the cause of the failure to meet standards.
2. The nursing staff meets established performance standards. If they do not meet performance standards, the staff's failure to perform adequately is due to conditions other than excessive work load.
3. Staffing patterns for nursing units adhere in practice to predetermined patterns. There is evidence of utilization of staff at predetermined levels. The daily variability of staffing is within ranges agreed upon in advance.
4. Based upon evidence gathered through a predetermined evaluation system to assess satisfaction, the nursing staff expresses satisfaction with the scheduling and assignments.
5. The cost of staffing is within the limits determined as a result of the application of the methodology.
6. The patterns for staffing have been re-examined for adequacy at regular intervals on the basis of current staffing standards, statistics, and changing needs, trends, and practices (ANA, 1977, p. 8).

NOTES

A full-time job—weekends only. *Business Week*, October 15, 1979, pp. 150–152.

American heritage dictionary of the English language. Boston: American Heritage, Houghton Mifflin, 1973.

American Nurses' Association Commission on Nursing Services. *Nursing Staff requirements for in-patient health services.* Kansas City: Author, 1977.

Ballantyne, D. A computerized scheduling system with centralized staffing. *Journal of Nursing Administration,* March 1979, *9*(3), 38–45.

Bennett, A. C. Administrator must share authority. *Modern Healthcare*, February 1980, *10*(2), 90.

Blome, M. (Vice President, Portland Adventist Hospital, Portland, Oregon) Unpublished interview, 1978.

Bower, K. *Management of professional orientation in nursing.* Aspen Systems Corp., ms. in preparation.

Cisarik, J. M., Higgerson, N. J., & Van Slyck, A. *A patient classification system for staffing and charging for nursing services.* Phoenix: St. Luke's Hospital Medical Center, 1978.

Cohen, A. R., & Gadon, H. *Alternative work schedules: Integrating individual and organizational needs.* Philippines: Addison-Wesley, 1978.

Computer expands staffing capabilities. *Modern Healthcare*, May 1979, *9*(5), 85. Reprinted with permission.

DiVincenti, M. *Administering nursing service* (2nd ed.). Boston: Little, Brown, 1977.

Ferguson, V. Critical considerations from the perspective of a nursing administrator. *Nursing Administration Quarterly*, Summer 1977, *1*(4), 49.

Friesen, G. & Silvin, R. Concepts of health planning. *World Hospitals,* Winter 1975, XI(1).

Frohman, A. L. More effective development for new nurses. *Nursing Administration Quarterly*, Summer 1977, *1*(4), 41. Reprinted with permission of Aspen Systems Corp.

Ganong, W., & Ganong, J. *101 tremendous trifles.* Chapel Hill, N.C.: W. L. Ganong Co., 1978.

Gots, R., & Kaufman, A. *The people's hospital book.* New York: Crown, 1978, pp. 78–79.

Hoesing, H. Memorial Hospital of Dodge County, 1978. Nursing Department Staffing and Scheduling Policies, 1978. Reprinted with permission.

Hughes, G. D. Can marketing help recruit and retain nurses? *Health Care Management Review,* Summer 1979, *4*(3). Reprinted with permission.

Kramer, M. *Reality shock: Why nurses leave nursing.* St. Louis: C. V. Mosby, 1974.

Kramer, M., & Schmalenberg, C. *Path to biculturalism.* Wakefield, Mass.: Contemporary Publishing, 1977, p. 21.

LaViolette, S. Does primary nursing offer solutions or cause problems? *Modern Healthcare,* August 1979, *9*(8).

LaViolette, S. Hospitals change registry game plan. *Modern Healthcare,* May 1979, (9)5, 38–39. Reprinted with permission.

Medicus Microsystems, Inc. Evanston, Ill.: Author, 1979.

Meyer, D. *GRASP: A patient information and workload management system.* Morganton, N.C.: MCS, Rt. 5, Box 326A, 1978.

Memorial Hospital of Dodge County. *Nursing Service Supplement to "Personnel Pointers".* Mimeographed, 1978, p. 1.

Price, E. M. *Staffing for patient care.* New York: Springer, 1970.

Price, E. M. *The Price plan for staffing and scheduling,* 1979. Privately printed and distributed by the author, 500 Evergreen, Inglewood, Cal., 90302.

Price, J. L. *The study of turnover.* Ames, Iowa: The Iowa State University Press, 1977.

Rowland, H. S. *The nurse's almanac.* Germantown, Md.: Aspen Systems Corp., 1978.

Tirney, T. R., & Wright, N. Minimizing the turnover problem: A behavioral approach. In S. Stone, M. S. Berger, D. Elhart, S. C. Firsich, & S. B. Jordan (Eds.), *Management for nurses: A multidisciplinary approach.* St. Louis: C. V. Mosby, 1976, pp. 219-228.

West, E. M. Manpower control system for the nursing division. Unpublished manuscript. Nashville, Tenn.: Hospital Affiliates International, Inc., 1979, pp. 3, 6, 7, 127. Reprinted with permission.

Zander, K. *Primary nursing: Development and management.* Germantown, Md.: Aspen Systems Corp., 1980.

Ziff, D., & Filoromo, T. *Nurse recruitment: Strategies for success.* Germantown, Md.: Aspen Systems Corp., 1980. Ms. in preparation.

Reading List

Books

Froebe, D. J., & Bain, R. J. *Quality assurance programs and controls in nursing.* St. Louis: C. V. Mosby, 1976.

National League for Nursing. *Nursing service in a specialty, a rural, and an urban hospital.* New York: Author, 1979.

Nursing staff requirements for in-patient health care services. American Nurses' Association, 1977.

Staffing: A JONA reader. Wakefield, Mass.: Contemporary Publishing, 1974.

Staffing 2. Wakefield, Mass.: Contemporary Publishing, 1975.

Staffing 3. Wakefield, Mass.: Contemporary Publishing, 1976.

Worstler, M. E. (Ed.). *Staffing: A journal of nursing administration reader.* Wakefield, Mass.: Contemporary Publishing, 1974.

Articles

Brown, B. (Gen. Ed.). Staffing: Part I. *Nursing Administration Quarterly,* Summer 1977, *1*(4), entire issue.

Ganong, J., & Ganong, W. Staffing and scheduling: "Numbers game" or nursing management? *Health Services Manager,* December 1978, pp. 6-7.

Giovannetti, P. Understanding patient classification systems. *Journal of Nursing Administration.* February 1979, *9*(2), 4-9.

Graham, R. Permanent part-time work. Review Magazine, April 1979, *4*(4), 44-63.

Liebmann, R. S. Resort hospitals use flexible summer staffing. *Health Care Week,* July 24, 1978, *2*(3), 9.

Miller, S. Letter from a new graduate. *American Journal of Nursing,* October 1978, *78*(10), 1688-1689.

Roehrl, P. K. Patient classification a pilot test. *Supervisor Nurse,* February 1979, *10*(2), 21-27.

Simendinger, E. A., & Gilbert, V. Flexible staffing. *Supervisor Nurse,* March 1979, *10*(3), 43-46.

Part IV

Human Resources Management

Chapter 10

Motivational Management in Nursing

THE IMPORTANCE OF MOTIVATION

Everyone is motivated. You, the staff, personnel, patients, clients, family members—everybody. All the people who enter the healthcare arena for reasons of work or care bring with them all their own motivations, values, needs, knowledge, and skills. They come as workers to do, to help, to learn; or they come as patients for diagnosis, treatment, care, prevention of future health problems, and (increasingly) to become involved in the planning, implementing, and evaluating of their own care. The healthcare agency is a complex mixture of individuals with needs, problems, talents, feelings, faults, abilities, interests, and life styles. Their motivations are vital to a discussion of human resources management.

Chapra (1976) reports on a study of several thousand managers, supervisors, and their subordinates designed to learn what makes some of them more successful than others in accomplishing what they set out to do. He found that a characteristic of the more successful groups was their high degree of motivation. This was evident in their enthusiasm and their high level of interest and commitment, regardless of the nature of the task. The members of such groups were motivated to *work with each other*. They seemed to find working with each other to be enough of a satisfying experience, and they were willing and able to tackle almost any problem. The nurse manager needs to be able to build on each individual's motivation, whether weak or strong, for the good of all concerned. This means understanding what motivation is all about.

THEORIES OF MOTIVATION

A theory is simply someone's idea about something, usually based on considerable experience, study, and research. Thus a theory of motivation attempts to provide a valid explanation of why people act the way they do. This is not the same as "causation." Causes may be many and varied, but motivation generally deals with a single class of events that determine behavior. Motivation is different from ability, which also influences behavior. You may be *able* to do something but not *want* to do it. Or you may *want* to do something but be *unable* to do it. For example, if while driving your car a crisis situation arises and you want to avoid an accident, you may be able to do so only if you can respond with the necessary mental and physical reflexes and skill. Thus both desire and ability combine to affect what you do. Undoubtedly you can name a variety of other factors that influence your behavior. Motivation is ordinarily indicated by such words as want, wish, desire, need, and striving.

The names of a number of researchers and scientists are identified with theories of motivation and human effectiveness. M. Scott Myers in *Every Employee a Manager* summarizes these theories by giving the name of the person identified with each theory, then grouping them in three categories. The first category includes those theories that focus on managerial styles and assumptions; the second describes combinations of managerial style and management systems; and the third describes the impact or consequences of styles and systems. In addition, the theories are presented on a low-to-high scale representing conditions ranging from those conducive to ineffective behavior at one end to conditions for greater effectiveness at the other (Myers, 1970).

For example, Douglas McGregor's "Theory X" (reductive assumptions) is included as a managerial style having its impact at the ineffective end of the scale. "Theory Y" (developmental assumptions) is shown as leading to greater human effectiveness. Rensis Likert's "System 1" (exploitative, authoritative) is in the same group at the ineffective end of the scale, with "System 4" (participative group) at the high effectiveness end of the scale.

Chris Argyris's "Autocratic Relationships" (conflict and conformity, alienation) is in the second grouping, and ineffective. "Authentic Relationships" (interpersonal and technical competence, commitment) is high effectiveness. Frederick Herzberg's concept of motivation-through-the-work-itself is also in the second group. "Environmental Comfort" (hygiene seeking) is ineffective; "Meaningful Work" (motivation seeking) is more highly effective.

David McClelland's achievement motivation concept is in the third grouping. "Low Achievement" (more interest in things like affiliation, security, money, possessions) is less effective than "High Achievement" motivation (achievement is its own primary reward, high challenges, moderate risks, independence). Abraham Maslow's need hierarchy is also in the third group. "Lower-Need Fixation" (halted growth) is seen as providing lower human effectiveness than "Self-Actualization" (realizing potential).

Others included in Myers's summary are Blake, Hall, Bennis, Pare, Fromm, and Glasser. The comparison is most useful since all of the theories have the common purpose of defining conditions which inhibit or enhance the expression of human talent. These theories, all of them carefully tested, can help nurse managers understand conditions for improved goal orientation and for the reduced—or more constructive—use of authority in achieving performance results.

All nurse managers need to have a personally comprehensible basis for their actions. They need to understand their own behavior. Just as important is the need to comprehend the behavior of others, to predict such behavior insofar as possible, and to make decisions and take actions that are most likely to produce the desired results in terms of goals and objectives. Your own education and experiences in living and working have provided you with some useful understandings about human nature and motivation. We suggest, however, that as a nurse manager you have a responsibility to yourself, your people, and your agency to have a well-founded personal theory of motivation based upon your own experiences as well as upon the best research findings available to you.

We find that Maslow's theory works well for us. This theory sees human needs as a basis for understanding human motivation. It rings true. It jibes with our experience. It is easy to use. It is positive in its impact. It also provides an explanation for other motivational theories. It gets good results for us, and it can do the same for you. For these reasons, and because developing a sound working knowledge of Maslow's motivational ideas may be more useful to you than a smattering of knowledge about many theories, we focus on Maslow's work throughout this book. And we believe you will be able to adapt Maslow's theory to your own purposes. (See Appendix I.)

Motivation is a very personal matter. It stems from the needs of the individual. This is as true at work as it is in other areas of life. In a very real sense, then, you cannot motivate others; they motivate themselves. This helps to explain the frustration of so many managers, getting poor results in spite of their own dedicated efforts. "Why won't they do what I tell them? Why don't people care anymore? How can I ever get good work out of my people?"

Have you ever attempted to motivate another person only to discover that the other person (employee or patient) simply shows no evidence of being motivated? Have you asked yourself why your people seem not to respond; why they do not become motivated to do what you expect of them? Yet employees *are* motivated! They do act on the basis of what they feel as a desire, want, yearning, wish, or lack. The problem, of course, is that too often their actions (insubordination, lack of interest, aggressive and unruly behavior, carelessness, quitting the job, joining the union), in response to what they feel as their needs, seem inimical to administrative goals and not in the best interests of patient care. What is the manager to do? How is the manager to satisfy organizational and patient-care goals and at the same time help individuals satisfy their own personal needs and goals?

THE NURSE MANAGER'S USE OF MOTIVATIONAL TECHNIQUES

A motivational technique is a way of encouraging actions that will assist others in meeting their needs while helping to achieve patient care objectives. The nurse manager who comprehends motivational technique has a potent force available for use. The technique involves identifying the currently felt needs of the other person, then helping that person to get what he wants—insofar as that is possible. Needs which are frequently unsatisfied—or poorly satisfied at best—include recognition, sense of achievement, enjoyment of the work itself, responsibility, advancement, and growth. All of these are manifestations of the five Maslow-identified needs with which you are familiar.

Herzberg, Mausner, & Snyderman (1959) found that certain factors contribute to job satisfaction. They called them the "motivators" or satisfiers. They found that other factors (organization policy and administration, supervision, work conditions, wages) contribute to job dissatisfaction. These they called the hygiene or maintenance factors. Note that an improvement in one or more of the maintenance factors may remove some causes for dissatisfaction but not contribute to job satisfaction! The opposite of job dissatisfaction in this case is not job satisfaction but no job satisfaction. Similarly, the opposite of job satisfaction is not job dissatisfaction but no job satisfaction. This distinction is significant in understanding the authors' findings and their impact upon motivational efforts by nurse managers and healthcare administrators.

They examined and summarized the factors affecting job attitudes reported in 12 investigations. They tallied those factors characterizing 1,844 events on the job that led to extreme dissatisfaction, as well as those factors characterizing 1,753 events on the job that led to extreme satisfaction. The major factors, listed in rank order based upon their percentage frequency, are as follows:

Extreme Satisfaction	*Extreme Dissatisfaction*
1. Achievement	1. Company Policy and Administration
2. Recognition	2. Supervision
3. Work Itself	3. Relationship with Supervisor
4. Responsibility	4. Work Conditions
5. Advancement	5. Salary
6. Growth	6. Relationship with Peers

The motivational factors are not mutually exclusive. One builds on another. If employees express to you their need for advancement, you may find ways to allow them to grow and to recognize their achievement by recommending advancement. Then more than one motivator is being used. In each instance the individuals are being helped to meet their own human needs—and so they are self-motivated.

The use of such motivational factors can be a positive force in staying union free or in providing a better working climate in a unionized setting. The motivational factors must be understood and cultivated by the goal-oriented nurse manager. They may well become a part of your value structure and be built into your own goals and objectives for yourself at work. In addition, they deserve consideration when your agency, department, or unit sets goals and objectives.

Because motivation is such a personal thing and people's needs vary from individual to individual, all people do not necessarily respond to the same appeals. Some people do not actively seek more responsibility or growth, for example. These same people may find satisfaction enough in the work itself. Such persons deserve continued encouragement; they may comprise a large segment of your workforce and meet their performance requirements satisfactorily.

The nurse managers, then, have to know their people. What works for one person at one time may not work for another person, or, indeed, for the same person at another time. Human needs shift in their priority. So you will need to be aware of such shifts and how they blend with the needs of your organization. People will be committed to your agency goals and objectives when they can identify how these tie in with their own needs. This is essential for the realistic application of motivational management concepts. Your use of motivational techniques must be genuine and open. The rewards can be felt in terms of job satisfaction for you and your people as well as better results in patient care and the delivery of patient care services.

If you agree with all of the foregoing, you may be wondering (as a pragmatic nurse manager) how to make it work for you. First of all, recall one of Maslow's early conclusions: "Success and reward have a far more powerful effect upon motivation than failure or punishment" (Wilson, 1972). Second, follow the admonition of Peter Drucker, who said, "You cannot build on people's liabilities; you can build only on their assets" (Drucker, 1974). Third, identify and help people satisfy their felt needs. When you comprehend, believe, and act upon these three motivational precepts, you can become a successful management motivator. You will be able to utilize the wisdom of Myers, who wrote, "People's behavior stems from their under-standing of what they think they perceive" (Myers, 1970, p. 1).

Skillful nurse managers use the six motivational factors summarized by Herzberg, et al. to help their staff members achieve optimum job satisfac-tion. The human needs are implicit in these factors. All three steps of plan/do/control in the motivational management cycle are action steps for the nurse manager: the nurse manager plans (mutually with the affected in-dividuals) what specific needs, assets, and opportunities exist now and in the immediate future for specific members of the nursing staff; the nurse manager interacts with the specific individuals, using the developed plan and related knowledge, and applies the three precepts cited above; the nurse manager gets feedback, measures results against expectations, and follows through (all with direct involvement of the affected staff members). The cycle continues for these and other staff members. As with other techniques, once the pattern is established and practiced it becomes semiautomatic and spon-taneous. But as with other techniques, the learning and initial implementa-tion phases require special attention and extra effort.

For example, one way to practice the motivational management technique is to set up for each of your people (by name, dated) a sheet on which you simply list the motivational factors (and perhaps a specific, current, un-satisfied need) together with your thoughts of how specific motivators can be used. Then keep a follow-through record. Such a sheet would include items like these:

1. Achievement (successful accomplishment). Provide a work assignment (named) more consistent with demonstrated capabilities (named assets), challenging, but with minimum risk of failure.
2. Recognition (acknowledgement, be aware of, sense of self-worth). Commend regularly for performance results. "You did a fine job of that (by name)." "That was really a great effort." "Good job." "Well done." "I appreciate your help. It means a lot to me." "You are really good at that." "What I like about you is...."
3. The Work Itself (intrinsic interest in and satisfaction with job content). Improve job content to include more planning, self-direction, and evaluation by (action). Coach the employee.
4. Responsibility (to be answerable for, accountability, sense of trust). Delegate responsibility and authority suitable to the individual (taking some calculated risks, allowing more freedom of action). Get feedback; be available, helpful, supportive as invited.
5. Advancement (to make progress; move forward; rise in rank, amount, value). Recheck person's own desires. Provide opportunities for special projects, new assignments as appropriate. Encourage person to qualify self for career-ladder opportunities. Use job enrichment concept in

present job assignment. (Seek help from informed management engineer, systems analyst, or psychologist.)

6. Growth (to develop; become more capable). Provide fair opportunities to attend inservice, continuing education, workshops, and related programs. Encourage further formal education and other learning opportunities based upon person's needs and expressed desires. Find ways to be able to say yes to requests. Seek assistance from inservice and staff development staff for on-the-job training designed for your own unit.

7. Social Need (affection, sense of belonging). An example might be a current unmet need because of recent separation and divorce. Give extra quota of special attention, as acceptable by person, during succeeding weeks and months. Possibly arrange invitation to home. Discuss options with personnel director or other interested persons.

An Employee Care Plan

The foregoing may be expanded into an Employee Care Plan. It may be as simple as the following, patterned after a patient care plan. (See Exhibit 10-1.)

Exhibit 10-1 Employee Care Plan

Care Plan for _____ Date _____
                    name of employee

Needs/Problems/Goals/Strengths	Action Plans/Progress Notes
List here what you recognize as current needs, problems, and goals: security, social status, self-actualization needs?...changes in life situation?...desires for growth and development? Use existing sources of information in personnel files, personal observation, discussion. Identify and number a few key items only—the ones that *mean* something.	For each numbered item in left column, decide upon an action plan. Write it as a short-term objective— "who will do what, when?" Consider ways you can make effective use of the motivational factors—achievement, recognition, work itself, responsibility, advancement, growth. Identify how to use resources, including identified strengths of the person. *Involve* the employee as appropriate—it is his/her plan!

Source: Ganong, J. and Ganong, W. *101 tremendous trifles: A collection of management mini-guides.* (2nd ed.) Chapel Hill, N.C.: W. L. Ganong Co., 1979, p. 32a.

Neither patient care plans nor employee care plans will work well unless they are considered important and receive adequate time and attention. But they also must be designed—and their users trained—so that they can be used expeditiously.

First of all, care plans must be used in a way that truly demonstrates *caring*. This has much to do with the skills of individual nurse managers. Second, care plans must be viewed as related to, and supported by, the components of "A Framework for Nursing Management." (See Chapter 2.) Especially significant are the ways in which career planning assistance and opportunities for growth (well-designed, in-house career ladder options) are provided for the nursing staff in all job categories.

Closely related to this is the need for an employee performance evaluation program that meshes with the qualification specifications for each level on your agency's career ladders. ROPEP, the Results-Oriented Performance Evaluation Program, is highly cost-effective, since the job performance descriptions developed for ROPEP serve two purposes: (1) they provide the behaviorally-oriented, criterion-referenced specifications for each job level in nursing, and (2) they provide the standards of performance for each of the key job responsibilities that serve as the basis for employee performance evaluation. Therefore there is no longer any need for a separate form and procedure for employee performance appraisal.

Seen in this perspective, employee care plans serve as the coordinating link between a well-structured nursing management program and the individual employees upon whom rests the success of the total patient care program. Together these components provide nursing administration with an excellent way to comply with the major requirements of Standard II of the JCAH standards for nursing services.

ORGANIZING FOR MOTIVATIONAL MANAGEMENT

Healthcare organizations are living, dynamic, changing entities. They may be cumbersome, slow moving, and traditional; or innovative, quick to respond, and attuned to environmental impact. While these words are used to describe organizations, they more accurately portray the agency director, administrator and other leaders who, more than anyone else, influence and project the image of the healthcare agency (and its major departments).

Maslow thought of creative management and creative education as developing the individual not only in terms of one's own identity—one's self—but also as part of one's community, team, group, and organization. In his writing on eupsychian management (i.e., human-oriented management enhancing psychological health), Maslow set forth 36 assumptions as preconditions to McGregor's theory of participative management (Maslow, 1965). The first of these is the assumption that everyone is to be trusted. Other assumptions are that people are not fixated at the safety need level, that people are improvable, that people prefer working to being idle, that all human beings prefer meaningful work to meaningless work. These assumptions, and the remainder of the list of 36, provide a provocative philosophical base for nurse managers in their discharge of their human resources management responsibilities.

It is obvious that some agency leaders will be more receptive than others to the management principles, concepts, and techniques presented herein. The attitudes and values of the chief executive influence also the organizational structure itself and whether or not the structure contributes to or hinders goal achievement. These views are supported and emphasized by John F. Mee, who points out that effective performance of a manager requires a way of thinking, not the occupancy of a position (Mee, 1974). Flexibility in adapting to change is essential in response to the changing economic, political, technological, social, and ecological environments. But the ability of managers to respond to change and to assist other members of their management team to adapt to changing concepts of management is heavily influenced by: (1) the values and philosophy of the managers, especially as these affect behavior and decision making; (2) the kinds of knowledge and information possessed by managers; and (3) the abilities, skills, and proficiencies possessed by managers. In fact, Mee asserts that managers of the future are likely to be evaluated more on the basis of their value systems than on their knowledge and proficiencies.

Managers more and more are being considered as resource persons for those striving to achieve results, rather than being looked upon as authoritarian decision makers operating from the apex of a system of authority (as shown in a typical organization chart) who put their emphasis on an activities-oriented approach. By contrast, goal-oriented managers help focus the achievement motivations of people toward accomplishing common objectives and realizing personal need satisfactions.

The tendency towards a broader based college education for the general population, coupled with the reduced need for unskilled workers, will result in significant shifts in occupational patterns (see Figure 10-1). The traditional pyramid occupational structure, with a large base of workers at the bottom and a small number of managers and well educated people at the top, is changing. The shape of the evolving structure is closer to a diamond form, with a reduction of the workers at the base and a substantial increase of well educated persons in the middle strata (Tomeski & Lazarus, 1975, p. 233). Compare the diamond form in Figure 10-1 with Figure 2-3 and the related discussion of organization structure in Chapters 2 and 4.

Kraegel, Mousseau, Goldsmith, and Arora supply a pertinent definition of organization as part of an introductory chapter to *Patient Care Systems:* "An *organization* is defined as a system of interrelated resources, including en-

Figure 10-1 Changing Organizational Patterns

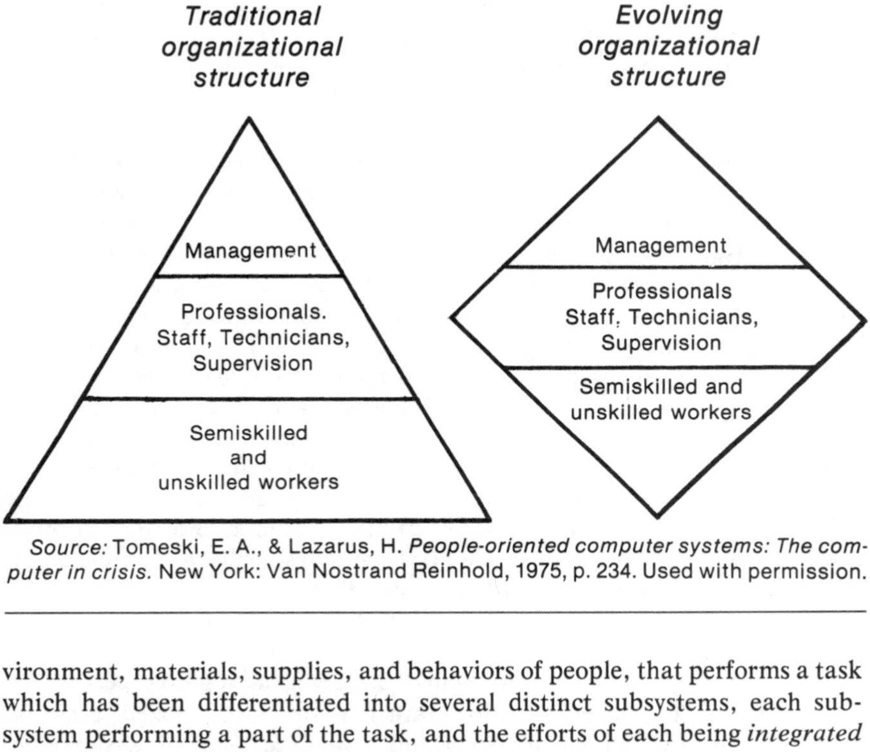

Traditional organizational structure   *Evolving organizational structure*

Management

Professionals.
Staff, Technicians,
Supervision

Semiskilled
and
unskilled workers

Management

Professionals
Staff, Technicians,
Supervision

Semiskilled and
unskilled workers

Source: Tomeski, E. A., & Lazarus, H. *People-oriented computer systems: The computer in crisis.* New York: Van Nostrand Reinhold, 1975, p. 234. Used with permission.

vironment, materials, supplies, and behaviors of people, that performs a task which has been differentiated into several distinct subsystems, each subsystem performing a part of the task, and the efforts of each being *integrated* to achieve effective performance of the total system" (Kraegel, et al., 1974, p. 7). The complexities of a hospital's interdepartmental and systems relationships dictate specific, purposeful action by top-level administration to establish the kind of dynamic integration that leads to unity of effort toward achieving the primary common purpose of meeting patients' needs. The problem-oriented nursing system is one of the vital systems contributing to the integrative plan.

When a nursing department decides to implement PONS, it is timely to carry out an objective review of the department's organizational plan and assignment of functional responsibilities. Some structures are better designed than others to provide the required support for a broadly based system such as PONS. What is usually called for is reorganizing the present structure, since the opportunity rarely exists to establish a new organizational structure from scratch. One of the dictums in architectural design is "Form follows function." The same principle applies in designing or redesigning the organizational plan of a hospital or a department of nursing: the plan of organization should fit the purpose of the organization and facilitate people's working together to achieve their goals and objectives. Problems and inefficiencies develop when an organizational structure, once adequate for an earlier time and environment, is no longer appropriate for today's demands. A "Model T" organization has no place on today's superhighway of modern healthcare. Yet some hospitals persist in attempting to adapt already outmoded organizational and systems models from general business or manufacturing industry in the name of modernization and progress. Results of such misguided attempts, predictably, often are more disastrous than they were when first developed for their original applications a quarter or half century ago.

Factors Influencing Organizational Structure and Performance

As a nurse manager, consider the variety of factors having an impact upon departments of nursing as they influence organizational structure and performance. Such factors include:

1. Increasing demands and expectations from other professional groups and departments, ranging from hospital administration and the physicians to the younger generation of employees and labor unions.
2. The new period of stress and transition in the nursing profession itself as leaders strive to influence legislation affecting licensure; reduce intergroup dichotomy and fractionalization within the profession; and consolidate several sources of power so that nursing speaks with a stronger, more unified voice.
3. Greater clinical demands due to continuing increase in the technologies affecting patient care.
4. Burgeoning requirements of governmental, accrediting, educational, institutional, insuring, and related agencies.
5. Critical necessity for cost containment through operational effectiveness in all areas.
6. The erosion of nursing's role in the delivery and management of patient care.
7. The pronounced thrust toward prevention rather than cure per se as the future emphasis in healthcare.
8. The human rights movement—here to stay in all of its manifestations—consumers, patients, employees, students, union members, managers, educators, doctors, nurses, and all the other interrelated groups of which people are members.

These eight factors are discussed in other chapters. In total, they represent a substantial set of challenges to nurse managers. Traditional departments of nursing—structured with responsibility, authority and accountability highly centralized in the director's position—are not well positioned for coping with these challenges. Such an organizational structure, tending to rigidity and morbidity, cannot respond successfully to the everchanging aspects of these demands, challenges, trends, and opportunities.

Criteria for an Effective Organizational Structure

Suppose a nursing department wants to become pro-active in relation to the eight factors cited. What kind of organizational structure would this department need? Our suggestions are based on assisting large numbers of nursing administrators and managers in moving their nursing departments toward a more viable plan of organization. We believe an effective organizational structure for nursing meets the following criteria:

1. The organizational design has its focus on aiding the implementation of diverse, individualized patient care programs using the problem-oriented nursing system.
2. The structure is adaptive rather than monolithic; each unit or unit cluster may have its own unique way of organizing to meet its patient and personnel needs. For example, key functions (such as patient care programs, staffing, cost control) may be handled by the unit clusters rather than being fully centralized in the nursing office or fully decentralized to individual units.
3. True decision-making authority is held by nursing personnel at every level, especially by those closest to the patients.
4. Responsibility is not considered as delegated downward, but as an inherent component of each person's self-worth.
5. Accountability is first to oneself; all other aspects of accountability to others stem from this concept.
6. Problem solving is facilitated horizontally and vertically throughout the organization—the matrix model.
7. Power and communication centers are varied and dispersed—the homeostatic biological model.
8. The structure demands the use of motive force and innovative action from the greatest possible number of persons.
9. Systems changes are easily accommodated.
10. Interdepartmental communication and collaboration occur at all levels.
11. Intradepartmental coordination and control require minimal attention, but are effective through use of the management process at all levels.
12. Widespread nurse manager involvement in utilizing the management functions and techniques at all levels permits meeting current objec-

tives while identifying and planning future goals for all three responsibilities of patient care management, operational management and
human resources management.

In an article on nursing organization and performance we have said:

> No single plan of nursing organization is appropriate for all
> healthcare agencies, or even for all hospitals. Each agency is
> unique. Each has its own special environment, history, purposes
> and people. Yet these special circumstances may become reasons or
> excuses for maintaining the status quo, for continuing an out-
> moded and unresponsive organization plan far beyond the point at
> which change is advisable. When this occurs, organizational
> changes may then have to be made in a crisis atmosphere with exac-
> erbated recoil/turmoil reaction—rather than in a planned, devel-
> opmental fashion with low initial impact and ample time for
> facilitative adjustment by all who are affected by the changes
> (Ganong & Ganong, 1979, p. 61).

There is no structural design that will meet the requirements of all
healthcare agencies. In one situation, for example, the department of nursing in a large state mental hospital redesigned their own organization and
met most of the stated criteria. These nurses accomplished their goal by
eliminating the position title of director of nursing and substituting a nursing
committee elected by the RNs with cochairpersons. For a period of several
years this committee form of elected leadership has met the needs of the
nurses for more involvement in directing their own affairs, improving communications, and in solving their own problems.

Figure 10-2 shows a decentralized schematic organization plan evolved by
the nursing department within a university medical center hospital. In this
situation there was a recognized need for strengthening the posture and performance of the nursing department at all levels, while securing the benefits
of productive dialogue, counsel, and guidance from other professional
university departments—notably the college of medicine, the medical staff,
and the college of nursing. The diagram is an adaptation of the matrix model
and provides the benefits of clearly defined channels of accountability within
nursing (the solid vertical lines) and the necessary input and cooperation of
the other professional departments (represented by the horizontal dash
lines). The concept portrayed by the chart is important at all organizational
levels, but especially so at the patient care unit level—which is "where the action is." Such a plan works most successfully when its purpose is understood;
when the doctors, nurses, and educators want to make it work; and when the
head nurses are strong, competent nurse managers who are skilled in all

Figure 10–2 University Hospital Department of Nursing Decentralized Schematic Organization Plan

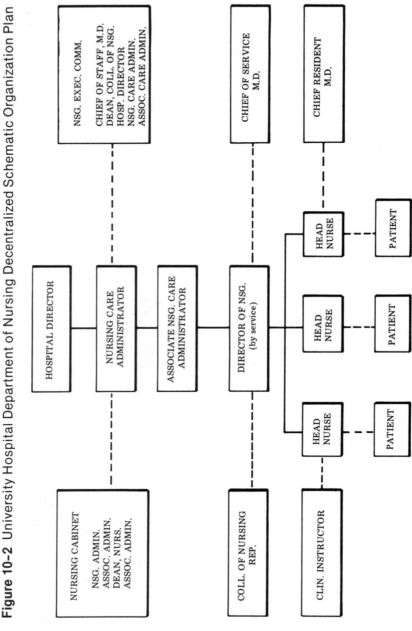

three areas of clinical, operational, and human resources management. When such conditions exist, there is the best possible environment to encourage nurse managers to become "excellent hospital integrators," as suggested by Marvin Weisbord (1976, p. 26).

A highly innovative approach to organizational change is recounted by Maas and Jacox in *Guidelines for Nurse Autonomy/Patient Welfare* (1977), which

> describes the activities of one group of employed professionals in their quest for organizational change. It is about a group of registered nurses who are engaged in the process of increasing their authority and accountability as employed professionals. ... The achievement of nurse autonomy and accountability is viewed as a necessary step on the way to nursing's full participation in collegial relationships with other disciplines in health planning and delivery (p. vii).

The authors point out that, "the development of nurse autonomy and accountability within an organization is a process of individuals behaving together; it involves both individual and collective behavior directed toward a common cause and the formation of new social relationships." The organization that was developed by the nurses in the above setting created a system for collective decision making.

MANAGING ORGANIZATIONAL CHANGE

Any change in departmental structuring involves the redefinition of position responsibilities. Even a single change in the structure has multiple ripple effects upon the interrelationships of many persons and groups. When the change embraces moving from an authority-oriented centralized structure to one that is goal-oriented and decentralized, care must be exercised to make the transition from one to the other as painless as possible.

Planning can help. Welch, in an excellent article on the theory of planned change, points out that planned change is

> initiated and carried out by a *change agent* who is skilled in the theory and practice of planned change. Planned change has a specific client system—which can be an individual, group, or institution—who is the focus for the change (Welch, 1979, p. 307).

The nurse manager as change agent needs to be aware of Lewin's work on field theory and his three stages of the change process—unfreezing, moving, and refreezing. (On pages 307–310 of Welch's article, she summarizes Lewin's change theory. See also Chap. 1 and Chap. 1 Notes—Argyris, Lewin, and Meissner—for more about Lewin's field theory.)

Despite careful planning, a change of any magnitude produces some degree of trauma. People don't resist change as much as they resist being changed by others. The nurse manager can help staff members respond to the requirements and risks of change by treating such requirements and risks as new opportunities for personnel growth and progress. Hirschowitz says that the failure of organizations to appreciate the complexity of human beings and their multiplicity of needs is a contributing factor in lack of adaptation to change (Hirschowitz, 1974). He cites three predictable sequential phases experienced by people going through change: (1) impact, (2) recoil-turmoil, and (3) adjustment and reconstruction. From experience with systems in transition, he suggests what does and does not help ease the difficulty of adjusting to change. Briefly, and with a few additions, these are:

WHAT HELPS	WHAT DOES NOT HELP
Involvement in planning and problem solving	Denial (by those who must face up to change)
Support and reassurance	Simplifying complexities
Guidance	Overspecializing, by trying to overdevelop functions and domains
Presence and proximity of superiors	Holding onto cherished habits, routines, and rituals
Talking about feelings	Hidden agendas
Clarification of roles	
Respect for values and dignity	
Hope, through communicative leadership	
Planning	
Timing	
Trust	

What Friedman says about changing behavior in therapy groups applies to people in any group:

> The facilitation of change involves an assessment of discrepancies. There may be discrepancies in the way the group member has organized his understanding of what happened in the past; discrepancies between his experience of himself and the way others perceive his actions in the present; discrepancies between where he is now, in relation to his needs, wants, and expectations, and where he would like to be. These discrepancies may be more visible or obvious to others than to the individual who experiences and maintains them (Friedman, 1979, p. 28).

A change as complex as restructuring a nursing department can begin with a review of the existing departmental structure. This can become an occasion for an exciting self-evaluation by each unit and can initiate the first item that Hirschowitz identified as helping the change process—*involvement*. One hospital has devised its own self-assessment program that includes having each patient care unit develop its own unit profile. This approach grew out of the collaboration between an associate director of nursing service and a non-nurse with responsibilities in the area of staffing and personnel utilization. They prepared an outline for the content of the profile, with guidelines for its development through the participation of all personnel on the units. Each profile includes the following topics:

1. description of unit (history, philosophy, types of patient, personnel mix)
2. financial status (budget comparisons, staff understanding and attitude)
3. quality of care (feedback, audit, opinion polls, incidents, errors)
4. personnel (age, education, needs, objectives, strengths)
5. clinical, operational, and human resources management (approach, relationships)
6. inservice education (activity, needs, hospital-wide involvement)
7. interdepartmental relations (supportive services)
8. medical staff (attitudes, expectations, rationale).

With the involvement and participation of every person who works on a unit, it is easy to see how this approach applies nurse manager concepts and principles. More than this, the project becomes a self-development and growth process for every member of the unit patient care team. It opens the door to requests for input and help from other departmental and institutional resources, ranging from inservice education to the business office and from the personnel department to other supportive services.

Barbara Donaho, Executive Director of Nursing at Abbott-Northwestern Hospital in Minneapolis,* accustomed to the appropriate use of power, commented as follows in an interview for *Modern Healthcare*:

> To make major organizational changes and move from a very autocratic model to a democratic model is a five to eight year process.
>
> The reorganization of nursing departments along democratic lines is being pushed by both better educated, more assertive nurses

---

*Hospital Week, in the December 21, 1979 issue, announced the appointment of Barbara Donaho to the board of commissioners of the Joint Commission on Accreditation of Hospitals—the first nurse named to that post in JCAH's 28-year history.

and hospital administrators, who are themselves being pushed by consumer and government groups (LaViolette, 1979, p. 62).

Figure 10-3 provides an example of a program performance plan in which we were involved as part of assisting one university hospital's department of nursing to meet its own particular needs. This plan is included as a pertinent example of how a director of nursing administration can effectively use a nurse management consultant in restructuring a nursing department to meet patient care and organizational goals. The three-phase plan is designed to build upon the existing structure and strengths; facilitate the change process through a maximum degree of involvement of nursing staff members, medical staff, the college of nursing, and other resources in the university setting; introduce the problem-oriented system; and strengthen the nurse managers' use of the managerial functions, techniques, and skills.

MOTIVATION AND POWER

Nurse managers are no strangers to the exercise of power. You, like everyone else, have been subjected to power in a variety of forms all of your life. And nurses as a group have been discovering ways to exercise power to achieve goals important to them. The nurse manager in the role of nurse administrator has authority by virtue of that position. In an article on power, Peterson (1979) states that:

> Through the acquisition of power, the nurse administrator *acts* rather than *reacts*, moves rather than resists, compels rather than bends. Effective leadership of the nursing service requires that the administrator view herself as an executive and the hospital as an organization. To assume another perspective is naive and detrimental to the administrator and to the nursing service (p. 10).*

Power, as seen by Peterson, is a positive force. This is a concept with which we heartily concur. Rollo May points out that power is the ability to cause or to prevent change (1972). There is potential power and latent power. Influence is a form of power. Power may be exploitative, as in using force to destroy choice. Power is competitive and may pit one person against another, productively or unproductively. Power is also manipulative. To the extent that this means to handle or control others in a skillful way, or to influence or manage others shrewdly or deviously, some nurse managers will believe that

---

*Reprinted from "Power: A perspective for the nurse administrator" by Grace G. Peterson as printed in the *Journal of Nursing Administration*, July 1979, vol. 9, no. 7.

Figure 10-3 Nursing Department Self-Development Project Program Performance Plan: University Hospital Department of Nursing

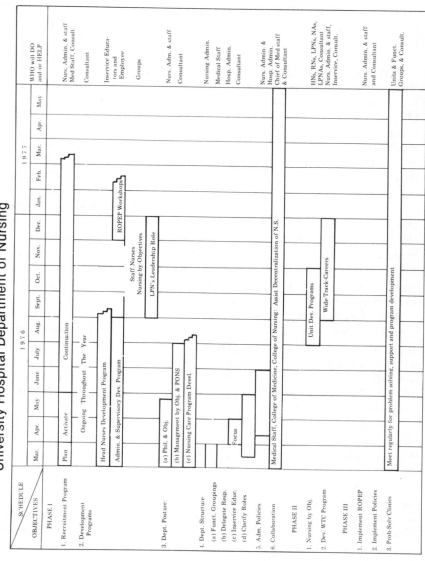

manipulation is motivation. In a limited sense this is true, because manipulation can cause others to be self-motivated so that they will do what you want them to do. The crux of the matter has to do with the manager's value system as well as the relevancy of the aims in terms of patient care needs and the needs of the person being manipulated or coerced through whatever uses of power.

Adolf Berle, Jr. writes about power from the viewpoint of political science and economics (Berle, 1959). He points out that power in any form implies at least two relationships: (1) the relationship of the individual or group with the power to the individual or group over which the power is exercised; and (2) the relationship of the particular power organization to the concurrent social-political structure. Little imagination or experience is required to relate these two considerations to the hospital and community environment with the diverse power groupings (political, medical, educational, administrative, managerial, labor union, and others) all having an impact upon individuals and groups.

The exercise of power requires organization plus the capability of delegation. The greater the power, the greater the need for delegating. Organization is essentially the mechanism by which decisions and instructions of a central individual or group can be made causative at distant points of application. Building an organization involves gaining and redistributing the power of individuals, a process permitted by the individuals for the benefits they obtain from the group activity.

Berle cites also the internal and external aspects of power. Internal power is that which the central group wields over individuals within the organization and those dependent upon them. The external aspect of power has to do with the capacity to affect others not part of the organization itself. Once again the implications are many for the hospital and nursing organization as related to nurse managers, employees, patients, families, and the assorted community groups.

Some understanding of power and its uses is important to nurse managers who are part of, and affected by, organizational power structures. James and Marge Craig offer another view of power as a positive natural force. Their idea of synergic power offers individual nurse managers and other people a way to generate creative cooperation in their personal relations, organizationally, and on a society-wide scale (Craig & Craig, 1974). The book shows how people can move away from mistrust and manipulation and begin to transform strangers or enemies into friends and allies. The Craigs build heavily upon Maslow's concepts to develop a simple and useful motivational model. The authors postulate that when a motivating gap is generated in a person, motivated instrumental behavior will normally follow. This relates to the earlier section of this chapter in which it is suggested you use a motivational factors sheet for each of your staff members. Nurse managers will find the Craigs' book especially helpful. Its thrust is suggested by the authors' use of a quotation from Albert Camus: "Ends do not justify means, but rather means justify means, and means have a way of becoming ends, so it is well to be scrupulous and uncompromising as to means" (Craig & Craig, 1974, p. ii).

Power and politics go hand in hand. Rogers (1977, p. 5) sums up his idea of politics as "the process of gaining, using, sharing or relinquishing power, control, decision-making. It is the process of the highly complex interactions and effects of these elements as they exist in relationships between persons, between a person and a group, or between groups."

There is a relevancy for the nurse manager in this definition of politics and the way it relates to power and to an organization such as a hospital or a healthcare agency. Rogers (p. 104) points out that:

> I have not often used the term "politics" in this description, but it should be clear that the politics of a person-centered organization is 180 degrees removed from that of a traditional organization. It is based on different values, works on different principles, achieves effectiveness through different operations. A person-centered organization is not a modification of a traditional one. It is a collective organism, totally unlike present-day organizations. It is a revolution in the achievement of human purposes.

Maslow expands upon this viewpoint in his book *Eupsychian Management* (1965).

An understanding of both power and politics is essential for the nurse manager who wishes to motivate patients and staff.

MOTIVATION AND ASSERTIVE BEHAVIOR

The nurse manager's behavior with others can affect individual motivation and can influence what happens in the internal and external environments of the nurses' workworld (described in Chapters 1 and 2). In its broadest sense, behavior includes anything the individual does or experiences (Chaplin, 1968, p. 54). Nurse managers need to be aware of their behavior as they work with the nursing staff, related personnel, patients, and others.

Robert E. Alberti and Michael L. Emmons provide a definition of assertive behavior in their book *Your Perfect Right: A Guide to Assertive Behavior* as "that behavior which enables a person to act in his own best interests, to stand up for himself without undue anxiety, to express his honest feelings comfortably, or to exercise his own rights without denying the rights of others" (Alberti & Emmons, 1974). The authors clarify nicely the distinction between nonassertive, aggressive, and assertive behavior. Nonassertive behavior is characterized by inhibitions, holding in your true feelings, being anxious and hurt, emphasizing your own inadequacies (real or presumed), not striving for your goals, letting others make decisions for you, and general dissatisfaction with the outcomes of your involvement with others. Aggressive behavior is characterized by extreme self-assertion, putting down others, hurting others while making choices for them, disregard for others' worth as persons, and achieving your goals at the expense of others. Assertive behavior is characterized by appropriately expressive, self-enhancing action; choosing for yourself; feeling good about yourself; and usually achieving your self-determined goals.

Table 10-1 summarizes the characteristics, feelings, and consequences that are typical for persons whose behavior is nonassertive, aggressive, or assertive. The chart also shows how such behavior is likely to affect others. Note that with nonassertive and aggressive behaviors, only one of the two persons involved is likely to achieve his or her desired goal. But using assertive behavior, both persons are likely to achieve their own goals.

Here are examples of three conversations, each exhibiting a different kind of behavior for handling the same situation. As you consider these interchanges, relate what you perceive to Table 10-1.

Situation: Insufficient linen has been delivered from the laundry for today's needs on the unit. More linen must be obtained to permit completion of A.M. care for patients. The laundry has to be called.

(First interchange, nonassertively.)

UNIT SEC'Y: "Joe? Hey, we're short of linen up here on Three West today. I've got to get some more somehow. Here's what I need. ...."

JOE: "Now wait a minute! Why are you calling me now? You know it's after 9 o'clock. When did you find out you are short?"

UNIT SEC'Y: "Just a little while ago. The staff is upset and blaming me. Can you help me?"

JOE: "Well, it's probably your own fault. I can't help you now; too busy. Try some of the other floors."

(Second interchange, aggressively.)

HEAD NURSE: "Joe? You've let me down again. We're short today, and we couldn't check it out earlier because you delivered too late. We'll make out OK, though, if you'll have six bed sets available for me in fifteen minutes. I'll send Jack down for them."

Table 10-1 Comparative Chart of Behavior Characteristics

Characteristics and Affect on Self[1]

Nonassertive Behavior	Aggressive Behavior	Assertive Behavior
Self-denying	Self-enhancing at expense of another	Self-enhancing
Inhibited	Expressive	Expressive
Hurt, anxious	Depreciates others	Feels good about self
Allows others to choose for him	Chooses for others	Chooses for self
Does not achieve desired goal	Achieves desired goal by hurting others	May achieve desired goal

Characteristics and Affect on Others[2]

Nonassertive Behavior	Aggressive Behavior	Assertive Behavior
Guilty or angry	Self-denying	Self-enhancing
Depreciates other person (1)	Hurt, defensive, humiliated	Expressive
Achieves desired goal at other's (1) expense	Does not achieve desired goal	May achieve desired goal

(1) Self, the initiator of the action.
(2) Other(s), the responder to the action.

Source: Adapted from Alberti, Robert E., PhD, and Emmons, Michael L., PhD, *Your Perfect Right: A Guide to Assertive Behavior* (3rd ed.). Copyright © 1978. Impact Publishers, San Luis Obispo, Ca. Reprinted by permission of the publisher.

JOE: "Darn it all, how can I do that? Two other units want more today too. I'm up to my ears...."

HEAD NURSE: "Look, I don't know about them, but you know we don't hoard the stuff up here. And we've just about had it with your slow delivery. Jack will be down soon."

JOE: "Don't blame me for the delivery schedule. We've got problems with the help I get. If my budget was what I asked for you'd get your linen."

HEAD NURSE: "So what else is new? We still have to get what we need for the patients. But all right, I'll go easy on you. I'll get by with five sets—no less! Don't let me down."

JOE: (sigh). "Don't do me any more favors. Have Jack here in twenty minutes." (Slams down receiver.)

(Third interchange, assertively.)

UNIT COORD: "Good morning, Joe. How's things in your sweatshop?"

JOE: "Lousy. Everybody wants everything two hours ago. So what's your problem?"

UNIT COORD: "Wouldn't you know, we had a few extra admissions and we're caught short. On top of that, I gave two sets yesterday to the second floor. I've got to have six sets, pronto."

JOE: "Have you checked with Four East?"

UNIT COORD: "No. I thought I'd better consult you first."

JOE: "O.K. Have Jack pick up three sets here in ten minutes; then I'll be able to tell him where to get the other three."

UNIT COORD: "Thanks, Joe. You're a gem!"

If you put yourself in Joe's position, you can imagine how he feels in response to each of the three approaches. You can visualize also the results of each type of behavior exhibited. A short summary of the evidence and the results might be as follows. The letters P (*parent*), A (*adult*), and C (*child*) are included in parentheses to add a consideration of Transactional Analysis (TA) in each interchange.

First interchange

Evidence of Behavior:
Unit sec'y (*C*, nonassertive). "Here's what I need. Can you help me?"
    Joe (*P*, angry, depreciatingly): "Why are you calling me now? It's probably your own fault."
Results:
    Unit sec'y's goal: Not achieved. No linen from Joe.
    Joe's goal: Achieved. He avoided the extra bother.
Second interchange

Evidence of Behavior:
Head nurse (*P*, aggressive): "You let me down again. You delivered too late. I'll go easy on you. I'll get by with five."
    Joe (*P*, denying, defensive): "How can I do that? Don't blame me. If my budget was what I asked for. ..."

Results:
   Head nurse's goal: Achieved (partially).
   Joe's goal: Not achieved.
Third interchange

Evidence of Behavior:
   Unit coord (*A*, assertively): "We're caught short. I've got to have six sets."
   Joe (*A*, self-enhancing): "Have you checked 4 East? Have Jack pick up three. I'll tell him where to get three more."
Results:
   Head nurse's goal: Achieved.
   Joe's goal: Achieved.

According to Clark (1979):

> Assertive behavior includes presenting oneself in a comfortable, clear, and confident way without trampling on others' rights; taking an active orientation toward work; using constructive work habits; being able to give and take criticism and help; and dealing with anxiety and fear so as to be able to function effectively. In the nursing care environment, it also includes assessing the rights and responsibilities in a nursing situation and acting on these assessments in a thoughtful, problem-solving manner.
>
> In contrast, aggressive behavior contains an element of trying to control or manipulate another person. The goal of aggressive behavior is to win, regardless of the price to others. It often results in negative feelings on both sides. The person who is manipulated feels humiliated and resentful, while the aggressor may be the target of active or passive counteraggression in the form of sarcasm, defiance, or passive resistance.*

The use of assertive behavior can enhance the nurse manager's efforts on behalf of motivation.

"TO BE, RATHER THAN TO SEEM"

The Latin phrase *Esse Quam Videri*, "To be, rather than to seem," appears on the Great Seal of North Carolina and expresses an ideal or goal that must have been in the mind of its original author and in the minds of those visionary persons who adopted it for the state. "To be"—to exist in actuality,

---

*Reprinted from "Assertiveness issues for nursing administrators and managers" by Carolyn C. Clark as printed in *Journal of Nursing Administration*, July 1979, vol. 9, no. 7.

have reality or life—rather than "to seem"—to give the impression of being, appear—we admit a liking for the value concepts implicit in the motto. The values we associate with the motto have to do with being a genuine person rather than a phony, open and honest rather than closed and devious, trusting rather than suspicious, creative and at times childlike rather than rigid and nonresponsive to the people and wonders around us.

The motto captures in its simplicity much of Maslow's philosophy and the humanistic psychology that was his life. Yet Maslow recognized the fact that progress is seldom, if ever, all sweetness and light. In *Eupsychian Management* he described how good eupsychian conditions may produce in some people a regressive, masochistic, or self-defeating tendency (Maslow, 1965, p. 43). When their organization or department is in transition from an authoritarian structure and style to a more participative one, some people do not know how to handle the new freedom. Lifting the rigid restrictions of authority may cause some chaos and release of hostility. It takes some time to convert and retrain authoritarian nurse managers. While this is taking place, some people may view their nurse manager's changed behavior as a form of weakness and attempt to take advantage of the situation. If managers and staff are not prepared for the transitional recoil-turmoil period that involves some disappointment, the temptation will be great to give up and change back to the authoritarian style before the accommodation and acceptance phase of change has been reached. Maslow, sought out by great numbers of people for counsel, had unvarying words of advice about values and goals: "Be stubborn!" This advice has served us well, as it has so many persons whose lives he touched during his lifetime and whom he continues to influence through his voluminous writings. We can do no better than to pass along to you that same advice: *Be stubborn*—appropriately!

NOTES

Alberti, R. E., & Emmons, M. L. *Your perfect right: A guide to assertive behavior* (3rd ed.). San Luis Obispo, Ca.: Impact, 1978, p. 11.

Berle, A., Jr. *Power without property: A new development in American political economy.* New York: Harcourt, Brace & World, Harvest Books, 1959, p. 79.

Chaplin, J. P. *Dictionary of psychology* (Rev. ed.). New York: Dell, 1975.

Chapra, A. Motivation in task-oriented groups. In S. Stone, Ed., *Management for nurses.* St. Louis: C. V. Mosby, 1976, p. 155.

Clark, C. Assertiveness issues for nursing administrators and managers. *Journal of Nursing Administration.* July 1979, 9(7), 20–24.

Craig, J. H., & Craig, M. *Synergic power, beyond domination and permissiveness.* Berkeley: ProActive Press, 1974, Chapters 1, 2 4, and 5.

Drucker, P. F. *Management: Tasks, responsibilities, practices.* New York: Harper & Row, 1974, Chapter 23.

Friedman, W. H. *How to do groups.* New York: Jason Aronson, 1979.

Ganong, W., & Ganong, J. Nursing performance reflects nursing organization. *Nursing Administration Quarterly*, Winter 1979, *3*(2). Reprinted with permission of Aspen Systems Corp.

Herzberg, F., Mausner, B., & Snyderman, B. *The motivation to work*. New York: Wiley, 1959.

Hirschowitz, R. G. The human aspects of managing transition. *Personnel*, May–June 1974, pp. 8–17. (*Notes & Quotes*, July 1974. Hartford: Connecticut General.)

Kraegel, J., Mousseau, V., Goldsmith, C., & Arora, R. *Patient care systems*. Philadelphia: Lippincott, 1974.

LaViolette, S. Hospital pressures trigger increased democracy in nursing departments. *Modern Healthcare*, May 1979, *9*(5).

Maas, M. S., & Jacox, A. *Guidelines for nurse autonomy/patient welfare*. New York: Appleton-Century-Crofts, 1977, pp. vii, 17.

Maas, M., Specht, J., & Jacox, A. Nurse autonomy: Reality not rhetoric. *American Journal of Nursing*, December 1975, *75*, 2201–2208.

Maslow, A. H. *Eupsychian management: A journal*. Homewood, Ill.: Richard D. Irwin and The Dorsey Press, 1965.

May, R. *Power and innocence: A search for the sources of violence*. New York: W. W. Norton, 1972, p. 99.

Mee, J. F. Changing concepts of management. *S.A.M. Advanced Management Journal*, October 1974, *37*(4), 22–34.

Myers, M. S. *Every employee a manager*. New York: McGraw-Hill, 1970, pp. 2–8.

Peterson, G. G. Power: A perspective for the nurse administrator. *Journal of Nursing Administration*, July 1979, *9*(7).

Rogers, C. *Carl Rogers on personal power*. New York: Delacorte, 1977.

Tomeski, E. A., & Lazarus, H. *People-oriented computer systems: The computer in crisis*. New York: Van Nostrand Reinhold, 1975.

Weisbord, M. Why organization development hasn't worked (so far) in medical centers. *Health Care Management Review*, Spring 1976, *1*(2).

Welch, L. B. Planned change in nursing: The theory. *The Nursing Clinics of North America*, June 1979, *14*(2).

Wilson, C. *New pathways in psychology: Maslow & the post-Freudian revolution*. New York: Taplinger, 1972.

Reading List

Books

American Hospital Association. *Employee-labor relations in health care institutions*. Chicago: Author, 1975.

Drucker, P. F. *The age of discontinuity*. New York: Harper & Row, 1968, 1969.

Goble, F. *The third force: The psychology of Abraham Maslow*. New York: Grossman, 1970.

Hersey, P., & Blanchard, K. H. *Management of organizational behavior: Utilizing human resources* (2nd ed.). Englewood Cliffs, N.J.: Prentice-Hall, 1972.

Jourard, S. *The transparent self*. Princeton: Van Nostrand, 1964.

Journal of Nursing Administration. *Motivating personnel and managing conflict: A Journal of Nursing Administration reader*. Wakefield, Mass.: Contemporary Publishing, 1974.

Maher, J. (Ed.). *New perspectives in job enrichment*. New York: Van Nostrand Reinhold, 1971.

Maslow, A. *Toward a psychology of being*. Princeton: Van Nostrand, 1968.

National Commission for Study of Nursing and Nursing Education. *An abstract for action*. New York: McGraw-Hill, 1970.

O'Neil, N., & O'Neil, G. *Shifting gears*. New York: Avon, 1975.

Perls, F. S., & Heffertine, R. F. *Gestalt theory: Excitement and growth in the human personality*. New York: Julian Press, 1951.

Renders, T. *Motivation: Key to good management*. New York: AMACOM, 1974.

Rubin, I. M., Fry, R. E., & Plovnick, M. S. *Managing human resources in health care organizations*. Reston, Va.: Reston Publishing, 1978.

Samples, B., & Wohlford, B. *Opening: A primer for self-actualization*. Menlo Park, Ca.: Addison-Wesley, 1975.

Selye, H. *The stress of life*. New York: McGraw-Hill, 1956.

Steers, R. M., & Porter, L. W. *Motivation and work behavior*. New York: McGraw-Hill, Inc., 1975.

Terkel, S. *Working*. New York: Pantheon, 1974.

Toffler, A. *The eco-spasm report*. New York: Bantam, 1973.

Articles

Anders, R. L. Matrix organization: An alternative for clinical specialists. *Journal of Nursing Administration*, June 1975, *5*(5), 11-14.

Charns, M. Breaking the tradition barrier: Managing integration in healthcare facilities. *Health Care Management Review*, Winter 1976, pp. 55-67.

Ciske, K. Primary nursing: An organization that promotes professional practice. *Journal of Nursing Administration*, January-February 1974, *4*(1), 28-31.

Fagin, C. M. Nurses' rights. *American Journal of Nursing*, January 1975, *75*, 82-85.

Fleishman, R. Human resource motivation. *Supervisor Nurse*, November 1978, *9*(11), 57-60.

Ganong, W. L., & Ganong, J. M. Good advice: Motivation and innovation—Concerns for nursing administration. *Journal of Nursing Administration*, September-October 1973, *3*(5), 7-9.

Ganong, W. L., & Ganong, J. M. Good advice: Organizational barriers—Real or imagined? *Journal of Nursing Administration*, January-February 1974, *4*(1), 7-8.

Ganong, W. L., & Ganong, J. M. Good advice: Patient care coordinators. *Journal of Nursing Administration*, September-October 1972, *2*(5), 9.

Hohman, J. Accountability: What it's all about. *Hospitals*, March 16, 1975, *49*(6), 145-150.

Hughes, E. Helping staff to manage conflict well. *Hospital Progress*, July 1979, *60*(7), 68-71, 83.

Johnson, G. V., & Tingey, S. Matrix organization: Blueprint of nursing care organization for the 80s. *Hospital and Health Services Administration*, Winter 1976, pp. 27-39.

Kalisch, B., & Kalisch, P. A discourse on the politics of nursing. *Journal of Nursing Administration*, March-April 1976, *6*(3), 29-34.

Maas, M., Specht, J., & Jacox, A. Nurse autonomy: Reality not rhetoric. *American Journal of Nursing*, December 1975, *75*, 2201-2208.

Parrish, W. Is fear a part of your management style? *Health Care Management Review*, Summer 1977, *2*(3), 17-29.

Schermerhorn, J. R., Jr. The health care manager's role in promoting change. *Health Care Management Review*, Winter 1979, *4*(1), 71-79.

Welch, L. B. Symposium on the nurse as change agent. *The Nursing Clinics of North America*, June 1979, *14*(2), 305-382.

Chapter 11

Labor Relations and Nursing Management

LABOR RELATIONS AS EMPLOYEE RELATIONS

This chapter and the others in Part IV will help you develop your own answers regarding your leadership responsibilities in respect to labor relations and personnel motivation. These subjects are vital to your third major area of responsibility as a nurse manager—namely, the management of your most important resource, your people. We provide some workable, tested guidelines for effective labor relations based upon an understanding of people and motivation. Labor relations is, after all, people relations—person-to-person relations. This is just as true in employee care as it is in patient care.

"Labor relations" in popular management usage denotes the responsibilities and activities related to maintaining a work force of hourly-paid employees within one corporation, healthcare agency, or industry group. Usually the connotation is that of a union-management relationship formalized by a contractual agreement reached through collective bargaining, with all of its attendant implications, requirements, and mystique. For better or for worse, nearly all segments of the healthcare industry have been caught up in learning about, fighting off, coping with, or adjusting to the labor relations of the past decade.

How did this happen? It came about largely through the kind of employee relations and managerial leadership practiced in healthcare agencies during the 1960s, 1950s, and earlier years. Individual agencies have remained union-free or have become unionized as a result of their response to the impact of a variety of factors—economic, cultural, political, community, environmental—that influence every institution. This will continue to be true in the years ahead.

In the light of the amendments to the National Labor Relations Act, hospitals have not stood still. They have taken positive actions to identify vulnerable areas in their employee relations programs. In its continuing struggle to work out the principles of its existence, the field of hospital labor relations looks to cooperation, communication, and dialog. Let us hope that all parties involved with hospital labor relations will not lose sight of their real reason for existence—the delivery of high quality patient care (Koncel, 1977, p. 73).

What is the current posture of your agency or organization? If you are union-free, does administration welcome the prospect of dealing with one or more labor organizations? Does administration vigorously resist organizational efforts? Or does administration passively accept the seeming inevitability of future unionization? If you already have one or more labor organizations representing employee groups, how does this fact influence administrative leadership? How is your administration's philosophy reflected in policies and procedures? How do these affect your own attitude and actions, and the managing of your department? This chapter will help healthcare agency department heads, supervisors, nurse managers, administrative staff, and members of boards of governance consider such questions and their implications for patient care and agency goals. Such searching inquiry, combined with skillful use of the human and technical modes of management described herein, will help give positive direction to your own—and your agency's—future.

"Labor relations" (or "industrial relations"), as already described, usually refers to all of the responsibilities and activities of management in maintaining an hourly-paid work force represented by a labor union (the bargaining agent). "Labor relations" may be used less precisely to refer to the broad field of personnel management as it applies to the labor force even when the employees are not members of a labor union.

In this chapter the term "employee relations" refer to the nurse manager's responsibilities and activities in maintaining either a unionized or nonunion work force in a specific healthcare agency. Our reasons are:

- "Employee" is an accurate term for every person on the agency payroll.
- It carries no negative connotations of rank or separateness—of being a group apart from management—as in "*labor* relations."
- It is a singular term referring to one person at a time, not to the amorphous group of personnel.
- Employee policies and practices apply to all persons on the agency payroll, with or without a labor union.
- Employees are motivated one at a time, individually, to act as they do.

These reasons are important to us and we hope important to you, for they relate directly to the content and message of this book. Our focus is on management as it applies to the coordination of human effort, of people working together as individuals to achieve common goals for mutual benefit. This kind of management, as previously emphasized, is the process of getting the right things done at the right time through and with the right people.

Our emphasis on the employee as an individual does not preclude a recognition of the fact that people in groups often respond to stimuli and behave in ways that are different from the ways the same persons might respond singly and apart from the group. Nurse managers need to recognize this fact and prepare themselves to provide leadership for groups as well as for individuals. For this reason we have included in this chapter the "Manager's Guide to Group Relations." It will help you understand some of the special characteristics of groups and how to cope with them.

THE 5M FORMULA

Every manager wants to do a good job. Our experience indicates that healthcare agencies are especially fortunate in having so many well-motivated department heads and nurse managers. And these leaders seem to want to learn more of the art and science of managing.

The 5M Formula is a simple way of looking at the function of a manager in any kind of an organization or department. This formula shows how the combinations of manpower, materials, machines, and management provide varying levels of patient care results. The word "formula" is one we would not ordinarily use in connection with the practice of management, since we believe that managing-by-formula is likely to be more mechanistic than humanistic. The best managers use an effective combination of the human mode and the technical mode. Thus "formula" is used here in a symbolic way, a model, an equation showing some logical relationships. With this in mind, let's examine the 5Ms.

Three of the Ms are arranged to show them in the form of simple addition, each being added to the other to get a result (R):

$$M + M + M = R$$

This shows a combination of manpower, materials, and machines (equipment) that added together in suitable combination produces a result that may be measured and evaluated. R may be reported as number of patient days of care, number of laboratory tests or x-rays per day, pounds of laundry per week, meals per month, or whatever units are appropriate. And it may be logical to assume that changing the input by some measurable amount will have a corresponding influence on the amount of output. Thus if manpower (number of hours of work/day by nurses on a unit, for example) is increased by 20 percent, we might expect to provide care for more patients, or provide more complete services for the same number of patients. The revised formula might look like this:

$$M^{(+20\%)} + M + M = R^{+}$$

If disposable dishware and utensils are introduced in food service, then less dishwashing might reduce workload and personnel in the kitchen (but with other effects in other departments):

$$M^{-2} + M^{-} + M^{-} = r$$

Similarly, other changes in one or more elements of staffing, supplies, equipment, procedures, facilities, and so on can be expected to influence results in some predictable way. But every experienced manager knows it's not that simple. It's not that simple because at least two influential elements have not been included in the formula up to this point. One of these is management. This is the department head, the head nurse, and all of the supporting supervisory and administrative staff who plan, coordinate, and implement whatever happens. So the big M is the manager—you:

$$\underline{M}(M + M + M) = R$$

Note that $\underline{M}$-for-manager is shown not just as another addition to the formula but as a multiplying factor. The manager's influence on results is pervasive; it permeates everything else, magnifying the outcomes—usually for the better, sometimes not. The comparison might be shown as follows, using units of 2 for each element in the formula. Example A shows the result if the affect of the manager were nothing more than to add the same amount of input units (2) as the other three M elements. Example B shows the greater result (12 instead of 8 units of output—quantity/quality measures) when the effect of a competent manager becomes a multiplying factor.

Ex. A:	Mgr. +	Mpr. +	Mat. +	Mach.	=	R
	2 +	2 +	2 +	2	=	8
Ex. B:	Mgr.	(Mpr. +	Mat. +	Mach.)	=	R
	2	(2 +	2 +	2)		
=	2 ×		6		=	12

But with a less capable manager (a factor of 1 instead of 2), results show as follows:

$$Ex.\ A: \quad 1 + 2 + 2 + 2 = 7$$
$$Ex.\ B: \quad 1 \quad (2 + 2 + 2)$$
$$= 1 \times \quad 6 \quad\quad = 6$$

The influence of the manager—symbolically as shown above, and realistically in day-to-day on-the-job practice—is profound.

There is yet another M—Money. It is an implicit and essential part of all elements in the formula. We include the financial component as follows:

$$\overset{\$\ \$}{M}(\overset{\$}{M} + \overset{\$}{M} + \overset{\$}{M}) = R$$

Money, therefore, ultimately must be included as the least common denominator, the bottom line on the agency's financial statement for the month and year that tells the end result of operating the institution in measurable input/ output terms—especially when reported as cost/patient-day. Other output reports are essential, too. These are the outcomes in human terms—the quantity/quality/personal data that identify how well the agency is fulfilling its human-service goals. Are these more important than the financial measures? The answer to this is not yes or no, because the question is misleading. Both are essential—the money and the service to people. One does not exist without the other. Adequate financing and a controlled budget are essential if services are to be provided—at any level of quality and quantity.

Some organizations have been experimenting with the human resources accounting method, described and introduced by Rensis Likert (1967). This method translates into dollars the human resources of the organization.

Admittedly, some managers are better than others in getting the maximum units of service (quality and quantity) out of each dollar of operating expense. One of the reasons for this is their skill in group relations. Group relations has to do with the human factors as they exhibit themselves in group behavior. The following pages examine the characteristics of people in groups and ways to maintain productive group relations.

UNDERSTANDING GROUP RELATIONS

People in groups are made up of individuals with their own skills, values, knowledge, and motivation. Each individual person is all-important. Remember, however, that each agency employs several, perhaps hundreds or even thousands, of employees. Each healthcare agency is actually a community. People live there nearly one-quarter of their lives. They must talk with others. They work with a partner or as part of a team. They may eat in the agency, too. And they joke and play there. Our modern agency employees are a far cry from the solo practitioners who ply their trades alone. They are part of a healthcare community.

What does each individual look like as part of the agency community, the agency society of which each employee is a part? Each person is one of a group. In its simplest meaning, a group is merely two or more persons who for some reason or other happen to be together. Nurse managers want people to be associated together in such a way that the resulting group meets a purpose and insofar as possible, does so effectively. A group in the healthcare industry, therefore, whether it be the state hospital association, the agency itself, the patient care committee, the planning department, housekeeping, personnel, or the noon-hour luncheon group, is more than merely a number of isolated individuals. Every member of a group has something in common with other members of the group. This common interest usually centers on the achievement of the group's purpose.

Definition of a Group

A group is a combination of individuals of similar interests who seek personal satisfaction through organized activity. This definition is sufficiently broad that we can apply it to any group. The personal satisfaction that comes from being a part of a healthcare agency (or a labor union) is in part measured by the economic and service justification of the agency (or the union). The organized activity is, of course, the method by which the agency (or union) is organized for the effective operation of the agency, society, or community (or union).

You live in a world of group activity. You have only to see the damaging effects of a strike of doctors, nurses, or other groups, or of a fire in the plant of one primary producer of supplies or the withdrawal of malpractice insurance by a national insurer to see the extent to which one industry group depends on the other. Within one agency, the same holds true. If purchasing does not get needed materials on time, if staffing can't supply the needed employees, if the laboratory does not have reports available before they are needed in the OR, or if any other of the many major groups does not do its part, all of the others will suffer.

Each of you fits into one or more of such groups. You cannot escape; you are all members of several groups. There was once a college professor who decided to disassociate himself from all groups. He resigned from his job, his clubs, fraternities, and even the church. After going to great lengths to become an individual, he found that he still belonged to the human race (he had a life membership in that) and he was a member of a small family group. He had no desire to resign from either. It is evident that most of your life is spent working or playing, inside the agency and out, with groups or members of groups. Actually, you spend most of your hours awake working or associating with others who share with you some similar interests.

Nurse managers can see that it is only through the groups with which persons work that they can satisfy their own basic individual needs and desires. It is through each person's group activity—through his association with others—that the satisfaction of needs and desires will result. Each person must satisfy many needs and desires through someone else.

But a group is not just a number of isolated individuals. In healthcare, a group is an association of people who by their combined efforts develop an effectiveness greater than the sum of the efforts of each separate individual. By group action, the combined result can be greater than the sum of the individual parts.

When you examine the individual persons in the group, you see the same things as when you examined them individually—skill, knowledge, values, and motivation. There is no reason to feel that individuals will change these when they join a group. However, when you look at the group, or at several groups, the first thing of note is that there are many different kinds of groups—the kinds which make up teams, associations, clubs, committees, unions, families, religious sects, audiences, federations, races, nations, conferences, and so forth. Within the healthcare agency there are many types of groups—administration, middle management, the medical staff, nursing, maintenance, dietary, housekeeping, and so on.

A second feature we see is that persons, while a part of several groups and loyal to them and their objectives, are still individuals. As both individuals and group members, their own interests and desires may not always coincide with those of the groups to which they belong. In each group we see individual persons. They, as individuals, are separately interrelated with the rest of the group. This can be identified as the Individual-Group Relation.

Listen to one such person, a nurses' aide. Note the relation of this worker's individual interests to those of various groups to which he or she belongs, and note the large number of different groups identified.

> Nurses' Aide (proudly): "I've been working in this department for twelve years, and there's no finer bunch of people. I wish we had a team like this running the union. They wouldn't cross us up the way those people do now. (Cautiously) Uh, oh—there's another new aide today. That's the third one they've replaced this month. I'd better watch my own step and not grab too much overtime. Those folks in personnel don't want us to get any time-and-a-half pay.

(Pause) (Friendly) Hiya, Jane! How'd you like the way that son of mine played ball at the high school Saturday? Sure put the family name in the news."

Note this worker's pride in the work group, fear for own security, antagonism to personnel department, and pride in family group.

Similarly, there must be relations among the several groups. Consider the intergroup relations as exhibited in the following comments:

Department head (complaining): "You people up there in the systems office always want us to change our procedures. We're out here on the firing line where the care is actually given. What do you people know about our operations?"

Licensed Practical Nurse (offhand): "We don't want any clinical specialists on our unit. They don't think the way we do!"

Mother (to husband): "I don't think we should let Junior play with those families down by the railroad tracks. Why don't you introduce him to those nice folks you ride to work with?"

Nurse on nights (with envy and feeling of injustice): "Those people on days always have more help. On this shift Louie, Alice, and I have to manage on our own."

In examining any group, you see still further that there are certain individuals who stand out from the rest. These are the leaders, the group representatives such as union stewards, department heads, and others. Listen to what some group representatives sound like:

The Community Fund Campaign Chairman (helping the group): "We've got to meet our quotas, folks, and you're the ones who have to do it. I'll give you all the help I can, but the real job is up to you."

Senior Nurses' Aide on evenings (challenging a newcomer): "What do you want to do, bust up a good thing? I've been on this job three years, and the others and me aren't going to have any young squirt come in and try to show us up with all your eager-beaver stuff."

Union Treasurer (persuading member): "Sure, you have to pay your dues on time; I can't finance you, and the local can't back you with national headquarters. Better let me have the twenty bucks now."

There is still another feature about every group. Each group has certain characteristics. These characteristics give a group a personality. They are common to all groups, though they vary in degree with each specific group. The Rotary Club begins a luncheon program with joint singing; a church service ends with the benediction; employee groups are identified with distinctive uniforms. You can name unique characteristics of your own groups. These will be examined shortly.

You have now looked at agency employees as individuals and as members of groups. How is it possible to improve people's relations to the various groups with which they come into contact? This can certainly be done with the individual agency group by setting a pattern of cooperative group action, by understanding the different groups in your agency, by noting the relations of the individual-group conflicts, by spotting the intergroup relationships, by properly working with group representatives, and through an appreciation of the general characteristics of groups.

By these means, group action can be improved and employees can be helped to meet their basic needs and desires. If you inform employees, train them, and match them to suitable jobs, you will be increasing their value and stature in the organization. Through this individual and group action you can help employees become more of what they want to be. And if you provide and develop people of greater stature (of greater value) for the 5M Formula, you will (in order to keep your equation balanced) obtain a greater R—in other words, the better patient care services you would like to provide. By increasing the value of your people (input), you increase your output.

Group Relations Guide

The Group Relations Guide Sheet (see Exhibit 11-1) provides a summary of some of the key points in the foregoing pages, expands the information about group relationships with additional facts about groups, identifies important general characteristics of groups, and then gives useful guides to managerial action in relation to groups. It deserves your careful reading, understanding, and application.

As you examine the guide sheet, consider its validity in the light of your own experience with or understanding of union-management relations. Labor unions exist because they fulfill needs—people's needs. Healthcare agencies exist also to fulfill needs—people's needs. When the methods of meeting people's needs cause conflict, at least part of the reason may be identified in the group relations guide sheet. Appropriate action by nurse managers can help prevent conflict or mitigate the results of such conflict.

Exhibit 11-1 Group Relations Guide Sheet

Part I

Good group relations is more than the absence of conflict; it is a positive condition of mutual reliance which the manager must build.

The Manager's Formula for Group Relations

A. Understanding *m.b.* Tolerance → Agreement
B. Responsibility *m.b.* Coordination + Incentive → Cooperative Action

---

m.b. = modified by   → = leads to

Basic Needs and Desires of Individuals	*Scientific Approach to Management Problems*
1. Survival	1. State or isolate problem
2. Security	2. Get facts
3. Social (love and belonging)	3. Restate problem
4. Status (self-esteem, pride)	4. Analyze
5. Self-actualization	5. Take action
	6. Follow up

These are satisfied through group activity. Earning the respect and confidence of all groups is the lifeblood of group relations.

The Common Aims of Every Group

1. an economic order favorable to the attainment of its objectives
2. cooperation, natural or imposed, of other groups in the attainment of its objectives
3. the right to utilize its skills to the greatest advantage
4. the maximum amount of freedom in the exercise of its skills
5. a maximum return for the skills of its members

The violation of accepted common law principles of justice in handling group relations is a manager's most fatal error.

Exhibit 11-1 continued

Part II

Group Facts	*Manager's Action*
A. Different Groups	
1. People belong to several different groups.	1. Identify your different groups and those of the people with whom you deal.
2. There are organized and unorganized groups.	2. Change unorganized groups into organized working teams.
3. There are friendly and hostile groups.	3. Create friendly working groups.
B. Person-Group Relations	
4. Group members have individual desires.	4. Harmonize members' individual desires with those of the group and vice versa.
5. Members move from one group to another according to satisfaction received.	5. Make your group an "in group" for its members.
6. Group membership results in conflicting loyalties.	6. Reduce (as far as possible, eliminate) conflicting loyalties in members.
7. Groups are not always satisfied with their members.	7. Fit yourself into your groups. Select members that fit and help them fit.
C. Intergroup Relations	
8. Conflict and antagonism among groups defeat groups' purposes.	8. Strive for cooperative action by all groups.
9. In intergroup conflicts, people align themselves with the group of which they feel most strongly a part.	9. Align yourself (get others also to align themselves) with group whose objectives offer greatest long-term benefits.

Exhibit 11-1 continued

D. Group Representatives
10. Effective group activity requires group leadership.
10. Lead your group and help representatives of your subgroups to be leaders.
11. Group follows its representative only when feeling that person works in group interest.
11. Stress interest in group to which you and your members belong. "Be on their side."
12. Most management groups comprise representatives of other groups.
12. Apply same principles and formula as to any other group.

General Characteristics of Groups

1. Group members will fight and sacrifice for their group and its objectives so long as the group serves its members.
2. Groups respond to emotional appeals.
3. Selfishness is dominant in group objectives.
4. Groups use distinctive methods and techniques.
5. Group thinking is simple and direct and may be more accurate than that of individuals.
6. Group effectiveness varies with the degree of intragroup balance.
7. Group effectiveness varies with the degree of active participation by group members.

Source: Ganong, J., & Ganong, W. *HELP with labor relations through motivational management.* Chapel Hill, N.C.: W.L. Ganong Co., 1976, pp. 35–36.

THE NURSE MANAGER'S ROLE IN COMPLAINTS AND GRIEVANCES

As noted in Chapter 1, nurse managers and other leaders have a responsibility to learn and use management terminology that is precise and appropriate. There is a distinction, for example, between a *complaint* and a *grievance*. A *complaint* is anything which is brought to your attention, or which you observe or sense, which is a possible cause for dissatisfaction or unfair treatment (real or imagined) of an employee. A *grievance* is a formal complaint presented in accordance with the provisions of the labor agreement (the union contract with the employer); or, in nonunion situations, based upon a violation of established personnel policies, and presented in accordance with a published grievance procedure.

You can usually decide whether a complaint is a genuine grievance by asking yourself two questions:

1. Did the employer violate the contract? If the answer is yes, you've got a grievance.
2. Has the worker been treated unfairly by the employer? If the answer is yes to this question, you've probably got a grievance, even though you're not sure that the contract has been violated. Sometimes this kind of grievance is hard to win, though, because of a loophole in the contract.

Usually a grievance is a violation of the contract. You may not think so at first, but if you read your contract carefully you can usually find some section of it that deals with the kind of problem your grievance involves.

"Complaint" is the broader term which can be used for all causes of dissatisfaction. Thus in the remainder of this chapter "complaint" is used as the all-inclusive term for complaints and grievances in both union and nonunion agencies. "Grievance" is used here only to mean a violation of the labor contract between the employer and the union.

It should be kept in mind, however, that "There is in plain fact, nothing wholly predictable—nothing cut and dried—about what takes place in situations of actual or impending conflict. Both responses and outcomes are various" (Overstreet & Overstreet, 1956, p. 22).

A complaint is not a threat. It need not be a problem. The most experienced nurse managers look upon a complaint as an opportunity. A complaint provides an opportunity for the nurse manager to:

1. Understand the reasons for the complaint. What's the real human basis for this complaint?
2. Evaluate the substance and value of a complaint. Has the employee been treated unfairly? Has there been a violation of agency or departmental policies?
3. Develop a consistent positive approach to the handling of complaints. Am I avoiding the danger of locking-in too soon?
4. Consider, in every complaint situation:
   a) The objective in handling it.
   b) The attitudes involved and their influence on the participants.
   c) The facts and assumptions involved.
   d) The relative costs of optional courses of action. What should I really want to achieve, and what are my options for action?

Your success in helping successfully resolve complaints is directly related to your ability to: (1) view a complaint as an opportunity for improving communication with your people; (2) avoid getting mad or disconcerted when you are presented with a complaint; (3) see how each complaint can lead to greater understanding, rather than be a chance to engage in a boxing match; and (4) avoid the danger of locking-in too soon; and make commitments only after checking feelings, facts, policies, and past practices.

Much may depend upon your own leadership style. Review the brief discussion of leadership styles in Chapter 1 in connection with your handling of complaints. For example, think about a recent complaint with which you were involved. Was it yours to handle? Do you feel you had the responsibility and authority to deal with it? What needs were in evidence—the employee's and yours? What assumptions did you make? What was your objective? Recall the facts, attitudes, and feelings as you identified them. What was the cost of that complaint? Was it a problem or opportunity? What were your feelings? Did they help or hinder a successful outcome?

Complaints that turn into grievances can be very costly. Some of the costs are direct and measurable and may be hundreds or thousands of dollars if arbitration is involved. Other costs are indirect, but expensive nonetheless in terms of group relations, motivation, and impact upon patient care services. Arbitration is a method of settling a dispute through recourse to an impartial third party whose decision is final and binding. Arbitration is voluntary when both parties of their own volition agree to submit a dispute to arbitration. It is compulsory when the two parties involved are required by law to submit the dispute to arbitration. Arbitration, costly yet sometimes justified, may be the end result of negligence by the nurse manager when a complaint first comes to light. The best time to resolve any complaint is when it is first made by an employee to the nurse manager. Thus our emphasis is upon ways to minimize the causes for complaints (through progressive policies, procedures, and management); to treat each complaint seriously and expeditiously when one occurs (resolving it fairly between employee and the nurse manager whenever possible); and if further steps are necessary, to resolve the complaint justly without arbitration.

Exhibit 11–2 presents a summary of a complaint that became a grievance which went to arbitration. It provides a typical example of the frustrating, lengthy, time-consuming, costly involvement of many people trying to resolve a case that, on the fact of it, seemed to deserve a decision to support the hospital's position. The arbitrator's award may have been wise and just; it's difficult to evaluate as just or not by the time the final decision is made. Sometimes the nature of the complaint itself seems to have changed because of all that happens in the often lengthy interval between initial complaint and the ultimate arbitrator's decision. The message is clear. To minimize the frequency and cost of complaints you can provide progressive leadership, minimize the causes for job dissatisfaction, maximize the conditions that lead to job satisfaction, build effective work teams using your understanding of group relations, focus on human needs and patient care goals, and resolve complaints promptly.

When your job requires your involvement in handling grievances, an excellent reference book is *Grievance Handling: 101 Guides for Supervisors* by Walter E. Baer. It presents the grievance machinery as "the formal process, preliminary to any arbitration, that enables the parties to attempt to resolve their differences in a peaceful, orderly, and expeditious manner" (Baer, 1970, p. 3). It includes among the 101 guides some helpful management suggestions for supervisors, a 50-item leadership checklist, what followers look for in a leader, and related tips on discipline and training.

Exhibit 11-2 THE FALSIFIED RECORDS ARBITRATION
The Confidential Case File on Millie Arnold
Case Number 292

The Grievance

Grievance No. 127 was filed October 26, 1974 by Millie Arnold, and read in part as follows:

Nature of Complaint—"I was unfairly terminated on Rules of Conduct, No. 26 which states, 'Deliberately falsifying employment records or other records such as time tickets or patient charts.' I am asking to be reinstated with pay for lost time as I am not guilty."

The Issue

Was the discharge of Millie Arnold for just cause?

The Hospital Position

The Hospital contends that the discharge was for just cause because the grievant deliberately falsified the record of her tardiness on Friday, October 20, 1974 and was properly discharged for violation of Rule #26 following a fair and objective investigation establishing the misconduct.

The Union Position

The Union contends that the grievant was the victim of harassment and discrimination; that the discharge was not

Exhibit 11-2 continued

for just cause, and requests her reinstatement with full seniority.

The Award

The grievance of Millie Arnold is sustained to the extent that the penalty of discharge is reduced to disciplinary suspension with loss of seniority beginning October 25, 1974 and ending as of the first payroll period following April 25, 1975, at which time she shall be reinstated in a position equivalent to the one she held on October 25, 1974. She shall retain all seniority earned prior to October 25, 1974.

The Reasoning

The full opinion and award of the Arbitrator in this case, and other related papers which describe the development of the grievance, total twenty-seven pages. They reflect the employee's record of former disciplinary actions for the same and similar infractions in the past two years. She appears to be a satisfactory worker when on the job. This arbitrator decided the award as stated, in spite of a decision to terminate another employee in an almost identical arbitration case a year previously.

Source: Ganong, J., and Ganong, W. *HELP with labor relations and motivational management.* Chapel Hill, N.C.: W.L. Ganong Co., 1976, p. 43.

Procedure for Handling Complaints

An effective procedure for handling complaints as opportunities involves five steps:

1. Let the employee talk.
   - Listen to the employee in private. Put the employee at ease. Allow the employee plenty of time to tell the story. Don't interrupt. Keep your temper.
   - Get all the details. Identify opinions and feelings.
   - Make certain the real complaint is the expressed one.
   - Repeat the complaint in your own words. State the opinions and feelings. Arrive at a common understanding.

- Tell the employee when you will give an answer.
2. Check the facts (including opinions and feelings).
   - Investigate the employee's story. Gather all the details you can about the complaint.
   - Refer to agency and department policies and past practices (precedents).
   - Know the employee and his/her needs.
   - Consult with others whose experience, knowledge, or observation may aid you in arriving at a decision.
3. Arrive at decision (considering alternative courses of action).
   - Base the decision on facts (including opinions, emotions, feelings), and on agency and department policy, procedures, and past practices.
4. Tell the employee the decision.
   - Plan when, what, where, and how you are going to tell the employee.
   - If complaint is justified, admit it graciously.
   - If complaint is unfounded, explain why.
   - Don't be bulldozed.
   - If the decision is adverse to the employee, prepare the case for possible appeal.
5. Follow through.
   - Take prompt action to correct the cause of complaint.
   - Check with the employee to see that the complaint has been eliminated.

This procedure is one which has been developed from the experiences of successful supervisors and managers, and also, as you can see, from a much older procedure, the scientific method in problem solving:

1. State the problem. (Put it in writing.)
2. Collect facts, opinions, feelings. (Recognize your assumptions.)
3. Analyze the facts. (Redefine the problem.)
4. Develop solutions. (Consider the options.)
5. Take action. (Be clear and direct.)
6. Follow through. (Assure expected results.)

Consistent use of the five steps in handling complaints helps prevent the temptation to give snap decisions, to take action precipitously, to let a complaint drag along, or to do those other human things that allow a complaint to fester, become a grievance, and turn an opportunity into a real problem for you.

PROBLEM SOLVING IN EMPLOYEE RELATIONS

Over the years since Public Law 93-360, 29 U.S.C. Section 152(14) became the law of the land, all private healthcare institutions (HCIs) have been subject to the provisions of the National Labor Relations Act. Problems that have developed between labor and management translate into problems between members of unions and nurse managers. Bryant points out that

> Problems and challenges to unions and HCIs have become more evident as differences occurred and were resolved, and as our consumer (the patient), third-party payors, and the community-at-large have come to realize and understand the role all must play in employee/management labor relations. The NLRB and the courts may continue to be called upon to regulate competing interests, for all activity must be tempered by the public's interest in the uninterrupted delivery of health care (Bryant, 1978, p. 37).

Using good judgment, always a goal of nurse managers, becomes especially necessary in the presence of a bargaining unit. Good judgment requires careful distinction between two kinds of ideas we have about the world around us. Such ideas stem from our observations and inferences. Observations are products of personal experience. To observe something we must see, hear, feel, smell, or taste it. Inferences are decisions about the meanings of our observations. Both kind of ideas are indispensable to our proper functioning; but when we mistake inferences for observations, we have trouble.

You may wish to test your own human tendency to make unwarranted inferences and assumptions. The Uncritical Inference Test in Appendix E provides such an opportunity. You may be surprised at your own level of assumptions. If you are like most people you won't agree with all of the answers as given for the two exercises. Even after discussion with others you may still be in disagreement, unable to comprehend the reasons for the "?" answers—or even some of the "T" and "F" answers. In fact, you may become upset, mad, and hostile. If so, then you have a complaint, but no grievance. The answers as provided are strictly in accord with the contract (the instructions, the "ground rules") provided for each exercise. Perhaps a cooling-off period is needed to permit you to take a fresh look at the exercises and your complaint. Perhaps part of the problem (opportunity?) has to do with an unclear understanding of the instructions and what T, F, and ? mean. If so, then your complaint is a true communications opportunity. These two exercises, like so many simple-seeming complaints, turn out to be quite complex when several persons get involved—with their various levels of understanding, values, motivations, feelings, and opinions. The message is clear—use the five-step procedure with skill and care.

Always be careful with "the facts." The definition of a fact is (1) something that exists and is supported by evidence, an actuality; (2) truth, reality; (3) an act considered with regard to its legality as in "after the fact." Transactional Analysis (TA) provides a helpful model for keeping facts in their proper place in relation to prejudgments (values, prejudices) and feelings (emotional reactions).

Edwin Bixenstine has written a scholarly and helpful description of "The Value-Fact Antithesis in Behavioral Science." In his introductory statement, Dr. Bixenstine poses a consideration of values and facts in a context that will be helpful to professional nurse managers:

> While values emerge ever more prominently for consideration in the reflective, scientific literature of our time, a stubborn cleavage remains in our construing of values and facts. This separation is encouraged by a 19th century construction of science which places limitations on humans as scientists, in an effort to preserve an unlimited and superhuman conception of science. The thesis of this article is that all knowledge resides in the human response to events, that this response is irreducibly subjective and evaluative, and that facts are a special class of (communicated) values distinguishable by intraobserver redundancy and interobserver consensuality (Bixenstine, 1976, p. 35).

The article with its generous listing of additional references will be rewarding for those nurses who want to pursue an understanding of the relationship between values and facts in a philosophical, scientific, and humanistic manner. As the author says in his summary comments, "Realism invites us to relax, to be both human and scientist" (Bixenstine, 1976, p. 55). Exactly! That is our theme in this book. The many nurse managers we know are—or want to be—both human and scientific in their contributions to patient care management.

Using Transactional Analysis (TA) in Handling Problems and Complaints

A transaction occurs whenever you are involved with someone else. TA is a way of analyzing, understanding, and improving your interactions with others. TA provides a simple way of talking about the complexities of human interaction based upon the study of ego states exhibited by human beings. This is explained in a very few words and with many pictures by Adelaide Bry in *The TA Primer* (1973). The author says everyone has three buttons inside them all the time waiting to be pushed. These are the PAC buttons:

(P) stands for the parent in you.

(A) stands for the adult in you.

(C) stands for the child in you.

You need all three of the PAC buttons. When you learn to push them selectively, on purpose, rather than randomly and irrationally, your results usually will be better. You will be able to give different strokes to different folks. And you find yourself in the happy situation of "I'm OK, You're OK." A variety of good books on TA are available in paperback editions. We suggest *The TA Primer* because it is so brief and easy to understand.

    The usual approach in solvng problems is to get facts about the problem situation, review the facts logically to identify the causes of a problem, then decide what action should be taken. This rational adult (A) approach is shown simply as follows:*

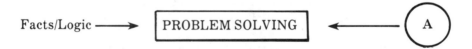

Facts/Logic ⟶ | PROBLEM SOLVING | ⟵ (A)

The experienced problem-solver recognizes a difficulty. People involved with a problem often are very emotional about it. They may ignore the facts. They let their feelings get in the way. They act more like a child (C) than as an adult:

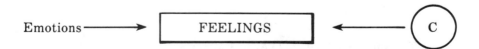

Emotions ⟶ | FEELINGS | ⟵ (C)

In addition, people often allow their prejudgments to affect their thinking. ("What can you expect from a person of that race, religion, or sex?" Or, "That's wrong." Or, "You should never do that." Or, "Listen to me; I know

---

*Biamonte, F. For this adaptation of TA to problem-solving we are indebted to Dr. Fred Biamonte, of the Graduate School of Pace University in New York.

best.") Prejudging a situation or person comes out of one's apperceptive mass. For better or worse, it reflects a lifetime of shaping one's values, beliefs, morals, and prejudices. It is the parent (P) in action.

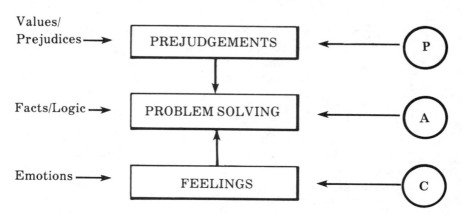

Values/Prejudices → PREJUDGEMENTS ← P

Facts/Logic → PROBLEM SOLVING ← A

Emotions → FEELINGS ← C

Every person has some of the parent, adult, and child in his or her personality. Some persons maintain a reasonable balance of P, A, and C. Others allow one to predominate, and seem to react consistently as P, A, or C. Recognizing this fact is helpful in your involvement with others, in solving problems, handling complaints, and in getting good results.

As you read more about TA you will learn how you can handle certain kinds of transactions that cause problems.

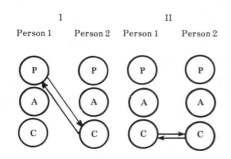

I   II

Person 1   Person 2   Person 1   Person 2

Examples I and II show complementary types of transactions. They may sometimes reflect a kind of game-playing, but are not so likely to cause the difficulties of Example III.

We know a fine operating room head nurse who learned TA and began to try it with the surgeons. She had always been accustomed to playing her parent (or tearful child) to the surgeon's emotional child and found her role demeaning and frustrating. At first, when she tried to change the relationship to that of adult to adult, she used the language of TA and didn't succeed. But when she learned to stay in her adult role and not talk about it, just

III
Person 1 Person 2

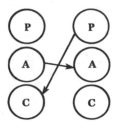

Crossed transactions cause problems. For example, in example III you may be Person 1 calling the food service department to ask, as one adult to another, "Will Mrs. Foster be able to have her special diet tray at 11:30 A.M.?" Person 2, in the kitchen, replies (from her parent), "Listen, Kiddo, we'll deliver what's ordered. We don't need any checking from you." This kind of crossed transaction is ready-made for fireworks. It should put up a warning sign to you: Danger Ahead — Proceed With Caution.

use adult behavior, it worked. She is justly proud of having been able to bring about an adult-to-adult relationship with the surgeons. In fact, she is now the OR supervisor.

As a nurse manager you observe and get involved in many kinds of transactions each day. You can enhance your value as a facilitative helper as you recognize P or C buttons (yours and others) being pushed at the wrong time and find ways to help untangle the crossed transactions. Such perception and skill will greatly enhance your ability to resolve complaints and grievances.

SKILLS AND TECHNIQUES IN EMPLOYEE RELATIONS

There are a variety of managerial skills and techniques, involving both the human and technical modes, that are necessary in carrying out your employee relations responsibilities as part of your management functions of planning, doing, and controlling. A technique, of course, provides a model which can be used repeatedly to aid in achieving your objectives. A skill is something you do with your head, hands, or body to carry out a technique. Here is a listing of some managerial techniques and skills you may use in carrying out your employee relations responsibility.

Techniques

- Handling Complaints
- Group Negotiation
- Management by Objectives
- Results-Oriented Performance Evaluation
- Transactional Analysis
- Wide-Track Career Planning
- Critical Incident Technique
- Crisis Intervention

- Third-Party Intervention
- Managing Change
- Securing Involvement

Skills

- Communicating (behavior, body language, eye contact, facial expression, listening, reading, silence, speaking, touching, writing)
- Conceptualizing
- Decision making
- Problem solving
- Instructing
- Day-to-day coaching

Techniques are likely to be only as good as the skills of the people who use them. The personal values and motivation of the manager have great influence upon the use of the skills and techniques. Your workworld as a healthcare manager is ultimately no more nor less than you choose to make it—for yourself, your employees, and your patients.

In our view, you are the key person in your employee relations situation. This is because you are the Big M in the 5M Formula. You have no need for gimmicks, crash campaigns, devious strategy, or behavior modification techniques for influencing employees. Progressive, businesslike, humanistic management is needed to permit and facilitate the need satisfaction of employees. When you create conditions that help your people meet their needs, their self-motivation is likely to be meshed with agency goals.

THE ROLE OF THE NURSE MANAGER IN LABOR RELATIONS

When a bargaining unit is first established, there is a tendency for much time and effort to be spent by all concerned in we/they, win/lose interchanges. We have observed that this carryover from the initial negotiating effort evidences itself in hospital settings in ways that are counterproductive to patient care. The newly awarded contract often weighs heavily as a stinging defeat to management and as a sweet victory to the bargaining unit members. The intricate ploys in a serious unionizing effort give way to the newly imposed rules and regulations established by the contract. The hours once devoted to the strategy of winning or losing the election are replaced by hours involved with the shop steward in union member problems, grievance procedures, living up to the letter of the agreement, educating all concerned in understanding and living within the contract, dealing with violations of the contract, and preparing for the next contract negotiations.

It is an exercise in futility for managers to maintain an attitude of hostile, controlled acceptance of the bargaining unit and for unit members to demonstrate smugness. The critical issues have been decided. The healthiest approach is to accept that fact and move toward developing positive relationships, healing old wounds, and working together. Accomplishing such a feat is easier said than done. The impact phase of this change from nonunion to union status within a department of nursing will begin to give way to a recoil/turmoil phase and eventually lead to acceptance and accommodation—or continued rejection by the individuals involved.

Once a bargaining unit is a reality, the role of the nursing administrator has several facets. The first of these is that of maintaining a facilitative leadership role in blending the contract provisions into the goals and objectives of the department of nursing. It is vital that the nursing administrator accept and not abdicate responsibility for sound management decisions. The nursing administrator and nurse managers at all levels within the department must deal openly with employee complaints and grievances as they arise. This is simply what nurse managers have been or should have been doing in the absence of a union.

Two major changes occur with the advent of the union contract. First, the nurse managers have an additional set of rules and guidelines which must be followed in handling grievances. These new rules are contained in the legal document which is the union contract. Second, the employee group is emboldened and empowered to pursue what they see as new expectations and rights which formerly may have received less-than-satisfactory attention in their view.

This combination of the contract provisions and the new feeling of group solidarity and power among the work force may cause the nursing administrator and nurse managers to feel that they have lost status, authority, and control. Such will be the case only if they permit it to happen. In some instances, whatever feeling they had previously of status, power, and influence may have been misplaced or misused. In these cases the union serves to bring about a more equitable relationship, the kind of participation and involvement achieved by the goal-oriented manager even without third-party intervention. In other situations where capable nurse managers or administrators experience a diminution of their management responsibilities and rights, adequate support and advice by the hospital administrator (or his counselors) can aid in renewing and maintaining the feeling of position, responsibility, and authority that is justly deserved.

It is pertinent to review once again the workworld of the nurse manager (Chapters 1 and 2). You remain the center of your workworld. What you know and how you feel has much to do with how you act and react. If you overreact to a significant change in your work environment—namely, the new presence of the union—then it may be because of a distorted perception of the influence of the union on your actions. You remain the manager with the same scope of legitimate functions. Necessarily, however, you must adapt to the new element in your workworld, the union. In many ways this is little different from your adapting to nursing audit, medicare documentation requirements, patients' rights, and similar regulations affecting healthcare management in your agency.

Another responsibility of the nursing administrator is careful preparation for contract negotiations. It is wise to go to the bargaining table well prepared to bargain in good faith about issues of major concern to management and employees. This means having facts and figures to support opinions and proposals. An informed forecast of the probable demands that will be brought to the bargaining table by the union representatives will permit preparation for a strong bargaining position. Management should not place itself in the position of simply receiving the union demands and responding thereto. Rather, management should prepare its own bargaining proposals for presentation to the union. The nursing administrator can be an important contributor to such proposals. One example of such action was a group bargaining situation in a midwestern city which resulted in establishing a three-month residency for recently graduated nurses with a new starting rate lower than the prior minimum rate for graduate nurses. This could not have happened without the initiative of the nursing administrators who worked together and bargained in good faith to secure it.

The goal-oriented nursing administrator wants what is best for the healthcare agency, the patients who are the recipients of care and services, and the nursing personnel who provide that care and service. Such an administrator goes to the bargaining table prepared to secure the best contract for all concerned.

NOTES

Baer, W. E. *Grievance handling: 101 guides for supervisors.* New York: American Management Association, 1970.

Bixenstine, E. The value-fact antithesis in behavioral science. *Journal of Humanistic Psychology,* Spring 1976, *16*(2), 35–57.

Bry, A. *The TA primer: Transactional analysis in everyday life.* New York: Harper & Row, 1973.

Bryant, Y. N. Labor relations in health care institutions: An analysis of public law 93-360. *Journal of Nursing Administration.* March 1978, *8*(3), 28–39. Used with permission.

Ganong, J., & Ganong, W. *HELP with labor relations and motivational management.* Chapel Hill, N.C.: W. L. Ganong Co., 1976.

Koncel, J. Hospital labor relations struggles through its own revolution. *Hospitals, JAHA,* April 1, 1977, *51*(7), 69–74.

Likert, R. *The human organization.* New York: McGraw-Hill, 1967.

Overstreet, H., & Overstreet, B. *The mind goes forth.* New York: Norton, 1956.

Reading List

Books

American Hospital Association. *Employee-labor relations in health care institutions.* Chicago: Author, 1975.

Bennett, D. *TA and the manager.* New York: AMACOM, 1976.

Cazalas, M. W. (Ed.). *Nursing and the law* (3rd ed.). Germantown, Md.: Aspen Systems Corp., 1978.

Ganong, J., & Ganong, W. *HELP with labor relations through motivational management.* Chapel Hill, N.C.: W. L. Ganong Co., 1976.

Gellerman, S. W. *Management by motivation.* New York: American Management Association, 1968.

Goble, F. *Excellence in leadership.* New York: American Management Association, 1972.

Harris, T. A. *I'm OK—You're OK.* New York: Harper & Row, 1967.

Herzberg, F. *Work and the nature of man.* Cleveland: World Publishing, 1966.

Jongeward, D., & James, M. *Winning with people: Group exercises in transactional analysis.* Reading, Mass.: Addison-Wesley, 1973.

Likert, R. *The human organization.* New York: McGraw-Hill, 1967.

Maslow, A. *Eupsychian management: A journal.* Homewood, Ill.: Richard Irwin and The Dorsey Press, 1965.

Myers, M. S. *Every employee a manager: More meaningful work through job enrichment.* New York: McGraw-Hill, 1970.

Myers, M. S. *Managing without unions.* Reading, Mass.: Addison-Wesley, 1976.

Nierenberg, G. *The art of negotiating.* New York: Cornerstone Library, 1968.

Render, T. *Motivation: Key to good management.* New York: AMACOM, 1974.

Rutter, W. A. *Labor law* (2nd ed.). Gardena, Ca.: Gilbert Law Summaries, 1974.

U.S. Department of Labor. *Important events in American labor history 1778-1968.* Washington, D.C.: U.S. Government Printing Office, 1969.

Articles

Bryant, Y. Labor relations in health care institutions: An analysis of public law 93-360. *Journal of Nursing Administration*, March 1978, *8*(3), 28–39.

Cleland, V. Shared governance in a professional model of collective bargaining. *Journal of Nursing Administration*, May 1978, *8*(5), 39–43.

Chapter 12

Education: The Nurse Manager's Role

THE TEACHING/LEARNING SPECTRUM

Learning and teaching are natural human activities. They are a part of everyday living and they are important components of a problem-oriented nursing system. Everyone caught up in the struggle for health—patients, families, significant others, healthcare professionals, and the myriad of related healthcare workers—is involved in the educational process revolving around the maintenance or regaining of health, the disease process, and even birth and death. There is so much to learn and so much to teach that it comes as no surprise to find education as an essential element in the foundation component of PONS (as presented in Chapter 3)—and as a component in and of itself.

Both teaching and learning are involved in all of the five components that make up the problem-oriented system. The assessment part of the nursing process includes the nurse's learning about the patient and those people important to the patient, as well as his problems, needs, and goals. In turn, the patient learns about himself, about illness, wellness, and about the healthcare system. Teaching is an integral part of the implementation phase of the nursing process. Patient and family teaching is built into the planning phase. It follows that the evaluation of results as part of the nursing process is also a time for learning what has resulted for the patient from the planning and doing.

The nursing record and the auditing components of PONS also provide teaching and learning opportunities—by both patient and nurse. During the nursing process, the patient sometimes is the teacher and the nurse is the learner; in other situations during the process, the roles are reversed and the nurse becomes teacher and the patient is the learner.

In a different context this teaching/learning process works in similar fashion for the nurse manager and the rest of the nursing staff. At times the manager is thrust into the role of learner by members of the staff. At other times the roles are reversed and the manager becomes teacher to the staff. This is true at all levels of management from the nurse administrator to the head nurse (or that person's equivalent).

The process of educating yourself and others is ongoing. It takes place in both formal and informal ways and settings. It happens in offices, classrooms, hallways, elevators, patient rooms, control centers, nursing stations, cafeterias, automobiles, streets. It takes place over the telephone; via tape recorder, radio, television; through the reading of books, periodicals, newsletters, patient records, memos, workbooks; by completing patient data bases and reviewing patient referral forms; through face-to-face conversation, discussion, argument, lecture; and in committees, meetings, reports, and presentations. Indeed, the nurse manager is bombarded by the educative process at every turn. It is as natural as breathing and just as essential. Since you cannot escape it, the best thing to do is to welcome it as a healthy part of the management process and put it to good use for yourself, your staff, your patients, and your colleagues.

Education has both cognitive and affective elements. In the writings of George Brown it becomes abundantly clear that knowledge and feelings are not separate entities moving along parallel paths that never meet or mingle. Brown defines "confluent education" as the flowing together of the cognitive and affective elements in individual and group learning (Brown, 1972, p. 3). People have feelings about what they know. Learning is a process that necessarily engages both your emotions and your intellect. Heart and mind, feelings and logic—all are continuously involved in the learning and teaching in which people engage.

Many persons find it easier to identify their thoughts than their feelings. Thoughts seem to relate to facts, to a framework of logic, to a rational relationship of things and ideas we know about. People can cope with matters of logic and usually can fit them comfortably into their own apperceptive mass, the associational area of the brain. But many people find it difficult to identify and cope with feelings. There are a wide range of emotions that people experience. Too often they pass unrecognized. You may feel confused, irritated, angry, amused, anxious, put down, enlightened, wondering, puzzled, excited, apprehensive, expectant, warm, cold, impressed, disaffected, apathetic, inspired, alarmed, thrilled, belittled, provoked, joyful, agitated, happy, sorrowful, or whatever. Your emotions, whether among those just listed or others, are all acceptable. They are neither good nor bad. They are simply yours and deserve to be recognized as such. And these emotions influence learning and teaching. This being the case, we hasten to explain a term that may not be a part of everyone's vocabulary.

Yin and Yang is the ancient (11 B.C.) polarity theory of two primal forces: the dark and the light, night and day, earth and heaven, female and male, the yielding and the firm. This is symbolized by a circle divided by a thin s-curve in which one side is dark and the other light to show the rotational interplay and flowing together of opposites. Confluent education can be seen as the interplay and flowing together of seeming opposites, the affective and cognitive aspects of the teaching/learning process. Unrecognized or unresolved emotions can affect the learning outcomes in unexpected ways. They can effectively sabotage, even if unwittingly, the best efforts of both teacher and learner—regardless of who may be experiencing the emotions. Or they can be utilized in a positive way, building upon the natural yin and yang relationship of learner and teacher, to achieve the educational objectives of both. There needs to be a careful, appropriate balancing of the cognitive and affective elements of education.

An exceptionally skilled California pediatrician has been discovering for herself something significant about the doctor-patient relationship and its influence upon the healing process. This physician had always assumed that a young patient admitted to the hospital realized it was for the purpose of curing the ailment, whether sore throat or broken leg. But when she began to ask the children themselves why they were in the hospital, she found that they had reasons quite at variance with her assumptions. Some answered, "Because I was naughty." Another said, "I stole some money; that's why I'm here." In terms of psychosomatic medicine, those may very well be significant reasons for the illness or accident and subsequent hospitalization, formerly overlooked or not understood by the physician, and hence having an effect upon the healing process or the lack thereof.

It is possible that the teacher/learner relationship in a healthcare setting can benefit from the approach used by this pediatrician and her patients. The pediatrician found that when she and her patient became colleagues in healing, the patient recovered faster. There is surely a message here for the nurse in modifying the traditional teacher and learner roles so that the educational process becomes more of a mutual adventure in learning shared by colleagues.

HUMANISTIC MEDICINE, NURSING, AND TEACHING

One of the more recent trends in healthcare is being identified as humanistic medicine. It applies the precepts and practices of humanistic psychology. One of its hallmarks is a holistic view of the patient. Patients are seen not as the "CVA in Room 428" or the "liver in Room 727," but as the complex human beings they are, with all of their physical, psychological, and spiritual components—the yang and yin interplay and flowing together of natural forces, sometimes in seeming opposition to one another. This trend toward humanistic medicine demands the implementation of more humanistic teaching. The holistic approach is not new in nursing. What is new to many nursing educators and managers is the confluent approach to teaching and learning. However, there is an ever increasing trend in nursing programs and healthcare agencies toward a flowing together of the cognitive and affective elements.

ATTITUDES AND VALUES IN PERSPECTIVE

Every nurse is a teacher. The nurse as a good teacher is often characterized by descriptive terms that connote positive attitude, strong sense of values, adherence to principles, vitality, enthusiasm, empathy, understanding of individual differences, and thorough knowledge of the subject. Undoubtedly the good learner also can be characterized by the same or similar terms. This matter of attitudes and values deserves further examination. Consider yourself, your contributions, and your opportunities in a broader framework of relationships of self and others in confluent education. You are at the center of these relationships, you and your apperceptive mass, made up of your values, motives, knowledge, and skills.

Ornstein (1972) attempts to reconcile two basic approaches to knowledge: one, the rational; the other, the intuitive. He explores the bifunctional brain, the differences between the right and left sides, and the psychology of consciousness. Ongoing studies hold considerable promise for greater self-direction and control, with significant implications for confluent education. Dr. Bogen, meeting in December 1975 with educators from 19 campuses of the California system, emphasized experience as part of the education process. He said, "We have neurologic evidence to favor the view that talking about something and writing about it are very inadequate ways to learn" (Ferguson, 1975, p. 3).

TEACHER/LEARNER VS. MANAGER/WORKER

The role of a teacher and the role of a manager (in healthcare, education, business, government, and other institutions) have many common characteristics. Both teachers and managers, for example, are responsible for:

- the persons (students, workers) whom they supervise.
- setting standards and goals.

- assigning work to be done.
- providing suitable supplies, tools, working environment.
- giving instructions.
- maintaining discipline.
- effectively utilizing resources (time, money, facilities, people).
- carrying out organizational philosophy, objectives, policies.
- solving problems and conflicts.
- evaluating the performance of students and workers.
- recommending advancement as deserved.

The foregoing list provides evidence of the similarity of the roles of teachers and managers. Further examination in depth will demonstrate how the two roles merge in other ways. One of these other aspects of role similarity is the characterization of leadership style. In Figure 5–3 entitled "The Role of the Manager" the left column headed "Authority-Oriented" lists eight identifiable behavioral patterns for this leadership style. The Plan-Lead-Control diagram shows how this type of manager sees the managerial role in contrast to the employee role of doing the work. In the righthand column headed "Goal-Oriented" are the same eight aspects of a manager's role, but now stated in behavioral terms that express a subtle but distinct contrast in role concept. The diagram illustrates an expanded job concept for employees, in which they have greater opportunity to plan and control their work activities in addition to doing the work itself. Now, change the title at the top of the page. Cross out the word "Manager" and change the title to read "Roles of Teacher/Facilitator/Learner." Read again each statement in the left column. Note how closely these same items apply to the traditional authority-oriented teacher. Similarly in the righthand, few words require changing (job incumbents to learners) to have the same descriptions apply for the learning facilitator role. The revised diagrams are shown in Figure 12–1. In the Teacher/Student diagram Model T, and the Facilitator/Learner diagram Model U, the letters "T" and "U" are used for several reasons. Visually, the two diagrams can be seen as a T and a U (on its side). And "T" stands for Teacher, the more traditional version. And while the Model T Ford was a great automobile and served its users well in its day, it has long since gone out of style—as have some teaching methods. The "U" represents the full impact of you that goes into the learning-facilitator role in confluent education.

The teacher/manager analogy deserves to be carried one step further. Among the ranks of professional managers, the real professionals are looked upon as those who are skilled developers of people, good teachers. People working with these managers grow and learn. They move up to broader management or clinical responsibilities because their managers have

Figure 12-1 Roles of Teacher/Facilitator/Learner

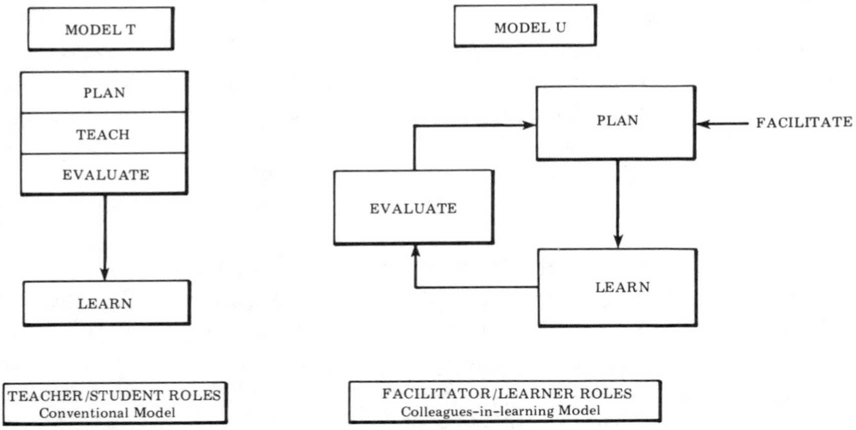

Source: Ganong, J., and Ganong, W. *HELP with innovative teaching techniques.*
Chapel Hill, N.C.: W. L. Ganong Co., 1976, p. 35.

facilitated their growth, have helped them to learn. In a similar vein, the best teachers are likely to be those who are good managers. As such, these teachers make sure that adequate tools, supplies, and facilities are available for use by the learners; encourage the learners to set their own goals; give access to information the learners want; aid their self-evaluation; recognize achievement; help the learners build on failures; and view themselves as facilitators of the learning process, as colleagues in learning.

Nurses who are in tune with the concepts of goal-oriented management and facilitative teaching can blend the two meaningfully in a patient care setting. Such nurses—in positions of administration, coordination, supervision, head nurse, or practitioner—bring to the nurse manager role a truly participative approach to the maze of daily problems.

KNEE GROUPS, IDENTITY GROUPS AND LEARNING BY INVOLVEMENT

A variety of useful learning-by-involvement teaching techniques may be used by nurse managers in their learning-facilitator role. One of these is the knee group. A knee group is defined as a discussion group of three to five people seated in a circle of chairs pulled so closely together that the knees of the participants touch. The purpose of such a group is to stimulate the maximum degree of informality and closeness among the participants so that a lively, productive interchange of ideas and feelings can occur in an atmosphere of trust and acceptance (Ganong, 1970, p. 10).

The knee group as a technique is an outgrowth of the Nurse Manager ACT-U-ARs, which are self-actualizing seminars we designed and conduct to help nurses in management positions sharpen their managerial skills and organizational effectiveness. The technique was utilized first because of the need to divide a workshop group of 30 nurse managers into small discussion groups of four or five in a meeting room with no tables and limited space. The unexpected benefits were so significant that it has since been used repeatedly with similar excellent results, regardless of the size of the room or the number in the total group.

The conference leader first provides a brief explanation of the knee group purpose and procedure. Usually the group members huddle their chairs in small circles so that their knees are in contact. This allows the people to get "in tight, not up tight," to share thoughts, feelings, and ideas through intense, personal contact with one another.

As participants begin to form the knee groups, their initial response usually includes humorous comments and joviality. The process of arranging the chairs and getting settled provides an opportunity for informal remarks and laughter which appear to relax the participants and ease them into goal-directed discussions.

A typical ACT-U-AR knee group session generally proceeds as follows:

- The group takes a few minutes to get better acquainted.
- A specific exercise, discussion question, or topic is agreed upon. The nurses focus their attention on the talking and listening aspects of the communication process. Distractions such as paper, pencils, and books are put aside.
- One person in each group volunteers or is selected to serve as recorder and jot down brief notes, when pertinent.
- The seminar leader promotes informality by his own attitude and actions.
- When appropriate, the leader may join a group briefly, getting into knee contact or not, depending upon the situation.
- At the end of the time period, the leader calls a halt to the discussion and takes a few minutes to wean the participants from their intense involvement.
- A spokesman for each knee group then presents the conclusions and salient points developed by each group.
- Additional comments are often volunteered by others in the groups.

- When all groups have reported, the ACT-U-AR leader builds upon the knee group conclusions to reinforce principles and concepts which are basic to effective management in nursing.

Since the inception of the knee group technique several years ago in the ACT-U-ARs, it has been adapted for use in a wide variety of healthcare and educational settings where the focus has been upon newer concepts of management in nursing. Nurse-managers have begun to use the knee group themselves for improving their own communications and problem-solving processes in a variety of settings. Some that have been reported to us include problem-solving by coronary care head nurses with their staff, personnel evaluation discussions by head nurses with staff members, and staff meeting discussions led by nurse administrators. Virginia Gierke, Director of Nursing Service, Memorial Hospital, Menomonie, Wisconsin, wrote:

> I have found knee groups very successful in my nursing staff meetings. R.N.'s, L.P.N.'s, Nursing Assistants, CSR. Techs and O.R. Techs are all included. They worked through their feelings about establishing priorities. Some of the feelings many Nursing Assistants and Nursing Staff expressed are:
>
> 1. "The patient pays so much per day—he deserves a complete bath every day."
> 2. "I just don't see why we can't have more staff—we can never complete all our work."
> 3. We just don't have time to work on Nursing Care Plans."
> 4. "After our work is done there is no time for a patient-centered conference."

In knee groups the following solutions were presented:
1. Start on the patient care plan at the time of admission. Involve the patient and his family in his plan of care.
2. Schedule patient-centered conferences three times a week at least and actively work at establishing priorities in order to find time for this most important part of the patient's plan of care. This will be scheduled early in the day, not after the "work is all done" (Gierke, 1976).

Times change, and ideas change, too. We now use the term *identity groups*. In any event they are a highly effective technique for securing involvement in establishing and achieving mutual goals for the improved management of nursing care and for problem solving. The close contact and intense concentration on matters of mutual concern promote feelings of genuine worth on the part of the nursing staff participants. They feel recognized as concerned persons with ideas and opinions deserving of consideration. Emphasis is upon sharing and experiencing rather than telling. The outcome is better problem definition and improved solutions with enthusiastic follow-through action. Thus identity groups provide a method for the nurse manager to secure wholehearted participation by others in the setting of goals and in implementing programs of managing by objectives.

Success by nurse managers with identity groups requires a basic belief in the worth of each individual and a willingness to perform within a framework of mutual trust and respect. Experience shows that in such a climate the nurse managers can improve team results by having their people get their heads together by getting their knees together.

The use of identity groups is especially valuable in structuring learning experiences that build upon the necessary intertwinement of the cognitive and affective components of the educative process. Following immediately is an example of a set of exercises designed to help participants better comprehend the significance of the five human needs. (See Exhibit 12-1.) The experiences are meaningful even when carried out not using identity groups. They carry extra impact, however, and achieve the objectives more successfully when the experiences take place in the small groups, and individual reactions are shared and discussed within each group. Your own experimentation with various ways of carrying out these learning exercises will prove exciting and help you develop your own innovative approaches to carrying out your learning-facilitator role for the maximum benefit of your patients and staff members.

Exhibit 12-1 Exercises in Experiencing the Human Needs

Time:　20–30 minutes.　　Group size:　Large or small.

Explain that the purpose of this exercise is to permit the participants to feel the needs and their influence on motivation and behavior.

1. Survival. Ask group to close eyes to minimize distractions. Instruct group, upon your signal, to take a deep breath and hold it for as long as possible. Tell them not to breathe again until you give the signal to do so.

(Allow 50–60 seconds to pass.)

Exhibit 12-1 continued

Ask:
- Why didn't you hold your breath longer?
- Why did you breathe again before I told you to do so?
- What was your basic need?
- What would all of you do if right now this room were sealed and the air extracted from the room?

Discuss implications. Point out (at this time as well as at end of entire exercise) that the other four human needs can be felt just as strongly, just as biologically, as the imperative need for air. (See Maslow, 1968, 1971.)

2. Security. First select a group member to stand close beside you as you explain this exercise to the group. Lean up against each other slightly, exerting modest pressure. Ask the other person to pull away from you abruptly at some time during your instructions to group.

Say to group, "Most human beings find security in their relationship to another person. That's just fine as long as the other person is there. But if one loses the support of the other (through leaving home, divorce, death) then one experiences the sense of loss. As is true with other needs, we are not conscious of its importance until it is no longer being satisfied."

Ask group to stand in pairs, side by side, and experience how it feels when the other removes the support. Allow group discussion of reactions and feelings.

3. Social: Love and Belonging. Instruct group to sit or stand in tight groups of six or seven persons, arms locked together, with one person on the outside. The group is to talk together and ignore the outsider completely, while he tries to join the group by whatever means possible.

(Allow several minutes, calling a halt as soon as appropriate.)

Allow group discussion of the experience. "How did it feel?" (To group members; to the outsider?) "If you got in (or didn't), how did you do it? What was group reaction?" Comment on the physical and emotional aspects of being an outsider. People must find a way to belong. This unsatisfied need sometimes leads to the formation of other groups, even if made up of the outsiders themselves.

4. Status, Esteem. Instruct group members, in pairs or in knee groups to tell each other, "What I like about you is . . . ." After a few minutes, when each person has told and been told, allow group discussion. Focus summary on implications for on-the-job employee relations and patient care.

5. Self-Actualization. Describe self-actualization as you understand it—a continuing reaching out for becoming more of what you can be, for peak experiences, for ongoing growth and development of oneself.

Ask knee groups to share personal examples of their own self-actualizing experiences, if any, as they understand it.

Conclude exercise by relating the experiences to confluent education, patient teaching, and the human and technical modes in patient care.

Source: Ganong, J., and Ganong, W. *HELP with innovative teaching techniques.* Chapel Hill, N.C.: W.L. Ganong Co., 1976, p. 61.

THE UNIQUENESS OF YOUR SETTING

The healthcare facility in which you find yourself is unique. It is the only one of its kind, solitary, sole, single. Its true quality of being the only one of its kind is conferred by the people, like you, who make it come alive. The people make it one of a kind. The same building with different people takes on a whole new character. Even a change of only one key person can influence the organization's personality.

In terms of confluent education, this uniqueness is the sum total of the flowing together of the thinking and feeling of all the people involved in the day-to-day operation of the institution. Your institution and the people involved in it have needs that cry out for innovative teaching techniques which will capitalize on the singular potential within each person—teacher/facilitator, student, worker, patient/consumer.

Innovative teaching in your unique setting calls for varying kinds of knowledge, skill, and ability put to use through two basic modes, the technical mode and the human mode. "Mode" refers to (1) a manner, way, or method of doing or acting; (2) a particular form, variety, or manner. The technical mode places its emphasis primarily on the techniques, systems, and procedures related to nursing, patient care, unit management, and teaching.

The main emphasis is on things rather than on people. The human mode has as its focus the people aspects of caring, planning, problem-solving, organizing, staffing, communicating, teaching, and learning. It includes the psychosocial aspects which involve understanding and awareness of self and others; attitudes, values, motivation, and personal attributes. The emphasis is on people rather than things.

Since all nurses are expected to be teacher/facilitators, they need to find a way to strike the necessary balance in the use of the technical and human modes in each setting. Both modes are necessary. Neither is independent of the other. They are, and need to be, confluent.

PRINCIPLES OF LEARNING AND TEACHING

There are available some useful roadmaps for the person who sets out upon the pathway to confluent education. These roadmaps are the learning principles, some traditional, others more innovative and in tune with recent advances in an understanding of Homo sapiens. Learning and teaching, you will recall, are two parts of the educational process. For the process to be meaningful, both the learner and the teacher need to share their feelings, skills, experiences, and knowledge. Both teacher and learner need to have feedback on their progress.

Consider now some of the more conventional concepts of learning. Margaret L. Pohl's *Teaching Function of the Nursing Practitioner* presents some useful principles as guides to action (Pohl, 1978).

1. Perception is necessary for learning.

This principle is pertinent in relation to the discussion of a learner's apperceptive mass in Section 1. People learn by relating new information and teachings to what they already know and have experienced. When experienced teachers say that they must begin from where the learners are, they are saying that they can build upon only what the learners have the ability to perceive; teachers cannot expect students to learn something not perceivable within their individual apperceptive mass. As we will soon see, however, there are ways to increase the ability to perceive, and hence to learn, within the apparent confines of current knowledge and experience levels.

2. Conditioning is a process of learning.

Conditioning is the process or result of inducing new or modified behavioral responses. To this extent, conditioning is learning. For example, in learning the Problem-Oriented Nurse System (PONS), it is necessary to become familiar with the five components of the system: The Foundation (Principles of Practice), The Nursing Process, The Problem-Oriented Nursing

Record, Nursing Audit, and Education (for Patients and Staff). Students can be helped to learn these steps by:

- writing them down on paper
- pairing off and explaining the steps to each other
- going to the board and writing them on the board
- repeating the foregoing steps, but including all of the elements for each of the five components of PONS
- practicing use of the components.

In such repetitive exercises, supported by suitable rewards and praise, the students remember and learn the PONS components and also the elements of each of the components.

3. People learn by trial and error.

Much learning is acquired through trial and error. This method works, often out of necessity. While costly, lessons learned in this way are often valuable. In certain situations where there is the need for immediate learning, such as an emergency, people do the best they can and learn from their doing. Making mistakes and correcting them as they are recognized is also a form of trial-and-error learning. People learn by doing.

4. People learn by imitation.

This is certainly one of the most common ways of learning. People tend to emulate and imitate those whom they admire and respect as well as others who have served as role models for them. They play the game of Follow the Leader. This is not just a childhood game, but one played by adults. Your nursing staff, your associates, and subordinates, observe you and say to themselves (often unconsciously), "My boss earned his/her job by being the way he/she is, by acting the way he/she does, by thinking the way he/she does. So if I become more like my boss, behaving, thinking, and doing like him/her, then I'll be a success, too." Sobering thought! Yes, people learn by imitation. The power of example is strong.

5. Developing concepts is part of learning.

A concept is an idea, especially an abstraction drawn from the specific. Thus a concept is a kind of mental picture a person develops about things in the world around him. This process of conceptualization, of concept formulation, takes place in a person's mind—just as all learning is accomplished by the learner, not the teacher. Thus concepts of a particular technique or nursing procedure may take on different characteristics in the minds of different learners.

For example, terms like "team nursing," "nursing by objectives," "performance evaluation," or "problem-oriented medical record" can mean different things to different persons. Their concepts vary according to how they were taught such techniques and how they have experienced them on the job.

One person's concept of the problem-oriented medical record is an acronym: POMR. Another person may visualize the file folder known as the patient's chart containing the carefully documented components: (a) Defined Data Base, (b) Complete Problem List, (c) Initial Plans, and (d) Progress Notes. A third nurse, however, when conceptualizing POMR, sees a whole system of quality nursing care integrated with medical care by the physician to provide the best possible patient care. A fourth person, a recipient of care, sees POMR as something that means better care for the patient, a shorter convalescence, lower cost, and an ongoing, readily accessible medical history of himself. Concepts, like perceptions, will continue to be influenced by the apperceptive mass and motivation of the individual. The cliches, "We see what we want to see," and "We hear what we want to hear," are meaningful. Thus the teacher—as guide, facilitator, and counselor—faces a real challenge in helping learners conceptualize reasonably consistent ideas about programs, techniques, and practices that affect organizational performance and patient care.

SOME NEWER PRINCIPLES OF LEARNING

Carl Rogers in *Freedom to Learn* offers a number of principles (or hypotheses) that he believes can be extracted from current experience and research. These are all related to newer approaches to learning designed to set students free for self-initiated, self-reliant learning. Here are some of his principles:

1. Human beings have a natural potentiality for learning.
2. Significant learning takes place when the subject matter is perceived by the student as having relevance for his own purposes.
3. Learning which involves a change in the perception of oneself is threatening and tends to be resisted.
4. Those learnings which are threatening to the self are more easily perceived and assimilated when external threats are at a minimum.
5. When threat to the self is low, experience can be perceived in differentiated fashion and learning can proceed (Rogers, 1969).

One can grasp quickly where Carl Rogers is coming from. He has over 40 years of experience as a teacher, experimenting and innovating in his approaches to his classroom students. He is renowned as a therapist, with unusual psychological insights and skills. He brings to his book a keen sense of urgency, deriving from his desire to help teachers and educators in a time of literally fearful crisis and incredible challenges in education. There is much of value for the nurse or teacher in what Rogers has to say. His focus is clearly on learning by doing, experiential learning, confluent education. Such learning is defined as having a quality of personal involvement, being self-initiated and pervasive (affects behavior, attitudes, even the personality of the learner), evaluated by the learner, and having its essence in meaning. This kind of learning requires a different concept of teaching. Rogers offers these precepts:

- Learning is facilitated when the student participates responsibly in the learning process.
- Self-initiated learning which involves the whole person of the learner—feelings as well as intellect—is the most lasting and pervasive.
- Independence, creativity, and self-reliance are all facilitated when self-criticism and self-evaluation are basic and evaluation by others is of secondary importance.
- The most socially useful learning in the modern world is the learning of the process of learning, a continuing openness to experience and incorporation into oneself of the process of change (Rogers, 1969).

THE CLINICAL CONFERENCE AS A LEARNING OPPORTUNITY

The clinical conference offers nursing personnel an opportunity to utilize in the work setting sound principles of teaching and learning. The clinical conference deals with real day-to-day patient care problems. It has many advantageous features as a learning environment. These features include the immediate nature of the problems and discussion topics, the intense personal involvement, the patient-focused concerns, the caring-sharing-doing tradition and the prospect of personal need satisfaction through participation and successful follow-through action. People want something to happen during, and as a result of, the clinical conference. Such desire, and the realization that each person is expected to contribute to a plan of action and its execution, helps to provide the kind of motivational climate so essential to learning. Conference participation promotes the kind of involvement that helps many persons satisfy some of their felt needs. Because a clinical conference demands participation at both cognitive and affective levels, there is an excellent opportunity for the nursing staff to observe, learn, and practice the skills of group leadership and problem-solving.

When patients (clients) are included in the clinical conference, there are benefits to them as well as to the staff personnel. Such benefits include: (1) pooling of subjective and objective information; (2) using everyone's creative potential in problem identification and problem solving; (3) raising of questions that may or may not have immediate answers; and (4) new kinds of learning as the patient and staff become colleagues in healing.

Carl Rogers indicates that "we are faced with an entirely new situation in education where the goal is the facilitation of change and learning" (Rogers, 1969). If, as Rogers states, the goal of education is the facilitation of change and learning, then the role of the teacher must be modified accordingly. What is now needed is a *facilitator* of change and learning. Such a facilitator role requires a different attitude and outlook than that of the traditional teacher. Compare the definitions of facilitate and teach. "Teach" means to impart knowledge, to instruct, to cause to learn. "Facilitate" means to make easier; to aid; to assist. The contrast between the two terms is striking. The orientation, the whole way of perceiving the teacher/learner relationship, is altered when the facilitative role is emphasized. This means a modification in how both teacher and learner think of their roles, their relationships, their expectations, and their methods of evaluating progress. Some newer techniques and methods are also required, and they are available.

One such technique is telelecture.

> Telelecture as a topic has received minimal space in the literature and/or research attention. Of that written and the research reported, only positive outcomes are depicted. In this article the use of telelecture in a continuing education course for registered nurses in two rural states is described. A critique of the author's experience in the use of this technology and an analysis of the use of cognitive learning theory in course design is presented. The author suggests that a major variable to success in the use of telelecture is the skill of the teacher/lecturer as a facilitator to solicit, organize, and present material in a manner most useful to the learner (Gosnell, 1978, p. 133).

SOME ADDITIONAL PRINCIPLES OF TEACHING AND FACILITATING

There are a number of principles of teaching conceived for the more traditional role concept of the teacher that are still useful and valid. They have served as helpful guides for many excellent teachers. Here are some of these principles:

1. The philosophy of the teacher affects teaching and learning.
2. Teaching requires effective communication and rapport.

3. Teaching requires planning and evaluation.
4. Teaching skills can be acquired through practice and observation.
5. The needs and objectives of the learner, the teacher, and the program must be considered.
6. Teaching must be relevant to the learner to be effective.

Every one of these principles is applicable to nurses in their role of teacher for staff and patients. Here are five additional guidelines for learning facilitators:

1. The facilitator has much to do with setting the initial mood or climate of the group or class experience.
2. The facilitator helps to elicit and clarify the purposes of the individuals in the group as well as the more general purposes of the group.
3. The facilitator relies upon the desire of each learner to implement those purposes which have meaning for him/her as the motivational force for significant learning.
4. The facilitator endeavors to organize and make easily available the widest possible range of resources for learning.
5. The facilitator regards himself/herself as a flexible resource to be utilized by the group.

These guidelines also apply to the nurse as teacher. The difference in emphasis between the two sets of guidelines is apparent. Each reflects a different orientation, a different way of thinking about—and attitude toward—the teacher/learner relationship. Even allowing for differing individual interpretations in what the words and sentences mean, the contrast is impressive.

HELPING THE STAFF TO LEARN

The educational process is an integral part of every nursing department's ongoing functional responsibilities. Over the years the nursing departments of healthcare agencies have created educational departments. These have been given a variety of names—Inservice, Staff Development, and Continuing Education—to name a few. These departments vary in the level of sophistication of their programs, the level of preparation of their directors and staff, their size, facilities, purpose, and budget. For some small healthcare agencies there may be one person who has the inservice function as a part of many other responsibilities. Others have centralized the educational function for the entire agency, sometimes under a director of human resources development with a registered nurse as part of the teaching staff.

There are all kinds of variations in between those two organizational extremes.

Before exploring ways to organize for the educational function of a nursing department that is supportive of a problem-oriented nursing system, there is a need to clarify some terminology with regard to the functions.

One way to examine the functions is to define them:

"Orientation," as one function, is defined as an organized program to acquaint new nursing personnel with the physical and social environment of the agency, the specific assigned work location, and the relationships within this environment of which they are now a part.

"On-the-job training," as another function, refers to that aspect of inservice education designed to help nursing personnel learn, or to improve their performance in doing, a specific task or procedure. It enhances the skill level of the individual.

"Inservice education," as yet another function, is defined as any educational experience that affects the work performance of nursing personnel. The focus is specifically job related.

"Continuing education," as still another function, is defined as organized learning experiences throughout life that contribute to individual growth and development. It is designed to help the nursing staff keep current with new concepts, knowledge, and techniques that relate to healthcare and nursing activities.

Each of these functions is appropriate to the role of education in a work setting. In a decentralized nursing department a considerable number of the activities within the first three functions take place at the patient-unit level under the overall direction of the nurse manager (by whatever title). In such a setting every nurse is accountable for the teaching part of his or her job. The nurse manager teaches the nursing staff, the staff teach other staff members as well as patients, families, and significant others. All learn from one another. Such a setting is readymade for the use of confluent education principles and guidelines.

Even a decentralized nursing department needs support and assistance from a staff development department (by whatever title). Some aspects of the educational functions are expediently handled by such a department while others rightfully are carried out at the patient-unit level. The following columns provide a typical division of responsibility between the staff development department and the patient care units for the educational functions:

Staff development department

Patient unit

1. For Orientation
    - To the agency and nursing department, and the overall organizational structure, philosophy, goals, objectives, policies, and rules.
    - To the layout of physical facility.
    - To the nursing department's patient care program.
    - To agency and nursing department systems and techniques.

    - To the unit and its specific organizational philosophy, goals, objectives, policies, and rules.
    - To patients, records, reports.
    - To unit personnel, staffing, patient assignments, unit meetings and conferences, performance responsibilities, and performance evaluation plan.
    - To the unit's physical layout details.
    - To the unit's patient care program.
    - To the unit's application of systems and techniques.

2. For Inservice
    - Plan, organize, coordinate, implement, and evaluate.
    - Agency and department-wide inservice programs—such as CPR, fire and safety, disaster, new procedures, systems, and techniques.
    - Clinical conferences of broad interest to the department.
    - Assist unit nurse-managers as needed and requested in unit-level inservice programs.
    - Collaborate with other agency departments in programs as appropriate.
    - On-the-job training for agency and department-wide procedures and tasks.

    - Knowledge and skill sessions specific to a unit.
    - Problem-solving clinics.
    - Clinical conferences specific to a unit.
    - On-the-job training for new procedures and tasks specific to unit.

3. For Continuing Education
    - Plan, organize, coordinate, implement, and evaluate

    - Assist with clinical experience aspects of residency program for

Staff development department	Patient unit
residency program for newly graduated nurses.	the newly graduated nurse.
• Clinical specialty development programs.	• Support and reinforce on the unit new learnings of self and staff for each of the programs conducted by others for unit personnel.
• Nurse-manager development program.	
• Nurse-educator programs.	
4. For Patient Education	
• Help update staff on current patient teaching principles and techniques.	• Offer direct bedside teaching.
	• Support patient learning sessions as part of nursing care plan.
• Provide resources for nursing staff and unit personnel.	

Whatever the division of responsibilities, careful planning and decision making is required so that there is mutual understanding about who is responsible for what. When everyone is responsible, then usually no one is. Managing the educational function requires an understanding of the philosophy upon which such a function is built. As one element of the foundation for PONS, there must be a stated purpose, clearly delineated objectives, and specific functions spelled out for the staff development department. The director of the department should be a nurse who can function as a facilitator, coordinator, teacher, and manager. Organizationally, such a person should be in a staff rather than a line position in relation to the rest of the nursing department. As such, he or she can be viewed by the nursing staff as a valuable resource person. Thus the job requires that this director be flexible, creative, and knowledgeable about current healthcare concepts, issues and trends as they relate to nursing; be able to listen to the needs and problems of others, and use confluent educational principles; and be attuned to the learning needs of both the staff development instructors and the nursing staff throughout the agency, using the results of nursing audit to help identify such current learning needs.

Another vital education-related function is selecting, maintaining, and encouraging the use of books and journals in a nursing library. This responsibility may be carried out by the staff development director in conjunction with the agency healthcare librarian (if any), the director of nursing, and the dean or director of the school of nursing. A new and highly valuable resource is the "Selected List of Nursing Books and Journals" updated on a regular basis in *Nursing Outlook* (Brandon & Hill).

PATIENT EDUCATION

Levin provides a useful analysis of the substantive distinctions between patient education and self-care education—the latter a concept which "challenges both the economic and philosophic lifelines of professional health care services" (Levin, 1978, p. 171). He cites and comments upon five areas of contrast. We summarize these as follows:

Patient Education	*Self-Care Education*
1. Assumes a sick person under the care of another; not usually directed toward reducing dependency.	1. Does not assume sickness; assigns a generic meaning to care—to look after; shifts decision-making control of healthcare to the lay person.
2. Deals largely with *insultive* diseases (biological, psychological, environmental), rather than *assaultive* diseases—those caused by the healthcare givers.	2. Emphasis on lay skills in the *management* of the professional care system, and control of iatrogenic illness.
3. Provides new knowledge and skills where patient has little or no experience.	3. Relies heavily on knowledge and skill person already has.
4. Focuses on individual's personal health behavior, activities over which he has control; may adopt a blame-the-victim posture.	4. Relates personal health status to forces in the environment; considers skills for social change; demystification of enviropolitics.
5. Uses methods suitable for teaching specific skills (active learner trials under supervision; problem solving; use of resources).	5. Uses similar methods—plus exercises designed to center health control in the individual; strategies to shift locus of health control from professional to lay person.

Levin believes that

> We are in an exciting era of transition in health and health care —a transition from a professionally dominated world of service to one of self-service. The process of demystifying medicine and demedicalizing society is just now rising to our consciousness as a profound turning point in the history of health. We must come to terms with changing patterns of morbidity, emerging pluralism in

> chronic disease care, less rigid and moralistic perspectives on
> avoidance of risk, recognition of iatrogenic effects, and apprecia-
> tion of the lay resource as the primary and least dangerous health
> resource. ... patient education and self-care education are ad-
> vocacy strategies which can contribute to the public's health com-
> petence at different points on the same continuum. Now is the time
> to clarify the mutuality of their values and to identify their special
> contributions to health education, uncompromisingly operating in
> the public interest (Levin, 1978, p. 175).

The level of satisfaction with patient education in most healthcare settings
can be improved. Many agencies are making strenuous efforts to upgrade
this vital aspect of patient care services. Patient education is more complex
than it may first appear to be. What is involved is a change process, actually
altering the way a person eats, exercises, sleeps, walks, bathes, uses various
parts of the body, adjusts to the wearing or manipulation of a prosthesis,
takes medication, and modifies the habits of a lifetime. These and other adjustments may seem complex and even frightening to the patient or client.
The problem is compounded by such things as the patient's values, cultural
background, religion, education, life style, the influence of family and
friends, past experience, superstition, misinformation, fear, and apathy.

> Effective teaching is an integral part of the nursing process, and the
> nurse is teaching, whether directly or indirectly, in every contact
> with potential learners. Sometimes teaching as a part of care is ob-
> vious. ... At other times it may appear that no teaching is being
> done. ... Actually the nurse is teaching through what is being
> done, by the way it is being done, and through attitudes expressed
> with or without words both to the patient and to visitors (Pohl,
> 1979, p. 126).

People change themselves and their habits only when they want to or need
to. Change, like motivation, is a personal thing. Change has much to do with
motivation. Learning has more to do with achieving personal change than
does teaching. Thus the nurse needs to be aware of what the patient is learning. Careful chronological documentation of a patient's learning progress
can prove to be an invaluable source of information to all nursing staff
members caring for that patient in preparation for discharge. The patient
teaching flow sheet previously described in Chapter 3 is an example of one
way to go about documenting the teaching objectives and learning
achievements as part of a patient's progress. This flow sheet is used as part of

the implementation phase of the nursing process. It is a part of the nursing plan of care and is used throughout the patient's entire care program.

Zander, Bower, Foster, Towson, Wermuth, and Woldum note that:

> There are times when nurses realize from their assessments that patients are unable to learn much of all of what must be taught. They may have physical limitations that prevent them from carrying out their care independently or they may be emotionally or intellectually unable to learn at the present time. In these instances the nurse seeks a responsible family member or friend, a "significant other," who is willing to participate in the care of the patient. The teaching process then proceeds, involving the patient as fully as possible but focusing primarily on a significant other (Zander et al., 1978, p. 3).

The HELP acronym has varied uses. We used it for our *HELP Series of Management Guides* to mean Healthcare Education and Learning Program. Children's Hospital in Columbus, Ohio, used HELP for its Homegoing Education and Literature Program. This is now available in book form—*Patient and family education: Tools, techniques, and theory* (McCormick & Gilson-Parkevich, 1979). For another patient education service, available in both English and Spanish, see *Patient information library*, 1980.

The use of the patient teaching flow sheet is an example of combining the technical and human modes for the benefit of patient care. The flow sheet itself is a technical mode: the form had to be designed and produced—simple enough for ease of use but complete enough for documentation purposes in connection with nursing audit. Plans had to be made for its introduction, acceptance, and use as part of the medical record. The human mode aspects were uppermost in considering the form in relation to its purposeful use by the patient care team—as part of the problem-oriented nursing system, discharge planning, and the patient's motivation to follow through during and after hospitalization. Well-designed tools and systems help make possible the effective use of the human mode; they never are substitutes for it.

A STEP-BY-STEP INSTRUCTIONAL GUIDE

The Job Instruction Training (JIT) program of years past helped many persons learn how to teach job skills to new employees. The four steps of "How to Instruct" are relevant to teaching patients certain skills such as injections, dressings, and other procedures they or their families will have to do at home. The following step-by-step guide for getting ready to instruct and then giving the instruction is adapted from the JIT program:

Get Ready to Instruct

Have a Timetable
   How much skill or knowledge is the learner expected to have, by what date?
Break Down the Task (or learning segment)
   List important steps.
   Pick out the key points. (Safety is always a key point.)
Have Everything Ready
   The right equipment, materials, and supplies.
Have the Workplace Properly Arranged
   Just as the learner will be expected to keep it.

How to Instruct

Step 1: Prepare the Learner
   Put him at ease.
   State the procedure (or learning segment) and find out what he already knows about it.
   Get him interested in learning the procedure.
   Place in correct position (if pertinent).
Step 2: Present the Procedure (or learning segment)
   Tell, show, illustrate one important step at a time.
   Stress each key point.
   Instruct clearly, completely, and patiently, but no more than he can master.
Step 3: Try-Out Performance
   Have him do the procedure (return demonstration); correct errors.
   Have him explain each key point to you as he does the procedure again.
   Continue until you know he knows—and can do it.
Step 4: Follow Through
   Put him on his own. Designate to whom he goes for help. Document progress.
   Check frequently. Encourage questions.
   Taper off extra coaching and follow-up.

The true worth of what the patient and family have really learned can be identified when the label "patient" is removed and the "person" once again joins the ranks of society outside the confines of the healthcare agency. The true indicators of successful patient teaching and learning are the changes the person decides to make in life style to continue recovery and to prevent or forestall further health problems and hospitalization.

This chapter has dealt with one of the three major responsibilities of the nurse manager, namely, human resources development for patients, families, and staff members. This responsibility deserves equal emphasis with the responsibilities for patient care management and operational management in the day-to-day delivery of healthcare.

NOTES

Brandon, A. N., & Hill, D. R. Selected list of nursing books and journals. *Nursing Outlook,* October 1979, *27*(10), 672–681.

Brown, G. I. *Human teaching for human learning.* New York: Viking, 1972.

Ferguson, M. (Ed.). University conference: Split-brain research and education. *Brain/Mind Bulletin,* December 15, 1975.

Ganong, J. W. Knee groups: Techniques for improving communications and achieving nursing objectives. *Supervisor Nurse,* December 1970, pp. 10–13.

Ganong, J., & Ganong, W. *HELP with innovative teaching techniques.* Chapel Hill, N.C.: W. L. Ganong Co., 1976.

Gierke, V. *The philosophy and objectives of the nursing service department.* Report submitted in a course on Patient Care Administration at the University of Minnesota, April 30, 1976. Used with permission.

Gosnell, D. J. $T^2 = 1$: Theory and technology combine for learning. *Journal of Educational Technology Systems,* 1978–79, *7*(2), 133–141.

Levin, L. S. Patient education and self-care: How do they differ? *Nursing Outlook,* March 1978, *26*(3), 170–175.

Maslow, A. H. *Toward a psychology of being* (2nd ed.). New York: Van Nostrand Reinhold Co., 1968, pp. 3, 23.

Maslow, A. H. A theory of metamotivation: The biological rooting of the value-life. *The farther reaches of human nature.* New York: The Viking Press, 1971, p. 316.

McCormick, R. D., & Gilson-Parkevich, T. *Patient and family education: Tools, techniques, and theory.* New York: John Wiley & Sons, 1979.

Ornstein, R. *The psychology of consciousness.* San Francisco: W. H. Freeman, 1972.

Patient information library. Daly City, Ca., 94015: Physicians Art Service, Inc., 1980 (updated annually, in English and Spanish).

Pohl, M. L. *Teaching function of the nursing practitioner* (3rd ed.). Dubuque: Wm. C. Brown, 1978.

Pohl, M. L. The teaching function of the nurse. In A. Marriner (Ed.), *Current perspectives in nursing management.* St. Louis: C. V. Mosby, 1979.

Rogers, C. *Freedom to learn.* Columbus: Merrill, 1969, pp. 157–164.

Silten, R. M., & Levin, L. S. Self-care evaluation. In P. M. Lazes (Ed.), *The handbook of health education.* Germantown, Md.: Aspen Systems Corp., 1979, pp. 201–223.

Travis, J. W. *Wellness workbook for health professionals* (Part IV). Mill Valley, Ca.: Wellness Resource Center, 1977.

Zander, K. S., Bower, K. A., Foster, S. D., Towson, M. C., Wermuth, M. R., & Woldum, K. M. *Practical manual for patient-teaching.* St. Louis: C. V. Mosby, 1978.

Reading List

Books

Bloom, B. *Taxonomy of educational objectives. Handbook I: Cognitive domain.* New York: David McKay, 1956.

Brown, G. I. *Human teaching for human learning: An introduction to confluent education.* New York: Viking, 1972.

Burton, W., Kimball, R., & Wing, R. *Education for effective thinking.* New York: Appleton-Century-Crofts, 1960.

Cyrs, T. E. *You, behavioral objectives and nutrition education.* Chicago: National Dairy Council, 1973.

Dewey, J. *Experience and education.* New York: Collier-Macmillan, 1963.

Ganong, J., & Ganong, W. *HELP with innovative teaching techniques.* Chapel Hill, N.C.: W. L. Ganong Co., 1976.

Gordon, T. *Teacher effectiveness training.* New York: Peter H. Wyden, 1974.

Gordon, T. *Leader effectiveness training, L.E.T.* New York: Wyden Books, 1977.

Highet, G. *The art of teaching.* New York: Random House, 1950.

Johnson, R. B. *Humanizing instruction or . . . Helping your students up the up staircase.* Chapel Hill, N.C.: Self-Instructional Packages, 1972.

Jonas, G. *Visceral learning.* New York: Viking, 1973.

Kübler-Ross, E. *Death: The final stage of growth.* Englewood Cliffs, N.J.: Prentice-Hall, 1975.

Lau, J. B. *Behavior in organizations: An experiential approach.* Homewood, Ill.: Richard D. Irwin, 1975.

Leonard, G. *Education and ecstasy.* New York: Delacorte, 1968.

Mager, R. *Developing attitude toward learning.* Belmont, Cal.: Fearon, 1968.

Mager, R. *Measuring instructional intent.* Belmont, Ca.: Fearon, 1973.

McCormick, R. D., & Gilson-Parkevich, T. (Eds.). *Patient and family education: Tools, techniques, and theory.* New York: John Wiley & Sons, 1979.

Medical self-care: Access to medical tools. Inverness, Ca., 94937: Medical Self-Care, P.O. Box 717. Published quarterly.

Moustakas, C. *Creativity and conformity.* Princeton: Van Nostrand, 1968.

Ott, H., & Mann, J. *Ways of growth—Approaches to expanding awareness.* New York: Viking, 1968.

Perls, F. S., & Hefferline, R. F. *Gestalt therapy: Excitement and growth in the human personality.* New York: Julian Press, 1951.

Pfeiffer, J. W., & Jones, J. E. (Eds.). *The annual handbook for group facilitators.* Iowa City: University Associates, 1972-1980.

Pirsig, R. M. *Zen and the art of motorcycle maintenance.* New York: Bantam, 1975.

Popiel, E. *Nursing and the process of continuing education.* St. Louis: C. V. Mosby, 1973.

Powell, J. *Why am I afraid to tell you who I am?* Niles, Ill.: Argus Communications, 1969.

Raths, L., Harmin, M., & Simon, S. *Values and teaching.* Columbus: Charles E. Merrill, 1966.

Samples, B., & Wohlford, B. *Opening: A primer for self-actualization.* Menlo Park, Ca.: Addison-Wesley, 1975.

Schechter, D. *Agenda for continuing education: A challenge to health care institutions.* Chicago: Hospital Research and Educational Trust, 1974.

Schrank, J. *Teaching human beings.* Boston: Beacon, 1972.

Simon, S. B., Howe, L. W., & Kirschenbaum, H. *Values clarification: A handbook of practical strategies for teachers and student.* New York: Hart, 1972.

Stevens, J. O. *Awareness: Exploring, experimenting, experiencing.* Moab, Utah: Real People Press, 1971.

Sutterly, D., & Donnelly, G. *Perspectives in human development—Nursing throughout the life cycle.* Philadelphia: J. B. Lippincott, 1973.

Thayer, L., & Beeler, K. (Eds.). *Handbook of affective tools and techniques.* Mimeographed. Ypsilanti, Mich.: E. Michigan University, 1974.

Tough, A. *The adult's learning projects: A fresh approach to theory and practice in adult learning.* Research in Education Series No. 1. Toronto: Ontario Institute for Studies in Education, 1971.

Wilhelm, R., & Baynes, C. *The I Ching or book of changes.* Bollingen Series XIX. Princeton: Princeton University Press, 1967.

Zander, K. S., Bower, K. A., Foster, S. D., Towson, M. C., Wermuth, M. R., & Woldum, K. M. (Eds.). *Practice manual for patient-teaching.* St. Louis: C. V. Mosby, 1978.

Articles

Calkin, J. D. Let's rethink staff development programs. *Journal of Nursing Administration,* June 1979, *9*(6), 16-19.

del Bueno, D. J. Patient education: Planning for success. *Journal of Nursing Administration,* June 1978, *8*(6), 3-7.

Ganong, W. L., & Ganong, J. M. Good advice: Training and education in health care organizations. *Journal of Nursing Administration,* May-June 1972, *2*(3), 8.

Ganong, W. L., & Ganong, J. M. Knee groups—In tight, not up tight. *Training and Development Journal,* July 1970, p. 27.

Levin, L. Patient education and self-care: How do they differ? *Nursing Outlook,* March 1978, *26*(3), 170-175.

Marenco, E., Jr. Health education: An alternative to illness. *Family and Community Health,* April 1978, *1*(1), 31-36.

Tranbarger, R. Continuing education in a rural hospital: Does it make a difference? *Journal of Nursing Administration,* August 1978, *8*(8), 39-42.

Wales, S., & Hageman, V. Guided design systems approach in nursing education. *Journal of Nursing Education,* March 1979, *18*(3); 38, 41-45.

Chapter 13

Wide-Track Careers
in Nursing

THE RATIONALE FOR CAREER LADDERS

Earlier chapters have referred to some of the needs, problems, and opportunities in connection with careers for nurses and other healthcare personnel. While much has been written and discussed about career ladders and planned job progression, specific examples of successful program applications are all too few. In fact, the requirements of the agencies which license, certify, and educate healthcare occupational and professional personnel sometimes seem deliberately designed to frustrate and discourage the person who seeks upward mobility in the field of healthcare. For many persons the time and economic considerations alone—in spite of governmental and labor union financial support programs—are enough to sidetrack their motivation to undertake the prescribed qualifying routine. And for nurses, as a capstone to this escalating educational edifice, is the discovery that after a four-year or even five-year program leading to a bachelor's degree with the privilege of taking an examination for state licensure as a registered nurse, the coveted and hard-earned RN has no more meaning legally or in being considered a nurse than does the RN earned by passing the same state board examination as a graduate of a two-year associate-degree program or a two- or three-year hospital school of nursing program.

In addition, the observant RN soon learns through experience that many long-service LPNs and some nurse aides are performing satisfactorily a significantly high percentage (80–90 percent) of the tasks and procedures once the responsibility of the registered nurse. At the same time, a trend in some hospitals has been to assign broad nursing management and administrative functions to nonnurse unit managers, coordinators, or assistant and associate hospital administrators. These trends over recent decades have in fact been encouraged and promoted by some nursing leaders and accepted passively by other nursing educators and practitioners. Current attempts to reassess the meaning of these trends and to evaluate their success in terms of patient care and their implications for nursing are long overdue, painful, and of great concern to all nurse managers. And well they should be!

In a May 1978 *AJN* editorial, Thelma Schorr wrote:

> It is now 13 years since the American Nurses' Association issued its famous position paper on educational preparation for nursing practice, which said that nursing education should take place in institutions of higher learning, that the minimum preparation for professional nursing practice should be a baccalaureate, and that the minimum for technical nursing practice should be an associate degree.
>
> The question of whether upper-division nursing education can be added to what nurses already know is causing new battles. The purists maintain that technical education (a term that never gained much acceptance or validity) is terminal (another idea that never really flew). Perhaps the high-quality minds of many of the students who have, for one reason or another, gone into associate degree programs helped to alter the original conception of the AD nurse as one who would not seek to further his or her professional education. Professionalism is the goal of all the diploma and AD nurses I meet, and most expect to move right along and earn their baccalaureates (Schorr, 1978, p. 823).

Nurses responded to the ANA position paper—individually and collectively. A widely-known response is the "85 Resolution" of the New York State Nurses Association, calling for legislative action to mandate a baccalaureate degree for nurse licensure (*RN Magazine,* 1976). A number of other states have similar proposals being considered. One response to these efforts is that of the American Hospital Association's Board of Trustees, which voted to oppose "with full vigor" legislative efforts underway in several states to limit by 1985 registered nurse licensure to graduates of baccalaureate programs (*Hospital Week,* May 28, 1976). (Also see Wilkinson, J. A. Hospital schools of nursing: Profits counterpoise costs. *Hospitals,* April 16, 1976, pp. 95-98.)

As we move into the 1980s, the marketplace is responding in its own way. Witness the degree requirements (*bachelor* and *master* levels) being specified in recruitment advertising. Recognizing this trend, nurses want to protect their license. And until such time as the BSN *is* the required degree, many nurses will continue to seek any routes to a nonnursing bachelor's degree as are available to fit their individual life situations. The one with which we are most familiar (as we have served as faculty members for the summer residency sessions) is the External Degree Program of St. Joseph's College in North Windham, Maine. We are impressed with the program's impact and results (Ganong & Ganong, December 1978). Gradually opportunities are becoming available for practicing RNs to earn the BSN degree without returning to *base one* and paying a heavy forfeit in their life/work situation.

For the future, we concur with the thrust towards professionalism in the interests of the consumer. Nurses will play increasingly varied professional roles in the clinical and management aspects of the promotion and maintenance of health—and in the prevention, cure-and-care aspects of illness. (See Chapter 12 for more extended discussion.)

Nurse managers by definition are leaders within their own agencies and are in a position to exert meaningful leadership in their professions of nursing and management. Unless you do so you have little reason to complain of the results of leadership provided by others.

The Nurse Practitioner

Other factors are at work too which influence nursing education and practice. An increasing number of master's and doctoral programs for nurses place their emphasis upon a high-skill level of clinical patient care for professional practitioners. Graduates of such programs are finding increasing opportunities as nurse practitioners in various clinical specialties in public health agencies, community centers, and medical practice groups, as consultants, and as independent general nurse practitioners. One hurdle to more extensive use of such nurse practitioners is the lack of payment for their individual services as part of third party payer contractual arrangements. This impediment is in the process of being resolved.

> The career ladder in nursing has some innovative rungs. .... the title, role, and qualifications of the "nurse practitioner" are still evolving and the advice of "go thou and do likewise" should prudently be offered to those contemplating practicing independently .... .
>
> Fee-for-service practice through individual contracts between nurses and patients, and in increasing instances through reimbursement by third-party payers, has been the economic base of private duty nursing in this country for years. Thus, while the idea of direct payment to a nurse for her services is not new, the nurse's being engaged in the independent practice of nursing is (Zimmerman, 1977, p. xiii).

Jacox and Norris, in this same book—a report of a two-day NMIH grant-supported conference of nurse practitioners—state that:

> They want to be responsible and accountable for their own patients or, as they say, their own "patient care load." They want to control their own practice, to provide primary care and have primary therapeutic responsibility in their areas of expertise. They want to be paid adequately and directly for the services they provide. They want a voice in health care legislation, recognition at all levels of government of the contribution professional nursing can make, and support for nursing built into new legislation in the same way it is built in for other professions. These nurses are competent in the business and economic aspects of professional practice (Jacox & Norris, 1977, p. 3).

A combination of actions by state legislatures, together with the entrepreneurial spirit of some nurses, is creating a new climate for nursing practice. In Maryland the state law now requires insurance companies to provide reimbursement for any services within the lawful scope of practice of a duly licensed healthcare provider (Reimbursement for all, 1979). In California nurses may own up to 49 percent of professional medical corporations, originally limited to physicians (California law lets nurses share, 1979). For nurses who wish to set up and manage their own practice, there are guides for doing so (Koltz, 1979).

Other Career Opportunities

Other advanced-degree graduates are finding opportunities in hospitals as clinical specialists, nurse clinicians, primary nurses, patient care coordinators, and related roles. Such well-educated clinical nurses sometimes encounter misunderstanding and lack of acceptance in the traditional hospital healthcare environment. The degree of acceptance varies with the caliber of orientation provided for the clinicians themselves and for the agency personnel for whom they are expected to become a valued resource. Much depends also upon the interpersonal skills of the individual clinicians and the particular nurse manager with whom they become associated. All too often neither party—the clinician or the nurse manager—has a clear conceptualization of the role relationships they must establish in an already complex socially layered organizational structure. With adequate planning, patience, and goodwill, a successful working relationship can be achieved so that the patient benefits.

One advantage of the primary nursing concept as an alternative method for the delivery of patient care is that it usually is an adaptation of the existing nursing process within the hospital. It becomes part of a transitional participative process, realigning and expanding the roles of present nursing personnel. Carefully introduced, it offers the possibility of achieving the patient-care goals sought through the introduction of nurse practitioner specialists, but with greater success. However, as with any innovation, success depends as much upon the process of implementation as upon the validity of the concept. And the success of the process in turn depends upon the knowledgeability and skills of the nurse manager in the three major areas of responsibility—clinical management, operational management, and human resources management.

The comments of the preceding paragraph apply also to the introduction of the problem-oriented nursing system. PONS is another example of how nurses can introduce and successfully implement an innovative management technique designed to enhance patient care through a planned transitional process. PONS builds upon the existing patient care medical model; it supplements and strengthens the nursing process as presently practiced; it accepts and functions within the established organizational structure and the realities of the ongoing medical-administrative-nursing staff relationships; it places faith in the nurse-as-manager for successful implementation; it permits nurses—from whatever educational program—to practice nursing in a manner commensurate with their visions of professional nursing; and PONS helps to provide the kind of inspirational environment that encourages nursing personnel to pursue their career inclinations and goals upon the wide track of nursing opportunities. (See Chapter 3.)

There has been a tendency during recent decades to create names to describe a variety of programmatic concepts for the delivery of nursing care. The names given to some of the popular approaches include functional nursing, team nursing, case method, and primary nursing. These kinds of nursing approaches and others as well have resulted from the natural striving of nursing leaders to improve nursing's contribution to patient care within our country's multifaceted healthcare delivery system. Problems arise, however, when enthusiastic followers and practitioners begin to espouse a particular brand name nursing method with missionary zeal and fervor. The time has come, we believe, for nurses to be able to refer to nursing in the same way that physicians refer to medicine. Nursing does not need, any more than does medicine, several brand name versions competing in this year's popularity contest. Hence our emphasis upon functions, techniques, and skills rather than upon a new way of delivering patient or nursing care.

THE WIDE-TRACK CAREER LADDER MODEL

A wide-track careers program in nursing is a viable system for providing selective career options with commensurate progression of responsibility and earnings on three main tracks in nursing—managerial, educational, and clinical—within a single healthcare agency; using agency-developed criteria for defining the progressive steps on each track, the necessary continuing education and training, and the related qualifying procedures; and opportunity to move from one track to another. Organizations other than general hospitals provide specific career opportunities that justify showing research as one of four main tracks open to qualified nurses—especially when career progress is being considered broadly in an interagency context.

Figure 13-1 shows the wide-track careers concept. First are the three main career pathways, with opportunities for nurses to move from one track to another—including research when that is a feasible option.

The concept is also presented as four career ladders with an ascending scale of progressive salary steps. The rungs on each ladder represent, at each level, equivalent salaries for equivalent performance responsibilities. (Such salary scales are commonly set by job and salary evaluation. For a discussion of the drawbacks of this technique and an explanation of another innovative method, see Jaques, 1979.)

Note carefully that salary progression depends on having prepared oneself for additional responsibilities through a qualifying procedure based in part on in-house availability of suitable education and training programs.

Actual salary adjustments occur (within the career ladder program) when the prepared person has been promoted into a higher-level job classification. This means having an expanded number of job classifications on all four tracks. At Rex Hospital, in the case example that follows, the levels of progression on the clinical track were set up in this way:

NA I
NA II
NA III
PN   Each of these performance levels was selected and
LPN I   defined to provide a meaningful career ladder. The
LPN II   number of steps from NA I through RN IV is af-
LPN III   fected in part by a pragmatic approach to how they
GN   will fit within the agency-wide wage and salary
RN I   system.
RN II
RN III
RN IV

It should be obvious that setting up a wide-track careers program in nursing is a major project. It has many ramifications which affect, and are affected by, the organizational characteristics of the entire healthcare agency.

Figure 13-1 A Model for Wide-Track Careers in Nursing

The Career Pathways

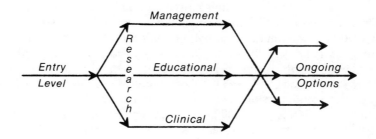

The Career Ladders

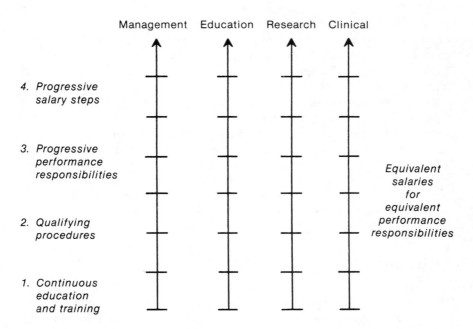

Source: Ganong, J., & Ganong, W. *HELP with wide-track careers in nursing.* Chapel Hill, N.C.: W. L. Ganong Co., 1977, p. 6.

Therefore, based upon experience, we recommend that any task force assigned to plan a career ladders program use the Nursing Organization Inventory Checklist as a first step. In fact, Exhibit 13-1 can be valuable as a detailed self-conducted management audit of your nursing department even if you are not yet ready to start planning for wide-track career ladders. (See also Ganong & Ganong, *HELP with Wide-Track Careers in Nursing,* 1977).

Wide-track careers in nursing must be considered in the context of one other set of facts about healthcare in this country. AHA statistics for 1977 indicated that approximately one-half (48 percent) of all community hospitals in this country had less than 100 beds, but these hospitals employed only 11.5 percent of all hospital personnel. All hospitals in the size category of less than 300 beds comprised 84 percent of all community hospitals, employing 47 percent of all hospital personnel in 1977. The remaining 16 percent of the community hospitals were over 300 beds in size, employing 53 percent of the personnel. However, the eleven-year trend from 1963 through 1973 showed a marked *decrease* in the less-than-100-bed hospitals. The *increase* was 72 percent for community hospitals in the 400-499 bed range, and 88 percent for those with 500 or more beds. These data—and other related statistical information connected with personnel utilization, costs, career opportunities, and nationwide trends in the delivery of healthcare—document the urgency of organized programs for facilitating career progress for all categories of personnel in hospitals both large and small. For nursing personnel, a wide-track careers program, as adapted to particular healthcare agencies or groups of agencies, provides an organized, effective plan for action.

One such example in a multihospital system is Intermountain Health Care, Salt Lake City, Utah. Career ladder steps are being developed for clinical nurses and include all 22 hospitals in the system, ranging in size from 15 beds to 587 beds. Verla B. Collins, Ph.D., corporate director of nursing and education, cites a number of advantages for nursing in such a multiunit system. These include resolving rural hospital staffing problems with a six-week to three-month job rotation program for nurses in the larger metropolitan hospitals (LaViolette, 1980). Another wide-track careers program as developed in a single hospital is described next.

REAP: THE REX HOSPITAL EXAMPLE

The Rex Employee Advancement Program or REAP is the name given to the wide-track careers program as it was implemented by the nursing department of Rex Hospital in Raleigh, N.C. This program proved to be an undertaking of major proportions. It was approved by Joseph E. Barnes, Director of Rex Hospital, and initiated after the nursing department had experienced a period of self-development and organizational renewal under the leadership

Exhibit 13-1 Nursing Organization Inventory Checklist

NURSING ORGANIZATION INVENTORY CHECKLIST
An Audit of Where We Are Now in Our Departmental Workshop

Prepared by _____ Title _____ Date _____

Instructions: *See accompanying description of each item. Use this checklist to indicate availability and adequacy of each item and whatever follow-through you decide is required. (Substitute your healthcare agency name for "hospital" in the item list.)*

ITEM	Available? Yes	Available? No (when?)	Reviewed (date)	Understandable? OK	Understandable? Not OK	Follow Through (What? Who? When?)
Hospital Organization Chart Nursing Organization Chart						
Support Personnel: Systems & Planning Coord. Staffing & Budgeting Coord. Nurse Recruiting Coord. Unit Instructors Clinical Specialists Quality Assurance Coord.						
Hospital Policy Manual Nursing Policy Manual						
Hospital Goals & Objectives Nursing Goals & Objectives						
Hospital Budget(s) Nursing Budget(s)						
Wage and Salary Scales Job Descriptions						
Performance Descriptions Performance Evaluation Plan						
Labor Union Contract Employee Handbook						
Workworld of Mgrs. Defined: Values Motivation Knowledge Skills Clinical Management Operational Management Ns. Mgr. as Hosp. Integrator Unit Profile						
Nursing Modality Defined Nursing Roles Defined						
Recruitment Orientation Staff Development Staffing Other: _____						

Source: Ganong, W. L., & Ganong, J. *HELP with wide-track careers in nursing.* Chapel Hill, N.C.: W. L. Ganong Co., 1977, p. 16.

of Sarah Hitchcock, Director of Nursing, in a most favorable professional environment for innovation. Organizational changes had included expanding to all patient care units the patient care coordinator concept which had been introduced earlier as a pilot project on one of the large patient care units. Not long thereafter the hospital school of nursing was phased out as another aspect of financial and program planning.

The initial planning and implementation efforts for REAP were carried out by the patient care coordinators and other staff personnel including the inservice education director and the staffing coordinator. This hard-working group produced the initial drafts of the lengthy task lists for the different job categories which serve as helpful criteria for the different job levels. These lists were later reviewed and refined by head nurses and other nursing staff representatives from the different units.

Another vital phase of the project was the writing of performance descriptions for all positions in the nursing department. These follow the format used in other chapters of this book (see Chapters 1 and 6). They replaced the existing job descriptions and serve not only to define the major responsibilities for the persons in each job category, but also to provide the basis for results-oriented performance evaluation.

The next section of this chapter presents the description of REAP as developed by the nursing department for its staff members, the membership and objectives of the REAP Committee, policy statements covering the program, and a sampling of the performance descriptions and task lists being used. As with any worthwhile program, continuing maintenance and updating is required. The REAP Committee meets as necessary to revise and refine important elements of the total plan. One such element is the criteria used for identifying the job levels in each position category and for evaluating the readiness of a person for promotion from one job level to another and from one position category to another. Work is being done to augment the task lists with criteria relating more directly to skill in using the nursing process and related patient care programs.

REX HOSPITAL NURSING DEPARTMENT

Rex Employee Advancement Program

The Rex Employee Advancement Program (REAP) was developed within Nursing Service to maintain and improve the caliber of patient care, to increase growth and income opportunities for Nursing Service personnel and to achieve these goals while decreasing the relative rate of operating expenses. It was felt that such a program should be implemented to assist in meeting the present and future staffing needs in the Nursing Department at Rex Hospital. The following factors have the potential for making these needs more acute:

1. The closing of diploma Schools of Nursing in North Carolina, including our own Rex Hospital School of Nursing, will greatly decrease the resources for recruitment.
2. The trend toward increased utilization of LPNs and graduates of Associate Degree programs will require that the employer provide for intensive and extensive orientation as well as continuing education.
3. The turnover rate among the Nursing Assistants is creating a cost factor that must be dealt with in terms of dollars and cents as well as the amount of Inservice Education time that must be spent in training. This time could be better utilized in the development of personnel already on the staff.

People have varied ideas of career planning and development. This is as it should be, since the subject is a matter of such personal concern. Yet it is also a matter of vital organizational concern, since the survival and well-being of Rex Hospital is dependent upon those who build their careers here. Thus, mutually understood concepts, assumptions, and procedures which best achieve the goals of all individuals and the organization are needed. A number of such concepts and considerations are set forth below:

1. People are one of the most important assets at Rex Hospital. This is a fundamental belief that forms the foundation for Rex's administrative philosophy and for its personnel policies and procedures.
2. "Career" means a person's lifework, profession, occupation. As the term "career" is used here, it means also "one's advancement or achievement in a particular vocation." Some persons may prefer the broader definition of "one's progress through life."
3. Each person's career is of mutual concern to him or her and to Rex Hospital. Both parties are making a substantial and often critical investment in the employment contract. Both have a right to expect some advantage, gain, and benefit from such employment. Both parties need to work actively and cooperatively together toward such benefit. Rex Hospital provides these types of self-development and personal growth opportunities which permit every person to advance as far as he/she is able.
4. Responsibility for an individual's career rests with the individual alone. This is a simple fact. As much as the hospital may wish to help with the progress of its employees, only they can be responsible for themselves. They are responsible for what happens in their progress through life

and occupation. As working plans are made, it is important to consider not only what you think you may *want* to do, but also what you *can* do (assets and liabilities), and what you *like* to do.

5. Each employee's supervisor has a responsibility to assist that employee in work and career development. Supervisors know that this is a key responsibility. They know that they help themselves when they help their people with their jobs and growth. They can suggest other sources of help when they feel it is needed and can be useful. Some of these sources are within the hospital. Others are outside the hospital, and some are within the employee.

6. The Rex Hospital concept of a satisfactory career accommodates everything from one with *no* job changes to one with many changes and promotions. Some persons are quite happy to do a good job of what they are already doing and do not seek promotion. Others want to feel that they can move along into more complicated clinical jobs or take on administrative responsibilities. Rex Hospital Employee Advancement Program for Nursing Service personnel makes room for many types of career success definitions within the framework of "advancement or achievement in a particular vocation." Together, these varied career successes contribute to keeping Rex Hospital "Tops in Patient Care" and "A Good Place to Work."

7. The Rex Hospital Employee Advancement Program offers many opportunities for job satisfaction and for growth if desired:

- on present job
- within technical specialty
- within nursing administration
- into other hospital functions
- outward to other healthcare agencies.

Rex Hospital Employee Advancement Program has the following features and benefits:

1. Identifies for *all* nursing service employees the pathways to earned promotions and merited increases in pay.
2. Provides both clinical and managerial promotional channels for qualified personnel beyond the present RN practitioner level.
3. Establishes standards of performance and a performance review plan for all job levels.
4. Provides additional promotional steps within specific job categories (NA, RN, LPN, WS).

5. Permits merit pay increases within job categories as promotions are earned from one step to another, based upon ability to satisfactorily perform additional tasks.
6. Assures qualified persons of Nursing Service positions.
7. Permits staffing each unit with the minimum number of qualified personnel with a resultant savings in wage costs.
8. Requires that persons who qualify for higher job levels be able to perform all tasks identified for lower-paid job levels and to actually perform those tasks when staffing emergencies occur.

At present there are approximately twenty levels for Nursing Service personnel. Each level is defined with established criteria and performance descriptions. These performance descriptions are utilized in the evaluation of Nursing Service personnel. Attached to each job description is a Task List which indicates the nursing tasks that can be performed by personnel at each level.

The REAP Committee

Primary Objective

To contribute to the improvement and maintenance of high caliber patient care by providing and evaluating increasing growth opportunities for all Nursing Service personnel.

Contributory Objectives

1. To assist in keeping the Rex Hospital Employee Advancement Program for nursing personnel up-to-date.
2. To evaluate recommendations received regarding the REAP Program.
3. To serve as a liaison between all nursing personnel and the committee.

Membership

Composed of at least one representative from each level of nursing personnel, with each nursing unit being represented. Members serve a one-year term, from January to January.

Statement of Policy (1)

Nursing Units Affected: All Units

Effective: July 29, 1974, the following Rex Hospital Employee Advancement Program policies will be activated:

1. The classification of Nursing Service personnel at Rex Hospital shall be determined in accordance with the criteria established in the Rex Hospital Employee Advancement Program. (It is expected that these employees will move through the classifications at different rates depending on such factors as academic preparation, previous experience, ability to apply knowledge, and motivation.)
2. The advancement of Nursing Service personnel from level to level will be determined by a meritorious performance evaluation with a subsequent recommendation from the Head Nurse and Patient Care Coordinator for the employee to begin preparation for the next level. When the basic criteria as established for that particular level in the Rex Hospital Employee Advancement Program have been attained, he or she is eligible for advancement with the appropriate salary adjustment being made.

Exceptions to the Above:

A. The practical nurse will advance to the LPN I level when licensure is obtained.
B. The graduate professional nurse will advance to the RN I level when licensure is obtained.
C. There shall be no ninety-day waiting period for the RN I and LPN I to be recommended by the Head Nurse and Patient Care Coordinator to begin preparation for the levels of RN II and LPN II.
D. The practical nurse may take the Medication Qualifying Examination before obtaining licensure; however, only after becoming licensed, may he or she pursue becoming certified in medication administration or participation in the Inservice Medication Course.
E. The graduate professional nurse may attend the certification programs offered through Inservice Education; however, supervision for certification in these procedures cannot be initiated until licensure is obtained.

3. The actual level advancement will occur only at the time a position for that specific level becomes available.
4. All Nursing Service employees whose qualifications fulfill the established requirements for each level as specified in the Rex Hospital Employee Advancement Program should become eligible for positions of advancement within the Nursing Service Department. In order to ensure every applicant the considerations that are due him/her, the following procedure will be followed.

A. Vacant positions for levels will be announced. A time limit will be established for receiving applications when appropriate.

B. Eligible applicants should submit a Special Request Form to the Director of Nursing stating his or her qualifications and reasons for seeking the position.

C. The applicant's form of request in addition to his or her evaluations and recommendations by the Head Nurse and Patient Care Coordinator will be reviewed by the Director of Nursing and Patient Care Coordinator from the unit with the existing vacancy.

D. The employee to fill the position will be selected with priority given to the one who has been prepared for the longest period of time for that specific level and whose qualifications are adequate for the position.

E. Priority for filling positions that would allow for level advancement will be given to the existing Nursing Service personnel before a new employee is hired for the position.

5. If an employee does not merit advancement through variable performance or lack of motivation, the preexisting classification status and the salary scale shall be maintained. If necessary, the employee may be reclassified to the level which best describes his or her current performance with the necessary salary adjustment being made.

6. The Programs stipulated as being necessary for level advancement in the Rex Hospital Employee Advancement Program shall be offered by Rex Hospital through the Inservice Education Department or through other health-related agencies. Programs provided by other agencies must be evaluated and recommended by the Inservice Education Department as meeting the pre-preparational needs of that specific level.

7. Any educational program attended prior to employment at Rex Hospital that appears similar in content to the program required by the criteria for a particular level must be deemed comparable by the Rex Hospital Inservice Education Department before credit will be granted.

8. The graduate professional nurse will be hired at Rex Hospital at the RN I salary scale; however, he or she shall be classified as a graduate nurse performing only those tasks assigned to the graduate nurse level as specified by the Rex Hospital Employee Advancement Program.

9. The graduate professional nurse at Rex Hospital will be allowed one year from the date the first State Board Examination is offered after his or her graduation to successfully obtain his or her licensure. If at

the end of this period of time, he or she has not successfully obtained licensure, he or she shall be reclassified into the LPN III salary scale; however, his or her level classification shall remain that of a graduate nurse and he or she shall continue to perform only those tasks specified for the graduate nurse level by the Rex Hospital Employee Advancement Program. If no position for this level employee exists on the unit assigned, a transfer to a unit with a vacancy for this level may be necessary.

10. The graduate professional nurse who has been unsuccessful in obtaining his or her licensure prior to applying for a position at Rex Hospital shall be hired at the LPN III salary scale if more than one year from the date the first State Board Examination was offered after his or her graduation has elapsed. However, he or she shall be classified in the graduate nurse performance level and shall be assigned only those tasks specified for the graduate nurse level by the Rex Hospital Employee Advancement Program.

11. The graduate practical nurse will be hired at Rex Hospital at the LPN I salary scale; however, he or she shall be classified as a practical nurse performing only those tasks assigned to the practical nurse level as specified by the Rex Hospital Employee Advancement Program.

12. The graduate practical nurse at Rex Hospital will be allowed one year from the date the first State Board Examination is offered after his or her graduation to successfully obtain his or her licensure. If at the end of this period of time, he or she has not successfully obtained licensure, he or she shall be reclassified into the NA III salary scale; however, his or her level classification shall remain that of a practical nurse and he or she shall continue to perform only those tasks specified for the practical nurse level by the Rex Hospital Employee Advancement Program. If no position for this level employee exists on the unit assigned, a transfer to a unit with a vacancy for this level may be necessary.

13. The graduate practical nurse who has been unsuccessful in obtaining his or her licensure prior to applying for a position at Rex Hospital shall be hired at the NA III salary scale if more than one year from the date the first State Board Examination was offered after his or her graduation has elapsed. However, he or she shall be classified in the practical nurse performance level and shall be assigned only those tasks specified for the practical nurse level by the Rex Hospital Employee Advancement Program.

14. Exceptions to the criteria established for the individual levels of Nursing Service personnel by the Rex Hospital Employee Advancement Program may be granted by the Director of Nursing based upon the

written recommendation of the Patient Care Coordinator who has evaluated the employee's knowledge and skills and previous experience.

15. A new employee whose education and previous experience based upon acceptable references meet the established criteria for a level with the exception of specific required certification programs may be hired into the level and be allowed ninety days to become certified in all the procedures. If at the end of ninety days, certification has not been attained he or she shall be reclassified into the appropriate level with the necessary salary adjustment being made.

16. A new employee may be hired into the level of Nursing Service established by the Rex Hospital Employee Advancement Program as is indicated by his or her education and previous experience based upon acceptable references for a ninety-day period of evaluation. At the end of this time, a written evaluation will be done and if he or she is functioning unsatisfactorily for that level, a reclassification in level may be necessary with the appropriate salary adjustment being made.

Origin of Policies: Department of Nursing
Originated: July 23, 1974
Revised: December 22, 1975

Signed: (Director of Nursing, Assistant Director of Nursing, Director of Rex Hospital)

Statement of Policy (2)

Nursing Units Affected: All Units

Effective July 9, 1975, the following policy will be activated regarding check-off of nursing tasks designed for each level in the Rex Employee Advancement Program:

A satisfactory check-off of all nursing tasks designated as core tasks on the REAP Nursing Activities Task List must be accomplished within ninety days of the completion of an Inservice Education class offered as preparation for a higher level. The action taken upon failure to accomplish this check-off will be at the discretion of the Patient Care Coordinator. Exceptions may be granted only upon the recommendation of the Patient Care Coordinator. Those other tasks designated as occurring infrequently or only in specialty nursing areas are to be checked off as they occur.

A satisfactory check-off is required on those tasks designated as occurring in specialty nursing areas only for nursing personnel assigned to those areas.

Nursing Service personnel who transfer from a medical-surgical area to a specialty area or from a specialty area to a medical-surgical area will be granted a ninety-day evaluation period at the time of their transfer. This will allow ample time for the check-off of necessary tasks and for an evaluation of performance in that area to be done by the Head Nurse and/or Patient Care Coordinator.

Origin of Policy: Patient Care Coordinators
                 Systems and Planning
                 Inservice Education
Originated: July 1, 1975

Signed: (Director of Nursing, Coordinator of Inservice Education, Director of Rex Hospital)

REAP: The Follow-Through

The Rex Employee Advancement Program was a lot of work—to develop, to introduce, to maintain. It happened because Sarah Hitchcock and her staff were committed to Concept A nursing and Concept A management. They believed in these concepts and have become a model for how to make them work—for patients, for employees, and for those who pay the costs (since they saved money in the process).

Close to five years after REAP was introduced, here are comments from employees directly affected (Hitchcock, 1978):

> I feel that I have greatly benefited from the REAP system. REAP has provided for me growth opportunities which have enabled me to advance to my present position of Unit Manager. The system also clearly defines the standard of performance expected of me. This helps me to evaluate for myself what kind of job I am doing. I like knowing where I stand.
>
> —Judy Russell, Unit Manager
> (formerly Ward Secretary)

> REAP offers the Rex Hospital employees a chance to advance and get credit for proficiency gained in their skills. This helps not only the nursing staff but applies to our nursing assistants and ward secretaries as well. By having set levels, staff members know the expectations of Rex for each job level and what they must do to move ahead.
>
> —(RN III)

Mildred Bartlett, RN III, relates her feelings about REAP:

> When I came to Rex Hospital four years ago, I found the Rex Employee Advancement Program (REAP) a new and interesting

concept. It gave me, as an experienced RN, a clear contract of the career opportunities that were available here. Promotional levels within my job gave me an incentive to work for both clinical and management expertise. Merit pay increases have long been a standard for recognition, but this program has additional benefits and features.

Another opinion about REAP comes from a nursing assistant:

When I applied for a job as nurse's assistant, I didn't realize the opportunity that you could have. I was in training for five weeks. I have been at Rex for one year and nine months. I have really enjoyed it. Since then I have taken other classes, which I have enjoyed and learned a lot from them. I also have been on the dress code committee for the nursing assistants.

It's been an honor and a pleasure to be asked to represent the REAP Committee from Pediatrics.

The purpose of the REAP Committee is to evaluate policies of the Hospital, job descriptions of each level, and electing new committee members. Also the REAP Committee presents a REAP Newsletter to assist in communicating information to the nursing staff. The newsletter has an advantage, particularly letting those affected by the programs know what the committee was doing and any changes made, etc.

The REAP programs us. Parliamentary procedure provides the protection of the right of the individual, the minority, the majority, and the rights of all these together. It allows everyone to be heard and to make decisions without confusion.

I have enjoyed being a member of the REAP Program for almost two years. It has been a pleasure and a sense of responsibility to myself and to the Hospital.

—Annette Carver, NA II
Pediatrics

Of course it is not all sweetness and light. Nancy Jones, RN II, sizes up the advantages and disadvantages as follows.

Advantages of REAP

1. Incentive for promotion.
2. Provides opportunity to participate in continuing education classes.
3. Task lists especially helpful if transferring to another floor—to

protect us so we don't have to do procedures we don't know how
to do.

4. Helps in knowing what other personnel can do so unqualified
person won't be doing procedure he/she shouldn't do—thus increases quality care.

Disadvantages of REAP

1. A lot of procedures do not pertain to specialty areas—OB, Peds,
etc.
2. Continuing education classes not held frequently enough.
3. Promotion should come sooner after classes completed.
4. Some material is just a review of material learned in nursing
school.

As Director of Nursing, Mrs. Hitchcock summarizes the REAP experience
this way:

> This system seems to be most attractive to the young graduate who
> is seeking clearly defined promotional routes. Problems occur when
> discrepancies exist between an individual's self evaluation of com-
> petency and that of his/her supervisor. Nurses with prior ex-
> perience have at times expressed negative feelings related to the
> levels but this has lessened as our coordinators have become more
> skilled in evaluating and placing people appropriately in the levels.

Here is another sign of the benefits accruing to Rex Hospital and its fortunate patients. During the summer of 1978, the Raleigh, North Carolina,
News and Observer wrote about the many problems caused by the shortage of
nurses in area hospitals—except Rex Hospital. Rather than a shortage, Rex
had a waiting list of RNs who wanted to work there. In other published
reports, Rex Hospital room rates are shown to be at the very low end of the
scale for hospitals in the Raleigh, Durham, and Chapel Hill areas. REAP has
certainly been a contributing factor.

These kinds of exceptional results can be had by other professional nurse
managers, too—if they really want them badly enough. Further details about
REAP are available at modest cost from Mrs. Hitchcock at Rex Hospital in
Raleigh, and from our publication *HELP with Wide-Track Careers in Nursing* (W.L. Ganong Co., Chapel Hill, N.C., 1977, 142 pp.).

A SUMMARY STATEMENT

The concept of wide-track careers reaches beyond the confines of a single
healthcare agency. Career ladders must necessarily allow the nurse to move

freely and to advance in a variety of work settings along the track or tracks available—clinical, education, or management. The number and variety of such growth and career opportunities continue to expand, and include the option of independent practice.

Golightly in *HELP with Career Planning, A Workbook for Nurses* states that:

> Nurses enter the world of work after completing their education, passing a state board examination, and receiving a license. They have a new professional identity and subsequently choose a setting within which to translate theory into practice. Why, you might ask, do nurses need to develop a career when they have already chosen a profession? There seems to be a lingering assumption that once a person chooses nursing, the nurse automatically knows how to develop that professional career. This assumption needs to be recognized as a myth, and dispelled. Too often nurses find themselves in positions which are not necessarily a result of their own careful planning but due to persuasive actions of others (Golightly, 1979).

Career planning, which is a personal matter for each individual nurse, can be enhanced through a program featuring well-developed career ladders. The use of the wide-track careers concept, by whatever name, is essential to help motivated nurses prepare themselves for advancement in responsibility, status, and remuneration.

AN INVITATION

We look upon nurses, especially nurse managers, as people with unique opportunities to live full and meaningful lives through their impact on the lives of others. We have attempted in this book to share with you a variety of beliefs, techniques, and skills that will enrich your own life and work through your helping relationships with patients, families, coworkers, and professional and community groups. No one can force you to use the suggestions in this book or in any other source. The motivation must come from you. By the same token, no one can prevent you from growing, from understanding the five basic human needs and how to utilize that knowledge, or from becoming skilled as a nurse manager. You, the nurse, are one of our most valued national resources—a resource that becomes enriched, rather than depleted, through use.

We invite you to full personal participation in the 1980s—*Decade of the Nurse.* Most certainly it is a highly personal decade for you. ANA welcomed it as a "Decade of Decision" for nurses and nursing (ANA, 1979). It is that—for you and all nurses. And you, more than you may realize, influence where you find yourself at the end of the 1980s in your life/work situation. We wish you well. Be stubborn! Godspeed!

NOTES

ANA Convention '80 notice. *The American Nurse*, August 20, 1979, *11*(7), 16.

California law lets nurses share in medical corporations. *The American Nurse* (ANA), September 20, 1979, *11*(8).

Ganong, J., & Ganong, W. *HELP with wide-track careers in nursing*. Chapel Hill, N.C.: W. L. Ganong Co., 1977.

Ganong, W. L., & Ganong, J. Letter to the editor. *Supervisor Nurse*, December 1978, p. 10.

Golightly, C. *HELP with career planning: A workbook for nurses*. Chapel Hill, N.C.: W. L. Ganong Co., 1979, p. 5.

Hitchcock, S. Personal correspondence, 1978 and 1979. Reprinted with permission.

Jacox, A. K., & Norris, C. M. (Eds.). *Organizing for independent nursing practice*. New York: Appleton-Century-Crofts, 1977, p. 3.

Jaques, E. Taking time seriously in evaluating jobs. *Harvard Business Review*, September-October 1979, *57*(5), 124–132.

Koltz, C. J., Jr. *Private practice in nursing: Development and management*. Germantown, Md.: Aspen Systems Corp., 1979.

LaViolette, S. Multiunits boost nursing's clout. *Modern Healthcare*, January 1980, p. 50.

Reimbursement for all wins approval. *RN Magazine*, September 1979, p. 26.

RN Magazine, May 1976, p. 10.

Schorr, T. M. Editorial: Entry into practice: Chapter two. *American Journal of Nursing*, May 1978, *78* (5), 823.

Zimmerman, A. Foreword. In A. K. Jacox & C. M. Norris (Eds.), *Organizing for independent nursing practice*. New York: Appleton-Century-Crofts, 1977.

Reading List

Books

Kramer, M. *Reality shock: Why nurses leave nursing*. St. Louis: C. V. Mosby, 1974.

Kramer, M., & Schmalenberg, C. *Path to biculturalism*. Wakefield, Mass.: Contemporary Publishing, 1977.

Lysaught, J. P. (Ed.) *Action in nursing: Progress in professional purpose*. New York: McGraw-Hill, 1974.

Articles

Anderson, M. I., & Denyes, M. J. A ladder for clinical advancement in nursing practice, implementation. *Journal of Nursing Administration*, February 1975, *5* (2), 16–22.

Bopp, W., & Rosenthal, W. Participatory management. *American Journal of Nursing*, April 1979, *79*, 671–72.

Bracken, R., & Christman, L. An incentive program designed to develop and reward clinical competence. *Journal of Nursing Administration*, October 1978, *8* (10), 8–18.

Colavecchio, R., Tescher, B., & Scalzi, C. A clinical ladder for nursing practice. *Nursing Digest*, January–February 1975, *3* (1), 5–9.

McClure, M. L. Entry into professional practice: The New York proposal. *Journal of Nursing Administration,* June 1976, *6* (5), 12–17.

Numerof, R. E. Expanded nurse role from the perspective of the new medicine. *Health Care Management Review,* Summer 1978, *3* (3), 45–51.

Reichow, R., & Scott, R. Study compares graduates of two-, three-, and four-year programs. *Hospitals,* July 16, 1976, *50* (14), 95–100.

Warren, J. G. Motivating and rewarding the staff nurse. *Journal of Nursing Administration,* October 1978, *8* (10), 4–7.

General Performance Responsibilities of Administrative and Management Personnel

PURPOSE: Deliver the required health care services consistent with the charter, philosophy, and objectives of your agency.

MAJOR PERFORMANCE RESPONSIBILITIES:	PERFORMANCE IS SATISFACTORY WHEN:

I. To Administrator or Manager

A. Organizational 1. Function within the general policies, stated beliefs and philosophy of Community General Hospital.	The hospital is represented to people within and without the organization with a general feeling of support and implementation of these policies and beliefs through both written and oral expression.
2. Maintain clear lines of authority and responsibility.	Up-to-date department policies and performance descriptions are maintained.
3. Obtain your own manager's approval of departmental policies and organizational plans.	Approval is obtained before establishing such policies or plans.
B. Operational 1. Prepare and administer departmental budget.	Department is operated within approved budgets; reasonable cost standards are developed and maintained; cost and budgets are periodically reviewed.

MAJOR PERFORMANCE RESPONSIBILITIES:	PERFORMANCE IS SATISFACTORY WHEN:
2. Perform or supervise record-keeping.	Records are maintained currently, are understandable to all personnel who use them, and meet legal or other requirements.
3. Establish specific goals and objectives for the department.	Such goals are in writing and include target dates for completion; and are prepared with the help of department personnel.
4. Plan, schedule and coordinate the day-to-day work activities.	The necessary work is accomplished effectively.

C. Communications
1. Keep your manager informed of current departmental activities, plans and developments through both oral and written reports.

Administration is informed of departmental objectives and plans, status of work and programs, personnel matters and performance of subordinates as appropriate; regular and special reports are accurate, complete, and submitted on time. "Never let your boss be surprised!"

2. Answer correspondence.

Correspondence is acted upon within 24 hours.

D. Developmental
1. Keep abreast of latest developments affecting your area of responsibility; keep own supervisor informed of such developments.

Your own manager is kept informed of new developments; recommendations are made as to how methods, procedures and quality may be improved through these developments.

2. Participate in research and experimental projects that are desirable and appropriate for the hospital.

Research and experimental projects improve patient care and services, employee relations, and the public or professional image of the hospital.

3. Plan and implement programs that improve the hospital's service to the community.

Provide written proposals for your manager's approval that:
(a) identify needs and issues concerning the department;
(b) structure issues in terms of alternative courses of action and cost factors.

MAJOR PERFORMANCE RESPONSIBILITIES:	PERFORMANCE IS SATISFACTORY WHEN:

II. To Department Personnel

A. Operational

1. Maintain an optimum staff of qualified personnel.

There are enough people to get the work done well, but no more than necessary. Those hired have the basic requirements to become productive workers.

2. Carry out the wage and salary administration program conscientiously.

Wage and salary increases are recommended as soon as justified. Dissatisfactions with pay are minimal.

3. Conduct personnel activities in accordance with hospital personnel programs and policies.

Policies and procedures are carried out effectively; necessary exceptions receive approval.

4. Maintain equipment in good operating condition.

Regular monthly inspections are conducted; needed repairs are effected; units are replaced when repairing would be inadequate.

5. Maintain adequate quality and quantity of materials and supplies.

No work interruptions occur because of "out-of-stock items."

6. Build a departmental environment which encourages maximum motivation of employees.

Employees show self-motivation rather than having to be pushed to get the work done.

7. Develop improved systems and procedures.

Evidence exists that these lead to easier ways of doing the work, to improved performance results, and minimum cost.

B. Training and Safety

1. Supervise training and orientation of subordinates.

Subordinates to be trained have been identified; types of experiences and training needed has been planned; subordinates are actively obtaining such experience or training; periodic evaluation is made of subordinates' progress; there is evidence of development of subordinates in terms of their results.

2. Supervise compliance of personnel with safety regulations and sanitation requirements.

Accidents do not occur to personnel or equipment because of violations of these regulations; the area is clean and orderly at all times; formal

MAJOR PERFORMANCE RESPONSIBILITIES:	PERFORMANCE IS SATISFACTORY WHEN:
	inspections disclose no violation of regulations.
3. Supervise training of personnel to cope with emergency situations such as fire, disaster, etc.	Personnel attend orientation and Fire & Safety Training Programs as scheduled; personnel are kept informed of procedures or developments that affect their performance in emergency situations.

C. Communications
   1. Keep subordinates informed of current changes that affect them.

Subordinates are informed promptly of hospital and departmental plans, policies, procedures, etc., that affect their work, welfare and morale.

   2. Maintain an effective upward flow of information.

Feelings, opinions and attitudes of employees are sought, obtained and used as a basis for management action.

   3. Resolve personnel problems.

Listening and counselling results in improved situation.

D. Developmental
   1. Evaluate employee performance.

Every employee "knows where he stands" at all times. Formal appraisals are carried out as scheduled.

   2. Encourage full self-development of all employees.

Ongoing training is planned and conducted to improve the quality of employee performance; there is evidence of improvement in work results. Employees are advanced to higher-rated jobs as they qualify for existing openings.

   3. Stimulate employee participation in planning for the immediate and long-range future.

Plans are made with the assistance of subordinates whenever possible; subordinates participate, within reason, in the setting of objectives.

III. To Other Departments

A. Operational
   1. Work cooperatively with other departments to accomplish hospital objectives.

Evidence exists that there are successful communications and harmonious working relationships among departments.

MAJOR PERFORMANCE RESPONSIBILITIES:	PERFORMANCE IS SATISFACTORY WHEN:
B. Communications 1. Participate in hospital meetings.	Attendance is regular and participation is meaningful.
C. Developmental 1. Provide instruction for other departments as required.	Appropriate instruction is provided as scheduled.

IV. To Other Organizations

A. Communications 1. Participate in activities of outside organizations to provide information on hospital activities and plans, explain the hospital's role and position in the health care field and in the community, promote the public image of the hospital; and to obtain for the benefit of the hospital such information and opinions as may be useful in guiding management action.	Suitable participation is provided to outside agencies as requested, or as sought; adequate feedback is provided and evaluated in time to be of value in influencing administrative planning and action.
2. Prepare reports as requested by federal, state, community agencies, hospital associations, etc.	Reports are accurate, complete and are submitted on time; duplicate copies are retained for hospital records.
B. Developmental 1. Participate in professional and technical society meetings pertinent to own areas of special interest.	Attendance and participation is meaningful.

Summary Worksheet
Our Principles of Nursing Practice

SUMMARY WORKSHEET
OUR PRINCIPLES OF NURSING PRACTICE

NAME _____   AGENCY _____

DEPT. or UNIT _____   DATE _____

As developed by: _____

OUR PHILOSOPHY

OUR GOALS

OUR CURRENT PATIENT CARE OBJECTIVES

DEFINITIONS FOR OUR UNIT

FUNCTIONS of OUR NURSING STAFF MEMBERS

OUR EDUCATION AND RESEARCH NEEDS

(Use additional pages as necessary)

Management by Objectives

An Instructional Model for Helping Others to Learn to Write Objectives

Advance Preparation: Have available examples of well written objectives that include the components and which are pertinent for your group and type of organization.

Step 1

Introduce written objectives in the context of the philosophy and goals of your organization. (Refer to Section 1 of HELP with Management by Objectives.) Use pertinent local examples of available statements of philosophy and goals.

Step 2

Explain briefly how written objectives help to focus attention on worthwhile projects; assist in setting priorities for action; and help in scheduling the necessary time and money.

Step 3

Write on the blackboard a specific statement of an objective that includes all or most of the components. Discuss briefly the meaning of this objective.

Step 4

Write on the board, "Components of a written objective." List three components. (See Section 2 of HELP study guide.)

1. *What* will be done (*includes* action verb)
2. *How much/how well*
3. *When* (Target date)

Step 5

Subdivide the group into pairs. Ask each pair working together to identify the components of the specific objective as written on the blackboard. Allow the group to work together in pairs, giving such help to each pair as may be necessary to assist them in identifying the action verb, what will be done, how well, how much, and how soon.
(Note: A second example of another objective may be used to repeat this Step #5. See example at end of steps.)

Step 6

Summarize for the group as follows: "Each written objective must have three main components as identified. In addition, the objective may include *who* will do the what *where*, and at what *cost*." Write these items on the board.

Step 7

Ask the group to just sit and look at the board to "drink in" these components. Then have the group members close their eyes, while the leader erases what is on the blackboard.

Step 8

Ask the group to write down on a blank sheet of paper exactly what they remember from the board information.

Step 9

As the first and second persons look up from their sheets giving an indication that they have completed the assigned task, ask them to come forward and have each reproduce on the blackboard what they have on their written sheets.

Step 10

Ask the rest of the group to make additions and corrections to what has been written on the blackboard.

Step 11

Erase the blackboard.

Step 12

Ask the group members to turn over their sheets and perform the same task of reproducing what was on the blackboard the second time.

Step 13

Break up the group into pairs again and ask one member of each pair to explain to the other member what are the components of a written objective.

Step 14

Ask each group member to use the specific objective as written on the board and mark over the specific words which are active verbs, what will be done, how much, how well, how soon. They may also mark if it is indicated who and where.

Step 15

Ask the whole group to give verbally, one more time, the components of a written objective.

Step 16

Ask group to break up into triads. People then write a specific objective for themselves based upon some area of real concern to them in their work situation.

Step 17

If some of the participants finish writing an objective before the rest of the group, ask those persons to write a second objective to keep them occupied and to avoid discussion while the rest are finishing.

Step 18

Ask members of each triad to exchange their written objectives so that each person is working with somebody else's written statement, and goes through the process of inspecting and correcting it to conform with the components checklist. People then receive their own written statement back and discussion ensues regarding the correct statements.

Step 19

The groups then reform into dyads, one person to be the boss and the other the subordinate. Each member of the dyad takes a turn at presenting the written statement to "the boss" and goes through the process of attempting to develop the written statement into a mutually-developed and agreed-upon statement of objectives to which both can subscribe.

Step 20

Entire group discusses what they have learned from the prior experience. "I learned that there is a cost attached to objectives."

Step 21

Group is asked to discuss how they now feel about writing objectives.

Step 22

Group members are asked to close their eyes and think about what they have learned.

Note: Here is an example of a second objective that may be used in Step #5. "Plan the allocation and scheduling of the nursing staff so that patient needs are met at all times on all shifts without varying more than five percent from the allocated number of nursing man-hours." Ask group members to identify again the components in this objective and to write in above the words the particular components. (This additional exercise may help to emphasize the fact that for some objectives the *how much* is just as important as the *how well*.)

Sample Performance Descriptions

**GUIDELINES AND WORKSHEET FOR PREPARING
YOUR OWN PERFORMANCE DESCRIPTION**

I. Consider your own performance responsibilities. What do you
    do, for whom? In the space below, list four of the persons
    (or groups of people) for whom you have to do something.
    Then list two things you have to do for each as part of your
    performance requirements.

Persons (or Groups of People)	What I Do For Them
1.	a.
	b.
2.	a.
	b.
3.	a.
	b.
4.	a.
	b.

II.   Now select one of the things you do for someone (as listed in
       the right hand column of Step I) which you think is easiest
       to measure. How do you know when you have performed satisfac-
       torily? When you have decided upon your answer, complete the
       following sentence:

My performance for item # ___ (from Step I) is satisfactory when

_____

_____

_____

_____

III.   Take the worksheet to your own manager. Show what you have
       written for Steps I and II. Ask your boss, "Do you agree
       with what I wrote down?" Discuss and modify as necessary
       to reach agreement.

       If you are prepared to do so, show your "measures of satis-
       factory performance" for another one or two things you do
       for someone else (your "performance responsibilities").
       Discuss, and reach agreement.

       Then soon after having had your discussion with your boss,
       write below your reactions as you recall them. What were
       your feelings during the discussion? What are your feelings
       now? How might this experience influence your use of per-
       formance descriptions with your staff members?

IV.   Follow through. What you do next is up to you, influenced
       by the reactions of your boss and your own feelings. Out-
       line below your follow-through plan of action.

SELF-EVALUATION OF PERFORMANCE

NAME: _____ DATE: _____

TITLE: _____

DEPARTMENT: _____ REPORTS TO: _____

PURPOSE OF YOUR WORK: (In your own words, tell the reasons for what you do.)

PERFORMANCE RESPONSIBILITIES: (In your own words, how well do you perform each responsibility? Include examples of results.

A. To Patients

B. To Medical Staff

C. To Your Own Manager (supervisor)

D. To Department Personnel

E. To Committees

F. To Personnel of Other Departments (or other organizations)

G. To Self

Note: Use Additional sheets as necessary. When completed, return the sheet(s) to your nurse manager (or supervisor).

COMMUNITY GENERAL HOSPITAL
PERFORMANCE DESCRIPTION

TITLE: R N   II   DEPARTMENT: Nursing Service

SUPERVISES: LPN's, Nursing Assistants, Orderlies, Technicians,
              Ward Clerks, Unit Service Aides

PURPOSE: To assess, plan and give nursing care at RN II level with a
              minimum of assistance. Functions as a team leader or may
              assume charge duties when adequately prepared.

MAJOR PERFORMANCE RESPONSIBILITIES: PERFORMANCE IS SATISFACTORY WHEN:

A. *To Patients*
1. Assist in formulating and carrying   1. Effective plan of care is imple-
    out patient care plans.   mented.
2. Evaluate care given to patients.   2. Care meets established criteria
                                               for quality and amount.
3. Assess the needs of the patient.   3. Needs are identified through
                                               skillful interviewing and obser-
                                               vation, and are recorded.
4. Act as liaison between patients,   4. Patient and family understand and
    physician and family.   carry out physician's directions.
5. Give direct patient care as needed.   5. Objectives of care plan are met.
6. Performs nursing activities as   6. These activities are carried out
    assigned for RN II on Nursing   safely, correctly and economically.
    Activities Task List.

B. *To Medical Staff*
1. Carry out physician's orders.   1. Orders are implemented with no
                                               mistakes.
2. Ask for clarification of physician's   2. Orders are clearly understood.
    orders as necessary.
3. Inform physician of changes in   3. Information is accurately recorded
    patient's condition.   and relayed.
4. Make rounds with Physician.   4. Rounds assist in formulating patient
                                               care plans and provide in-depth
                                               comprehension of patient's condition.

C. *To Own Nurse Manager*
1. Report on and off duty as assigned.   1. Established schedule is met.
2. Keep up-to-date in nursing   2. Competence in performing procedures
    procedures.   is demonstrated.
3. Conduct and participate in team   3. Greater understanding of patient's
    conferences.   condition is achieved by team members.
4. Communicate appropriate information.   4. Necessary communications are passed
                                               on. (Never let your boss be
                                               surprised.)
5. Make out patient-care assignment.   5. Skills of team members are
                                               recognized and utilized.

MAJOR PERFORMANCE RESPONSIBILITIES:	PERFORMANCE IS SATISFACTORY WHEN:

D. *To Unit Personnel*
1. Maintain harmonious relationship with other team members.
2. Participate in unit teaching and orienting as needed.

3. Encourage proper technique and procedures.
4. Function effectively as a professional team member.

1. Own efforts contribute patient-care team work.
2. Patient care team works effectively with favorable response to instruction.
3. Safe nursing care is rendered.

4. Own performance sets desired example and facilitates team work.

E. *To Committees*
1. Actively participates in assigned committee work.
2. Attend regular meetings of appropriate unit of Nursing Service Personnel Organization.

1. Committee objectives are met.

2. Active participation is evident and there is a feeling of satisfaction with the Unit meetings.

F. *To Other Departments*
1. Carry out interdepartmental assignments and communications.

1. Positive feedback is obtained.

G. *To Other Organizations*
1. Participates in appropriate professional nursing and community organizations.

1. Such activity aids in meeting personal and hospital goals.

H. *To Self*
1. Maintain sense of personal satisfaction.
2. Participate in continuing education programs.

1. Personal goals are met as related to job performance.
2. Progress is made in preparation for promotion, and in updating job knowledge and skills.

Qualifications

1. Graduate of Accredited School of Nursing.

2. Current State Registration   (or in process of licensing).

3. Certification of those procedures required for R.N. II; certification for special procedures.

4. Completion of the Community General Hospital orientation program within thirty days of employment.

PERFORMANCE DESCRIPTION WORKSHEET

NAME: _____ DEPT: _____

JOB TITLE: _____ DATE: _____

Name of your supervisor: _____

Name of your department head: _____

Names and titles of persons you supervise (if you are a supervisor or manager):

_____   _____
_____   _____
_____   _____
_____   _____
_____   _____

> INSTRUCTIONS: You can help prepare an up-to-date Performance
> Description of what you do in your work. Please be as complete as
> possible. Do not be bashful; list everything you think is part of
> your job. If you need more space, use additional sheets.

1. The purpose of my work is _____
   _____
   _____

2. For whom are you doing your work? _____
   _____
   _____

3. How do you know whether or not you are performing your work satisfactorily? _____
   _____
   _____

4. List anything you are doing which you think should not be part of your work: _____
   _____

5. List anything you are not doing which you think should be part of your work: _____
   _____

6. Who taught you your work? _____

7. When you started on your present job, how long did it take you to learn to do the work
   satisfactorily? _____

8. COMMENTS AND SUGGESTIONS: Add anything else that will help your work and how you feel
   about it. (Use additional sheets if you need more space): _____
   _____
   _____
   _____
   _____
   _____

Uncritical Inference Test

Let me begin the first of our patterns of miscommunication by inviting you to test yourself.*

INSTRUCTIONS

Read the following little story. Assume that all the information presented in it is definitely accurate and true. Read it carefully because it has ambiguous parts designed to lead you astray. No need to memorize it, though. You can refer back to it whenever you wish.

Next read the statements about the story and check each to indicate whether you consider it true, false, or "?". "T" means that the statement is *definitely true* on the basis of the information presented in the story. "F" means that it is *definitely false*. "?" means that it may be either true or false and that you cannot be certain which on the basis of the information presented in the story. If any part of a statement is doubtful, make it "?". *Answer each statement in turn, and do not go back to change any answer later and don't reread any statements after you have answered them. This will distort your score.*

To start with, here is a sample story with correct answers:

SAMPLE STORY

You arrive home late one evening and see that the lights are on in your living room. There is only one car parked in front of your house, and the words

---

Source: Haney, W.V. The inference-observation confusion. *Communication and interpersonal relations* (4th Ed.). Homewood, IL: Richard D. Irwin, Inc. 1979. Used with permission.

"Harold R. Jones, M.D." are spelled in small gold letters across one of the car's doors.

Statements about Sample Story

1. The car parked in front of your house has   (T)   F   ? lettering on one of its doors.
   (This is a "definitely true" statement because it is directly corroborated by the story.)
2. Someone in your family is sick.   T   F   (?)
   (This could be true and then again it might not be. Perhaps Dr. Jones is paying a social call at your home or perhaps he has gone to the house next door or across the street.)
3. No car is parked in front of your house.   T   (F)   ?
   (A "definitely false" statement because the story directly contradicts it.)
4. The car parked in front of your house belongs to a man named Johnson.   T   F   (?)
   (May seem very likely false, but can you be sure? Perhaps the car has just been sold.)

So much for the sample. It should warn you of some of the kinds of traps to look for. Now begin the actual test. Remember, mark each statement *in order*—don't skip around or change answers later.

THE STORY[1]

A businessman had just turned off the lights in the store when a man appeared and demanded money. The owner opened a cash register. The contents of the cash register were scooped up, and the man sped away. A member of the police force was notified promptly.

Statements about the Story

1. A man appeared after the owner had turned off his store lights.   T   F   ?
2. The robber was a *man*.   T   F   ?

---

[1] The story and statements are a portion of the "Uncritical Inference Test," copyrighted, 1955, 1964, 1967, 1972, by William V. Haney. The full-length test is available for educational purposes from the International Society for General Semantics, P.O. Box 2469, San Francisco, California 94126.

3. The man who appeared did not demand money.   T   F   ?
4. The man who opened the cash register was the owner.   T   F   ?
5. The store owner scooped up the contents of the cash register and ran away.   T   F   ?
6. Someone opened a cash register.   T   F   ?
7. After the man who demanded the money scooped up the contents of the cash register, he ran away.   T   F   ?
8. While the cash register contained money, the story does *not* state *how much*.   T   F   ?
9. The robber demanded money of the owner.   T   F   ?
10. A businessman had just turned off the lights when a man appeared in the store.   T   F   ?
11. It was broad daylight when the man appeared.   T   F   ?
12. The man who appeared opened the cash register.   T   F   ?
13. No one demanded money.   T   F   ?
14. The story concerns a series of events in which only three persons are referred to: the owner of the store, a man who demanded money, and a member of the police force.   T   F   ?
15. The following events occurred: someone demanded money, a cash register was opened, its contents were scooped up, and a man dashed out of the store.   T   F   ?

1. ? Do you *know* that the "businessman" and the "owner" are one and the same?
2. ? Was there *necessarily* a robbery involved here? Perhaps the man was the rent collector—or the owner's son—they sometimes demand money.
3. F An easy one to keep up the test-taker's morale.
4. ? Was the owner a *man*?
5. ? May seem unlikely but the story does not definitely preclude it.
6. T Story says the owner opened the cash register.
7. ? We don't know who scooped up the contents of the cash register or that the man necessarily *ran* away.
8. ? The dependent clause is doubtful—the cash register may or may not have contained money.

9. ?   Again, a robber?
10. ?   Could the man merely have appeared *at* a door or window but did not actually enter the store?
11. ?   Stores generally keep lights on during the day.
12. ?   Could not the man who appeared have been the owner?
13. F   Story says the man who appeared demanded money.
14. ?   Are the businessman and the owner one and the same—or two different people? Same goes for the owner and the man who appeared.
15. ?   "Dashed?" Could he not have "sped away" on roller skates or in a car? And do we know that he actually left the store? We don't even know that he entered it.

Corporate Goals

I. Continue to maintain, expand and improve our corporate hospital leadership position in providing comprehensive quality health care services to the region.

General Objectives

A. Establish Nebraska Methodist Hospital as a "Tertiary" level hospital.

B. Construct a new tower for patient services and beds at the 84th Street location.

C. Establish a formal on-going system for short and long range medical and management planning.

D. Expand management, systems, and services to other hospitals.

E. Encourage medical staff to expand their efforts to provide programs, and services to the region.

F. Develop the corporate organizational structure and provide for adequate manpower.

G. Strive to gain more visibility and recognition for achievements in providing health care service.

II. Assure the continued financial viability of the Nebraska Methodist Hospital.

Source: Reprinted with the permission of J. W. Estabrook, Administrator, and Ralph L. Morocco, Jr., Manager, Planning and Program Development, the Nebraska Methodist Hospital, Omaha, Nebraska.

General Objectives

A. Expand and develop sources of revenue other than normal hospital services.

B. Encourage the medical staff to develop their referral patterns on a regional basis.

C. Develop management, systems, and programs to increase employee productivity.

D. Develop management, systems, and programs to improve cost containment and effectiveness.

E. Develop an internal financial reporting system that will measure achievement in productivity and cost containment.

III. Continue to provide and expand an environment for employees to experience involvement, pride, security, and self-fulfillment.

General Objectives

A. Develop training, communications, reporting systems, and financial incentives to strengthen and improve middle management from the lead-man through the departmental director.

B. Keep employees informed of the achievements of their department and of the hospital.

C. Maintain a comprehensive wage, benefit, and personnel program that will encourage and reward productive employees and remove non-productive employees.

D. Develop training programs for employees and management aimed at improving technical and managerial skills.

IV. Provide sufficient and properly allocated resources to consumers of health care services in the region at a competitive price.

General Objectives

A. Develop reasonable standards for all aspects of patient care and treatment that will properly meet the needs of the patient and reflect favorably on the "image" of the hospital.

B. Identify, and evaluate new services, in conjunction with corporate planning activities, quantifying manpower, equipment, and supplies, necessary to develop the service.

C. Monitor and improve all aspects of patient scheduling from admission, through the coordination of technical services, to dismissal.

D. Evaluate present patient services and programs to determine whether they should be maintained, expanded, improved, diminished, or discontinued in relationship to the needs of the community, the needs of the medical staff, and the resource of the hospital.

V. Provide sufficient and properly allocated resources committed to quality health education for the governing board, physicians, students, employees, patients and the public.

General Objectives

A. Continue to develop the School of Nursing and other formal educational programs in order to meet the needs of the hospital and the region.

B. Develop a comprehensive program to provide continuing education to employees throughout the organization with emphasis toward technical and managerial education.

C. Provide for improved programs and methods to inform and educate the governing board, medical staff, and house officers and medical students affiliated with the hospital.

D. Continue to expand and improve patient education and the health education of the public in coordination with the medical staff.

VI. Develop strategies designed to preserve the high quality private practice of medicine and high quality hospital services in the face of increasing social and governmental interference and regulation.

General Objectives

A. Continue to monitor governmental activities
    and develop methods to communicate these to
    the governing board, medical staff, and
    management of the hospital.

B. Develop a mechanism to maximize the
    corporation ability to influence legislation.

C. Provide leadership in forming associations or
    affiliations with individuals or groups external
    to the hospital to communicate and develop strategies
    for countering undesirable regulation or
    interference.

D. Develop programs to react or to adjust to new
    or impending regulation.

Performance Descriptions—Nursing Department

TITLE: Coordinator of Systems and Planning

Department: Nursing Service

Responsible to: Director of Nursing

Definition: The Coordinator of Systems and Planning is a qualified professional nurse who is responsible for developing and implementing systems and procedures that will benefit patient care, personnel who perform them and promote cost effectiveness.

Performance Responsibilities

Performance is Satisfactory When:

A. TO PATIENT:

1. Evaluate and develop nursing procedures affecting direct patient care for their effectiveness and safety.

1. Procedures are reviewed on a periodic basis. Ineffective procedures are identified and revised as needed.

2. Evaluate nursing care related to ancillary department procedures and assist with recommendations, revisions and clarifications.

2. Ancillary department procedures related to nursing care are reviewed periodically. Nursing care aspects are clarified and communicated to appropriate persons for revision.

Performance Responsibilities	Performance is Satisfactory When:
3. Minimize the cost of delivering quality patient care through the evaluation of systems for safety, quality and therapeutic considerations.	3. Demonstrable savings are recorded and verified. Such results are communicated to appropriate departmental and administrative personnel.
4. Implement change in procedures, policies and/or equipment effectively.	4. Appropriate personnel are informed of changes prior to their implementation.
5. Evaluations of products are conducted in a systematic manner.	5. Product evaluations include product demonstration for staff on trial units, written evaluations and summary of results which is presented to appropriate groups for consideration. Plans for appropriate inservicing for products are made.

B. TO MEDICAL STAFF:

1. Assure that the systems and procedures for carrying out the patient care plans are safe and effective.	1. Recommendations from Medical Staff regarding specific systems or procedures are evaluated with appropriate actions taken.
2. Recommend and help to implement new systems and procedures which will contribute to more effective patient care programs.	2. New systems and procedures are presented to appropriate Medical Staff for review. Appropriate physicians are consulted in their development.

C. TO DIRECTOR OF NURSING:

1. Suggest specific analytical studies of systems, methods, procedures and/or activities which offer significant potential for improvement.	1. Documentation of such recommendations and follow-up exists.
2. Submit monthly reports itemizing status of current projects and future projects to be undertaken.	2. Monthly reports are submitted within 7 days after the end of each month.

Performance Responsibilities	Performance is Satisfactory When:
3. Represent the Director of Nursing in contacts with other hospital departments on matters related to systems and procedures.	3. Such contacts are carried out skillfully so that cooperation is secured. The Director is requested to aid in such contacts when judgment so dictates.
4. Inform the Director at once of matters which she needs to know.	4. There is never an oversight in following the dictum "Never let your boss be surprised."
5. Assist Nursing personnel in implementing Nursing Unit objectives.	5. Assistance is rendered to nursing personnel in accordance with current priorities.
6. Develop an annual action program with objective to be accomplished by Systems and Planning.	6. Objectives are submitted prior to beginning of each fiscal year.

D.   TO OTHER DEPARTMENTS:

1. Assist other departments in improving methods, systems and/or procedures that may affect patient care directly and/or indirectly.	1. Interdepartmental contacts are made promptly when problems arise affecting patient care.
2. Provide special services if approved.	2. Cooperation rendered to other departments upon request.

E.   TO SELF:

1. Maintain an up-to-date knowledge and practice of nursing trends and new developments in the health field.	1. Participate in professional and clinical meetings pertinent to areas of special interest. Recommend, implement and/or share new knowledge and trends which effect and/or enhance patient care.
2. Continue to improve own skills in methods and procedures analysis, systems engineering, and business planning.	2. Achieve a sense of growth and increasing satisfaction in Systems and Planning accomplishments.

Performance Responsibilities	Performance is Satisfactory When:
3. Visit other local hospitals and business organizations with a reputation for success .n improving problems similar to those being faced here.	3. Results of visits can be directly applied to current projects or to those planned for next year.
4. Become familiar with outside resources and services which can be utilized to help achieve objectives.	4. Resources contribute to cost effectiveness and achievement of objectives.

F.   TO COMMITTEES:

1. Participate on appropriate committees as member and/or resource person.	1. Committee membership responsibilities are accepted. Committee objectives are met.
2. Keep Systems and Planning committee informed of projects needing their consideration (ex. equipment, procedures, etc.)	2. Systems and Planning committee have opportunity to review projects and to make recommendations.

QUALIFICATIONS:

1. Graduate of an accredited School of Nursing.

2. Satisfactory references (personal and professional).

3. Current state licensure.

4. Advanced preparation in supervision, management, and research.

5. Demonstrate skills in establishing interpersonal and interdepartmental relationships.

6. Demonstrate working knowledge of hospital operation.

COMMUNITY GENERAL HOSPITAL

TITLE: Head Nurse

Department: Nursing Service

Supervises: RN, LPN, Nursing Assistant, Orderly, Ward Secretary, Technicians and Unit Service Aides.

Purpose: Coordinate management and clinical activities on a patient unit so that optimum quality of patient care is delivered at minimum cost.

Performance Responsibilities   Performance is Satisfactory When:

A. TO PATIENTS:

1. Plan safe, economical and efficient nursing care.

Relevant standards (i.e.) JCAH, ANA, NLN, governmental agencies) are met; and costs are controlled.

2. Plan and assist in patient teaching.

Patient demonstrates comprehension and performs satisfactorily.

3. See that quality patient care is given to each patient in accordance with quality standards.

Documentation on care plans and records, together with feedback, indicate that standards are met.

4. Give direct patient care as required.

Individual patient care needs are met, as in #3.

5. Formulate and utilize patient care plan to assist in resolving patient problems.

Documentation on the care plan indicates action on problems and progress toward discharge.

6. Act as liaison between patient, physician and family.

Patient and family understand and carry out physician's directions; feedback is provided to the physician.

B. TO MEDICAL STAFF:

1. See that physician's orders are carried out.

Orders are carried out promptly and accurately.

2. Act as liaison between physician and patient care team.

Communications are clear, as documented and used on patient care plan.

Performance Responsibilities

Performance is Satisfactory When:

3. Question physician when communication is not clear.

No documented errors; no negative feedback.

C.   TO OWN NURSE MANAGER:

1. Share appropriate communications with unit personnel.

Such communications are utilized and understood.

2. Assure adequate staffing.

Personnel are assigned for adequate coverage and optimum utilization.

3. Keep own nurse manager informed of unit activity, personnel problems and patients' conditions.

Appropriate information is communicated to own nurse manager.

4. Make out patient care assignments.

Assignments are made based upon competency of available personnel to meet patient care needs.

5. Seek assistance from nurse manager as necessary in solving clinical and management problems.

Specific instances of seeking and using such help occur.

6. Help with budget planning; operate unit within budget.

Budget is realistically related to patient care programs; and costs are within budget.

D. TO DEPARTMENT PERSONNEL:

1. Act as leader, model, and innovator.

An example is set by using conferences, demonstrations, available resources, and the problem-solving method.

2. Delegate responsibilities within scope of personnel abilities.

Personnel and patients' needs are met.

3. Hold regular unit personnel meetings.

Active participation is evident and there is a feeling of satisfaction with unit meetings.

4. Promote an environment in which the patient care team can work cooperatively toward objectives.

Cooperative relationship exists among members of unit team.

5. Provide an opportunity for personnel staff development.

There is evidence of participation in continuing education activities.

Performance Responsibilities	Performance is Satisfactory When:
6. Assist staff with development and usage of nursing care plans.	Every patient care plan is current on a daily basis.
7. Counsel personnel when necessary.	Counseling is used for problem solving.

E. TO COMMITTEES:

1. Participate actively in selected committee activities.	Committee objectives are met.

F. TO OTHER DEPARTMENT PERSONNEL:

1. Aim for intra-departmental cooperation.	Good working relationship exists.
2. Keep open communication contact as needed to plan patient care.	Cooperation between departments exists and such cooperation favorably affects patient care.

G. TO OTHER ORGANIZATIONS:

1. Current membership in appropriate professional organization.	Participation proves satisfying and productive.

H. TO SELF:

1. Maintain sense of personal satisfaction; keep skills up to date.	Personal goals are met as related to job performance.
2. Participate in continuing education programs.	New learnings provide sense of growth and competency.

QUALIFICATIONS:

1. Graduate of Accredited School of Nursing; current state license.
2. Satisfactory performance in top staff nurse classification for a minimum of one year.
3. Demonstrated competence in management and leadership skills.
4. Successful completion of a management program for head nurses.

Cumberland County Health Department Sample Forms

Exhibit A

MATERNAL CHILD HEALTH INTERAGENCY REPORT
CUMBERLAND COUNTY HEALTH DEPARTMENT
FAYETTEVILLE, NORTH CAROLINA

FOLLOW-UP:
( ) Emergency   CFVH Room #_____
( ) 1-2 Weeks   Clinic #_____
( ) 3-4 Weeks
( ) High Risk

Mother's Name_____ Race W ( ) NW ( ) B ( )
      Last   First   Maiden
DOB___ __ _____ Marital Status: M S W D Sep.   Education Level_____

Name_____ Relationship_____
    Head of household unit patient lives with

Address_____Telephone #_____

Directions_____

Previous Address (if changed)_____

Financial Resource: ( ) Medically Indigent ( ) Medicaid ( ) Employed ( ) Insurance

Antepartum:
Date of clinic adm._____ # of visits_____
Obstetrical history: Gravida_____ Para_____
Deaths_____
Hgb E_____ RH_____ R/Titer_____
GC_____ STS_____
AP complications_____

Infant's Name_____Sex M F
DOB_____Time_____Dr._____
Birth: ( ) Single ( ) Twin #1 ( ) Twin #2
Birth Wt._____Discharge Wt._____
Measurements: Length____Head____Chest____
Physical Exam: ( ) Normal Appar_____

Postpartum:
Delivered by Dr._____
Weeks of gestation_____ L&D Length_____
Episiotomy_____ Laceration_____
Complications_____
_____
_____

Problem:_____
_____
_____
Hearing Screening_____
Circumcision: Yes_____ No_____
Discharge date:_____
Plan for medical supervision:

Anesthesia_____ BP_____ Hct._____
Surgery: (specify)_____
Discharge date_____
BP_____ Breast_____ Lochia_____
Clinic appt._____

CHC_____
_____
Pvt. Dr._____
Date referred to PHN_____
Signed:_____

Notes by MCH Nurse:

CLOTHING	NUTRITION	FPM DESIRED	BABY CARE KNOWLEDGE	CLASSES ATTENDED
___Diapers (#)	___Bottles	___BCP	___How to feed &	___Baby care
___Cloth	___Formula	___IUD	prepare formula	___Discharge
___Pampers	___(type)	___Diaphragm	___Bathing &	interview
___T Shirts	___Breast feeding	___Foam & condoms	handling	___Other
___Gowns	___Food Stamps	___Sterilization	___Take temperature	
___Sleepers	___WIC	___Undecided	___Circumcision &	BED
___Blankets		___None	cord care	
___Other		___Consent signed		___Crib
				___Bassinet
				___Other

Primary Care Taker of Child:_____
Other (specify)_____
_____
_____

(Original copy to district PHN
 Pink copy to Child Health Clinic   Signed_____
 Yellow copy to Maternity Clinic)
CCHD 7/78

CUMBERLAND COUNTY HEALTH DEPARTMENT
MCH Form Part II

I.   Purpose: First PP Visit   0 - Normal
II. Observation: X - Problem/Explanation

A. Mother_____Weeks PP_____ BP_____

1. Breast   2. Bladder   7. ___FP Method
    ___Lactating   ___No frequency   8. ___Appt. PP Cl.
    ___Clean, non-irritated   ___No pain   9. ___Diet adequate
    ___Good support bra   3. Bowels   10. ___Vitamins/iron
    ___Non-breast feeding   ___Normal   11. ___Exercise
    ___Breast feeding   4. ___Lochia   12. ___ADL
    ___Nipples erect   5. ___Routine pericare 13. ___Mother/infant
    ___Rotation of breast   6. ___Episiotomy   interaction

Problem/Nursing Action:_____
_____
_____
_____
_____
_____

B. Infant_____DOB_____ Age_____

1. _____Skin   14. Abdomen   19. _____Spine
2. _____Head   _____soft   20. _____Normal BM's
3. _____Ant. Font.   _____umbilical cord 21. _____Normal voiding
    _____Post. Font.   _____hernia   22. Diet
4. _____Scalp   15. Genitalia   _____type formula
5. _____Eyes   _____vag. os patent   _____amt./24 hrs.
6. _____Ears   _____penis circumcised   _____water
7. _____Nose   _____foreskin retractable _____preparation
8. _____Mouth & throat   _____uncircumcised   _____following recom-
9. _____Palate   _____scrotal sac   mended diet
10. _____Neck   16. _____Fem. pulse felt   23. _____Mother gives child
11. _____Chest   17. _____Upper extrem.   care
12. _____Heart   18. _____Lower extrem.   24. _____Nec. equipment
13. _____Breast   25. _____Own bed

Problem/Nursing Action:_____
_____
_____
_____
_____

C. Surroundings:_____
_____
_____
_____
_____

III. Plan:_____
_____
                                            _____R.N.
(Original copy to district PHN
Pink copy to Child Health Clinic
Yellow copy to Maternity Clinic)   _____
CCHD 7/78   Date

_____
Used with permission

Exhibit B

CUMBERLAND COUNTY HEALTH DEPARTMENT
Fayetteville, North Carolina

Nursing Standards for First Postpartum Home Visit

CONDITION	STANDARD	NURSE'S ACTION
I. Mother-Physical Assessment Objective:	To determine health status of mother, promote awareness of health state, and provide nursing intervention as needed on first home visit two to four weeks postpartum.	
A. Normal Breasts 1. Non-lactating	Dry, soft, nipples non-irritated, firm support bra.	Support present care routine.
2. Lactating	Good quantity milk, firm nipples, erect and non-irritated, breasts rotated, adequate support bra.	Support present care routine.
B. B/P	Within range of 100/60 to 120/80 (?)	Check BP and record.
C. Elimination 1. Bladder	No urgency or frequency, good bladder control, painfree emptying.	Reinforce mother's knowledge of bladder function.
2. Bowels	Pre-pregnancy patterns resumed.	Reinforce mother's knowledge of bowel function.
D. Involutional Process 1. Lochia	Absent to scanty amount, color brownish to white, free of odor.	Teach patient re: normal involutional lochia.
2. Episiotomy	Healing, non-painful.	Support present routine.
3. Abdomen	Non-painful, free of cramping (except during breast feeding).	Patient teaching re: Fundus check.
4. B.C. Method	Knowledge of two acceptable methods.	If necessary PHN discusses each.
5. Patient teaching	Prevention of perineal infection, intercourse frequency, p.p. physiological changes, p.p. clinic appointment.	If necessary PHN discusses each.
E. Nutrition	Review basic diet and iron rich diet.	Modify for individual patient. Refer to p.p. diet standards.

CONDITION	STANDARD	NURSE'S ACTION
F. Physical Activities	Begin to resume normal daily activities, use p.p. exercises, and adequate rest.	Discuss progressive resumption and types of p.p. exercises, and rest needs.
II. Infant-Physical Assessment Objective:	To determine health status of infant, promote awareness of health state, and provide nursing intervention as needed on first home visit, two to four weeks after birth.	
A. Skin	Clean and clear (free of rash).	Reinforce skin care. Observe & record size & location of birth marks and/or mongolian spots.
B. Head	Normal shape & size in relation to other body proportions. Ant. fontanel open, flat. Post fontanel closed (or small opening) & flat.	Condition recorded. Size recorded. Size recorded.
C. Scalp (hair area)	Clean, washed at least every other day.	Reinforce scalp cleansing.
D. Ears	Top surface in line with external corner of eye, and symmetrical. Clean and normal in shape.	Reinforce bathing instructions including behind and in ears. (No Q-tips to be used.)
E. Eyes	Clear, clean, and tearing.	Reinforce correct cleansing.
F. Nose	Both nostrils patent and free of discharge.	Reinforce care.
G. Mouth & Throat	Mucosa clear and palate closed.	Reinforce oral care including water offered following formula to reduce milk coating and lukewarm temperature of formula.
H. Neck	Supple, free of masses and irritation.	Reinforce cleansing instructions including folds of neck.
I. Chest	Non-retracting respirations. Breasts non-enlarged.	Condition recorded.
J. Abdomen	Soft, and no palpable masses.	Condition recorded.
K. Umbilical Cord	On and dry, off and healing. Absence of herniation.	Reinforce umbilical care.

Exhibit B continued

CONDITION	STANDARD	NURSE'S ACTION
L. Genitalia		
1. Female	Vaginal os patent, folds non-swollen, area clean and free of irritation.	Reinforce vaginal care.
2. Male	Testicles descended and scrotal sac non-swollen. Circumcized penis healed, clean, and fore-skin easily retractible.	Reinforce continued ob-servance of sac for swell-ing and record. Record position of testicles. Re-inforce retraction of fore-skin.
	Uncircumcized penis clean and able to visualize meatus.	Reinforce retraction of fore-skin.
M. Extremities		
1. Upper	Simultaneous movement and full ROM. Hands—normal appearance, shape, and size.	Record findings.
2. Lower	Hips-bilateral full ROM. Legs-straight and equal with symmetrical poste-rior folds. Feet-straight.	Record findings.
N. Spinal Column	Straight, spinal process palpable and free of masses and/or sinuses.	Record condition.
O. Bowel	Anal os patent, free of tags and irritation. Stools—color, consist-ency, and frequency relate adequately to type of formula intake.	Reinforce mother's daily observance of bowel hab-its and knowledge of thermometer use.
P. Bladder	Voids every ½ hour, stream continuous not intermittent, urine stains yellow and has ammonia-like odor.	Reinforce frequent diaper changes and genital cleansing. Thorough diaper washing methods.
Q. Reflexes	Infant demonstrates grasp, startle, sucking, and head turning (fenc-ing) reflexes.	Record findings.
R. Nutrition		
1. Formula	Identify formula brand, 24-hour quantity, and fre-quency of feedings. Identify preparation method of choice to pa-tient.	Modify for individual pa-tient. (Refer to infant formula procedure.) Re-view method chosen (aseptic, terminal).

CONDITION	STANDARD	NURSE'S ACTION
2. Solids	Identify type of solids and frequency, if already introduced.	Discuss introduction and progression of solids. (Refer to infant feeding procedure.)
S. Safety	See Section III Environment.	

III. Environment Objective:	Evaluate physical and emotional environment and determine mode of child care.	

A. Physical (Dwelling)	Adequate water source.
	  1. Clean well water and pump.
	  2. Indoor plumbing.
	Adequate heating and cooking source.
	Screens on windows and doors.
		Record findings.

B. Emotional	Mother holds child securely, with ease, and relates to child. Family accepts child. Father supports family emotionally and financially.	Record observations. Reinforce.
C. Child Care	Adequate care given.	Determine and record who gives care and where.
D. Safety	Measures appropriate for age.	Record and reinforce.

IV. Equipment Objective:	Determine number of care items and inform mother of additional items needed.	
A. Mother	Firm support bra & sanitary pads.	Record findings. Reinforce usage.
B. Baby 1. Clothing	Diapers-24 cloth and/or Pampers, tops-6, receiving blankets-2.	Record findings. Reinforce usage.
2. Hygiene	Soap-Ivory, Dial, Safeguard, personal towel.	Record findings. Reinforce usage.
3. Formula	6 bottles, nipples, and caps (formula and water), can opener, refrigeration, formula container and cover.	Record findings. Reinforce usage.

Exhibit B   continued

CONDITION	STANDARD	NURSE'S ACTION
4. Foods	Personal spoon and dish. Solids appropriate for age level.	Record findings. Reinforce usage.
5. Sleeping	Separate bed with firm pad or mattress. Bed linens-crib sheets, puddle pads, mats or plastic pads, blanket.	Record findings. Reinforce usage.

Exhibit C

RETROSPECTIVE AUDIT SHEET

First Postpartum Home Visit   Patient's Name _____

Code: YES = Present
    NO = Not present   Date of Home Visit _____
    NA = Not assessible
    V   = Variation

	YES	NO	NA	V	Comments
I. Mother					
A. Breasts 96%*					
1. Condition of non-lactating breasts					
2. Condition of lactating breasts					
B. Recording of BP findings 100%					
C. Elimination 96%					
1. Bladder elim. noted					
2. Bladder control noted					
3. Bowel pattern noted					
D. Vagina 90%					
1. Description of lochia					
2. Condition of episiotomy					
3. Perineal self-care noted					
4. Perineal teaching including:					
a. hygiene					
b. intercourse frequency					
c. family planning					
d. next clinic visit					
E. Diet and exercise 100%					
1. Teaching re diet noted					
2. Teaching re PP exercises noted					
II. Infant					
A. Skin condition noted 96%					
B. Head notations re: condition of:					
1. Shape 96%					
2. Size 96%					
3. Size of Ant. Fontanel 96%					
4. Size of Post. Fontanel 96%					
5. Eyes 96%					
6. Ears 96%					
7. Nose 96%					
8. Mouth/Throat 96%					
C. Condition of neck 96%					
D. Chest 96%					
1. Condition of respirations					
2. Condition of breasts					
E. Abdomen 90%					
1. Condition of tone					
2. Condition of cord					

*See text for explanation of %.

Exhibit C   continued

First Post-Partum Home Visit

Patient's Name _____

Date of Home Visit_____

Audit Sheet	YES	NO	NA	V	Comments
II. F. Genitalia 96%					
1. Female-appearance normal					
os patient					
2. Male-circumcised & condition 96%					
uncircumcised & foreskin					
retractibility testicles &					
scrotal sac app. normal 96%					
G. Extremities					
1. Upper movement noted 96%					
2. Lower movement noted 96%					
position noted 96%					
H. Spinal position noted 96%					
I. Bowel					
condition of anal os 96%					
bowel activity noted 100%					
taught use of thermometer 50%					
J. Bladder					
diaper condition when changed 96%					
K. Remaining primary reflexes noted 96%					
L. Diet 100%					
1. Formula type noted					
Quantity of intake					
2. Type solids noted					
Teaching re progression noted					
Freq. of feedings noted					
M. Teaching re safety noted 96%					
III. Child Care 100%					
A. Who gives noted					
B. Where care given noted					
IV. Equipment					
A. Mother during 1st 2 wks PP. 100%					
peri-care noted					
pads used noted					

Exhibit C continued

First Post-Partum Home Visit   Patient's Name _____

                                      Date of Home Visit _____

Audit Sheet	YES	NO	NA	V	Comments
B. Baby					
1. Clothing items noted					
2. Hygiene items noted					
3. Formula items noted					
4. Solid food items noted					
5. Sleeping arrangement items noted					
V. Environment					
A. House					
1. Water source noted					
2. Heating source noted					
3. Window and door screens noted					
4. Cooking source noted					
VI. Emotional Climate					
A. Mother's handling of child					
B. Mother's relationship with child					
C. Family acceptance of child					
D. Type of support from father					

Exhibit D

QUALITY CONTROL CHECK: PUBLIC HEALTH NURSING AUDIT

Data must be held in STRICT confidence and MUST NOT BE FILED with patient's record.

All entries to be completed by trained clerk.

1. Name of patient: 2. Sex: 4. Admission date:
                                                              type:
(Last)   (First)   3. Age: 5. Discharge date:

6. Nursing Agency: 7. Number of visits to patient by agency:

8. Complete diagnosis(es):

9. Was patient hospitalized immediately   10. Medical supervision:
   prior to PHN service:

Yes No. Days No Unknown N/A   Private Ward OPD/Cl. N/A
☐   ☐   ☐   ☐   ☐   ☐   ☐   ☐   ☐

11. Patient referred to PHN by:
    Hospital Hospital   Patient's   MCH   Other
    Nurse   Soc. Wkr.   M.D.   Family   Nurse   Specify: N/A   Unknown
    ☐   ☐   ☐   ☐   ☐   ☐   ☐   ☐

12. Patient discharged from PHN to:
    Self-   Family   Rehospit-   Other PHN   Not dis-   Other
    Care   Care   alized   Died   Agency   charged   Specify: Unknown
    ☐   ☐   ☐   ☐   ☐   ☐   ☐   ☐

13. All nursing entries signed by   14. Nursing entries show whether made by
    name and dated: public health, professional, practical,
                                               student nurse, physiotherapist, other:
         Yes   No   Yes   No
         ☐   ☐   ☐   ☐

15. Plan of care is recorded: Yes   No
                                           ☐   ☐

                                                              Yes   No
16. Were there any accidents or special incidents?
    a. If yes, chart indicates report was submitted to administration   _____   _____
    b. Or, report is part of the chart   _____   _____
17. Nursing admission entry shows assessment of patient's condition:
                                              physical_____   _____
                                              emotional_____   _____
18. Nursing discharge entry shows assessment of patient's condition:
                                              physical_____   _____
                                              emotional_____   _____

EXPLANATION OF EXHIBITS

Exhibit A: The Interagency Report Form

The maternal child health interagency report is initiated by the maternal and child health nurse working in the hospital who completes Section 1 (as well as the top of Section 2). Section 1 serves as the data base on mother and infant for the district public health nurse who makes the first postpartum visit to the mother and infant.

Section 2 of the maternal child health interagency report serves as the progress notes and plan of care for mother and infant. The lower half is completed by the district public health nurse after the initial visit to mother and infant.

Exhibit B: Standards for First Postpartum Visit

Qualitative standards were established for the physical assessment and care of both mother and infant and for child care, equipment necessary for care in the home, the physical environment of the home, and the emotional climate in the home.

Exhibit C: Retrospective Audit for First Postpartum Visit

The same standard (Exhibit B) serves also as the basis for the retrospective audit for the audit topic: First postpartum home visit. A Retrospective Audit Sheet was designed to retrieve the necessary data (Exhibit C). The percentages on this form indicate 96% or below as acceptable for many elements. A 100% standard for data gathering on home visits is felt by the district public health nurses to be unrealistic due to occasional presence of neighbors and friends. Every effort is made by the nurse to avoid embarrassing the mother or family members.

Exhibit D: Quality Control Check of First Postpartum Visit

An audit of the nursing process is carried out for the same mother and infant. A quality control check form, Exhibit D, is used for this purpose. It is adapted from the form provided by Maria C. Phaneuf in *The Nursing Audit.*[1]

NOTES

1. Phaneuf, M. C. *The nursing audit: Profile for excellence.* New York: Appleton-Century-Crofts, 1972, p. 22.

Maslow's Theory of Human Motivation

Abraham Maslow

Abraham Maslow was born April 1, 1908, in a slum district of Brooklyn, New York. His early years of schooling were spent in New York city schools. His college years were spent at City College of New York, then Cornell, and later Wisconsin, where his interests turned to psychology. He was a shy, studious, brilliant student ... an achiever, following his own learning inclinations. After graduation, he worked for E.L. Thorndike, the Watsonian disciple (and developer of intelligence tests) at Teacher's College, Columbia University. Later he taught for fourteen years at Brooklyn College—until he moved to Brandeis University near Boston, Massachusetts. During his Brooklyn years he was able to learn much from his contacts with Max Wertheimer (the founding member of the gestalt school), Erich Fromm, Karen Horney, Kurt Goldstein, Ruth Benedict (the renowned anthropologist), and Alfred Adler.

In the early thirties, after studying human learning, he concluded that success and reward have a far more powerful effect than failure or punishment. Later, he became disenchanted with the kind of clinical psychology that was based upon the study of abnormal personalities—of sick people. So he decided to study the healthiest people he could find—the most creative, productive, happiest human beings. The result made history.

Maslow's findings are widely published, interpreted, and used throughout the world. He presented the need hierarchy and its relations to motivation in his now-classic book, *Motivation and Personality.* Though widely acclaimed by many, it met with skepticism from a wide spectrum of the traditional psychologists. Maslow was seen as a renegade and was virtually ostracized by the American Psychological Association. Later, however, in the mid-sixties, he was elected to the presidency of APA.

He became a founder of the Association for Humanistic Psychology and the recognized leader of "The Third Force"—the name he gave to the serious and fast-growing movement he fathered that challenged the most basic precepts which for a century had formed the basis for the study of personality. It challenged Freud's dictatorship of the unconscious and the mechanistic world of the behaviorists. In their stead, it proposed a new philosophy of behavior, an optimistic human awareness that sets people free to be themselves, to create and grow, to control their choices and goals.

Maslow died of a second heart attack, in California, in June 1970. He lives on in the hearts, minds, and work of a great host of people whose lives he touched in so many ways. He remains a force for good in a world coping with so many forms of the bad.

Henry Geiger, who wrote the introduction to the Maslow book, *The Farther Reaches of Human Nature*, explains the deserved popularity of Maslow's works.

> People who read him understand why. He has a psychology that applies to them. . . . All through his work one finds exposed nodes open to intuitive verification, good enough for any man of hungry common sense. These "insights" make people keep on reading Maslow. . . . Nearly all his writing gives off sparks.

Exhibit A Maslow's Theory of Human Motivation

The Hierarchy of Needs

The human being is motivated by a number of basic needs. It is the unsatisfied needs which have the greatest influence on behavior. Once a need has been gratified it has little effect on motivation. A want that is satisfied is no longer a want. The first two needs are basic needs, the latter three are growth needs.

1. Survival (Physiological) needs represent our needs for food, clothing, shelter, and other things which are essential to our existence. So long as these needs go unsatisfied, the individual is little concerned with other needs and his efforts will be directed toward satisfaction in this area.
2. Security (Safety) needs. Once the individual's survival needs are satisfied to at least a minimum degree, his dominant needs become security needs. His efforts are directed

toward satisfaction in this area. Security needs include physical safety, job tenure, insurance, pensions, etc.

3. Social (Love, affection, belonging) needs. When the individual has minimum satisfaction of his survival and security needs, belongingness needs become important to him. These are the needs for love, acceptance, and approval by others—his family, his friends, those with whom he works.

4. Status (Esteem, self-worth) needs. The individual whose survival, security, and belongingness needs are satisfied in at least a minimum fashion then becomes concerned with esteem needs—the need for recognition and status. Whereas belongingness needs are more or less passive, esteem needs involve the active favorable reactions of others. The esteem need also includes the individual's need for self-respect or self-esteem.

5. Self-Actualizing (Self-Fulfillment) needs. If the survival, security, belongingness, and esteem needs are all satisfied to at least a minimum degree, the individual's dominant need becomes self-fulfillment. This need is the individual's desire to become his best self, to realize his capabilities to the fullest, to know that he is making his greatest contribution to humanity.

Adapted from Maslow, A. H. *Motivation and personality* (2nd ed.). New York: Harper & Row, 1970; and Goble, F. *The third force* (The Psychology of Abraham Maslow). New York: Pocket Books, 1971.

Exhibit B Understanding Motivation

Why I Do What I Do

I HAVE FIVE HUMAN NEEDS; I DO WHAT I DO BECAUSE I MUST SATISFY MY NEEDS.

To Survive
I need to get food, shelter, air; things I need to stay alive.

To Feel Secure
I need to feel secure at home, on my job, in my life situation . . . within myself.

For Meaningful Social Contacts
I need such contacts to give me a sense of belonging, to share love and affection, to know I am wanted.

For Status
I need a sense of self-esteem, the respect of others, pride in my ability and accomplishments, a sense of self-worth.

For Self-Actualization
I need to continue growing toward becoming my best possible self and greater self-realization.

Beyond these needs I have *metaneeds*, the search for the "being values" ("B" for short), the ultimate values which are intrinsic. I need meaning in my life, to worship, to satisfy the human values of being including truth, beauty, goodness, simplicity, wholeness, and others.

Exhibits B and C are adapted from Maslow, A. H. *Motivation and personality* (2nd ed.). New York: Harper & Row, 1970; idem, *The farther reaches of human nature.* New York: The Viking Press, 1971; idem, *Toward a psychology of being.* New York: Van Nostrand Reinhold, 1968. For more information on metaneeds see idem, *Religions, values, and peak experiences.* New York: The Viking Press, 1970.

Exhibit C Why My Needs Are Never Fully Satisfied

I CAN UNDERSTAND MYSELF AND OTHERS BETTER WHEN I RECOGNIZE THE RELATIONSHIP BETWEEN MY NEEDS AND MY MOTIVATION.

If my survival is threatened, other needs become less important. I do what I must do to stay alive.

When I know I will survive, my need for security and safety becomes important. I act in ways which I think will help me to reach at least a minimum level of security.

Then, with survival and security needs satisfied to some degree, I begin to seek more social satisfactions (belonging to a group; giving and receiving affection).

I seek also more of a sense of status, esteem, and self-worth. And I reach out for greater self-actualization and personal growth.

Having attained a sense of satisfaction for all of the foregoing, I still want more. I strive for a higher level of aliveness, uniqueness, justice, order, perfection, self-sufficiency, playfulness, richness, effortlessness, and the other "B" values—the metaneeds.

I behave this way because I am a human being with human needs that must be satisfied. Other people are like me, all striving to satisfy their needs too. That's why we act the way we do.

If I can't meet the need that I feel most, then I hurt. When I satisfy a need, I feel good—but immediately another need takes its place. When I satisfy a need it is no longer a motivator for me, but another need is.

I am motivated when I feel desire or want or yearning or wish or lack.

Guidelines for Developing Mutual Expectations

Hospital Administrator ← → Nursing Director (PCA)

PURPOSE:

To clarify, through discussion, what the hospital administrator (HA) and patient care administrator (PCA; Director of Nursing) expect of each other and themselves in their role relationships—and thus avoid costly misunderstandings and unwelcome surprises.

PREPARATION:

- HA— Write brief statements of:
    1. what you expect from your PCA
    2. what your PCA can expect from you as HA.
- PCA—Write brief statements of:
    1. what you expect from your HA
    2. what your HA can expect from you as PCA.

Examples:

The HA might state these expectations of the PCA:

"(1) monthly progress report; (2) daily update on nursing matters of interest; (3) written budget requests with justification." And these statements of what the PCA can expect from the HA: "(1) support for personnel decisions and actions; (2) periodic evaluation of performance."

The PCA might state these expectations of the HA: "(1) to be kept informed of Board decisions affecting nursing; (2) support for decisions affecting patient care that involve nursing." And these statements of what the HA can expect of the PCA: "(1) adherence to the written philosophy, goals, and objectives of the agency; (2) effective cost-containment efforts, consistent with written objectives and patient care quality goals."

SHARING:

Set aside a generous amount of time for sharing the written statements of mutual expectations.

Note: If agreed upon, you may wish to invite a mutually-respected third party (staff development director, personnel manager, management consultant) to act as observer and keep the discussion on the topic without participating in the sharing.

At end of the session, both the HA and the PCA may summarize any new insights and helpful clarifications that have emerged during the discussion.

Set a date for another session if that appears to be necessary.

We acknowledge with appreciation our introduction to this Mutual Expectations sharing technique by Prof. John R. Malban, MSHA, at the Independent Study Program for HAs/PCAs, School of Public Health, University of Minnesota, Minneapolis.

Accreditation Standards for Nursing Services Purposes and Historical Review of JCAH

Exhibit A

PRINCIPLE: There shall be an organized nursing department/service that takes all reasonable steps to provide the optimal achievable quality of nursing care and to maintain the optimal professional conduct and practices of its members.

STANDARD I: The nursing department/service shall be directed by a qualified nurse administrator and shall be appropriately integrated with the medical staff and with other hospital staffs that provide and contribute to patient care.

INTERPRETATION: *Direction*—The administrator of the nursing department/service shall be a qualified, registered nurse with appropriate education, experience, and licensure, and demonstrated ability in nursing practice and administration. It is desirable, but not required, that the nurse administrator have at least a baccalaureate in nursing. The nurse administrator shall be employed on a full-time basis and shall have authority and responsibility for taking all reasonable steps to assure that the optimal achievable quality of nursing care is provided. When a hospital nursing department/service is decentralized and each clinical department/service has a director of nursing, there shall be one administrator to whom the directors shall be accountable for providing a uniformly optimal level of nursing care throughout the hospital.

A qualified registered nurse shall be designated and authorized to act in the nurse administrator's absence. The organizational structure of the nursing department/service shall provide for appropriate administration of nursing services on all shifts.

The nurse administrator shall have authority and responsibility for assuring that nursing care objectives are established and met, and, in accordance with delegated authority, shall assure that the policies, procedures, and practices of the nursing department/service are consistent with the hospital's goals and with the policies and procedures of the hospital and the medical staff. The development, allocation, and administration of the nursing department/service budget is necessary for the accomplishment of objectives and programs.

Integration—The relationship of the nursing department/service to other departments/service/units of the hospital shall be specified within the overall hospital organizational plan.

The nurse administrator, or an individual designated by the nurse administrator, should represent the nursing department/service in institutional planning and, when requested, should provide periodic reports on the status of nursing care. The nurse administrator should provide any formal liaison required between the medical staff and nursing department/service. Qualified registered nurses shall participate in other patient care activities, including, but not limited to, the infection control committee, the pharmacy and therapeutics function, the medical record function, the hospital safety committee, and when such exist, the professional library committee, special care unit committee, and emergency care committee. The role of the nursing department/service in the hospital's internal and external disaster plans shall be defined.

When the hospital provides clinical facilities for the education of nursing students, there shall be a written agreement that defines the respective roles and responsibilities of the hospital nursing department/service and of the educational program.

STANDARD II: The nursing department/service shall be organized to meet the nursing care needs of patients and to maintain established standards of nursing practice.

INTERPRETATION: The nursing department/service shall have a written organizational plan that delineates lines of authority, accountability, and communication. The manner in which the nursing department/service is organized shall be consistent with the variety of patient services offered and the scope of nursing care activities.

The nursing department/service shall be organized to assure that nursing management functions are effectively fulfilled. Nursing management functions shall include at least the following:

- Reviewing and approving policies and procedures that relate to the qualifications and employment of nursing department/service members.
- Establishing standards of nursing care and mechanisms for evaluating such care. This shall include the conduct of nursing monitoring functions and any review and evaluation performed to assess the quality and appropriateness of nursing care provided.
- Accounting for professional and administrative nursing staff activities. This includes receiving and, as necessary, acting upon the reports and recommendations of nursing department/service committees and other committees concerned with patient care.
- Implementing the approved policies of the nursing department/service.
- Appointing committees, as needed, to conduct nursing department/service functions. The purpose and function of each standing committee shall be defined and a record of its activities shall be maintained.
- Encouraging nursing staff personnel to participate in staff development programs and attend required meetings.

Appropriate nursing department/service personnel should meet as often as necessary, but not less than six times a year, to identify problems in the provision of nursing care, taking into consideration the findings from relevant nursing care and propose solutions monitoring and evaluation activities. This function may be performed on a department/service/unit level and should be carried out in a manner suitable to the hospital. A record shall be maintained that documents any resultant recommendations or proposed actions.

The nursing staff shall be involved in the accreditation process, including participation in the hospital survey and the summation conference.

All individuals, including graduates of foreign nursing schools and nursing personnel from outside sources, utilized in a registered nurse capacity shall be fully licensed in the state or shall have a current temporary license with a stated expiration date. There shall be a method for follow-up on temporary licenses.

Performance appraisal—A written evaluation of the performance of registered nurses and ancillary nursing personnel shall be made at the end of the probationary period and at a defined interval thereafter. An annual evaluation is recommended. The evaluation must be criteria-based and shall relate to the standards of performance specified in the individual's job description. Job descriptions for each position classification shall also delineate the functions, responsibilities, and specific qualifications of each classification, and shall be made available to nursing personnel at the time they are hired and when requested. Job descriptions shall be reviewed periodically and revised as needed to reflect current job requirements.

Outside sources—When outside agencies, registries, or other sources of temporary nursing personnel are used by the nursing department/service to meet nurse staffing needs, the registered nurses and ancillary nursing personnel from such outside sources ordinarily shall be evaluated by the hospital nursing department/service through its designated mechanism. If evaluation is performed by the outside source, the mechanism for evaluation and verification of its use must be available and acceptable to the hospital. When an appropriate evaluation has not been accomplished prior to the individual's working in the hospital, the assignment of such nurses shall be limited to units that are supervised by an experienced registered nurse from the hospital nursing staff on duty at the time.

STANDARD III: Nursing department/service assignments in the provision of nursing care shall be commensurate with the qualifications of nursing personnel and shall be designed to meet the nursing care needs of patients.

INTERPRETATION: A sufficient number of qualified registered nurses shall be on duty at all times to give patients the nursing care that requires the judgment and specialized skills of a registered nurse. Nursing personnel staffing shall also be sufficient to assure prompt recognition of an untoward change in a patient's condition and to facilitate appropriate intervention by the nursing, medical, or hospital staffs. In striving to assure optimal achievable quality nursing care and a safe patient environment, nursing personnel staffing and assignment shall be based at least on the following:

- A registered nurse plans, supervises, and evaluates the nursing care of each patient.
- To the extent possible, a registered nurse makes a patient assessment before delegating appropriate aspects of nursing care to ancillary nursing personnel.
- The patient care assignment minimizes the risk of the transfer of infection and accidental contamination.
- The patient care assignment is commensurate with the qualifications of each nursing staff member, the identified nursing needs of the patient, and the prescribed medical regimen.
- Responsibility for nursing care and related duties is retained by the hospital nursing department/service when nursing students and nursing personnel from outside sources are providing care within a patient care unit.

The nursing department/service shall define, implement, and maintain a system for determining patient requirements for nursing care on the basis of demonstrated patient needs, appropriate nursing intervention, and priority for care. Specific nursing personnel staffing for each nursing care unit, including, as appropriate, the surgical suite, obstetrical suite, ambulatory care department/service, and emergency department/service, shall be commensurate with the patient care requirements, staff expertise, unit geography, availability of support services, and method of patient care delivery. The hospital admissions system should allow for input from the nursing department/service in coordinating patient requirements for nursing care with available nursing resources.

Only qualified registered nurses shall be assigned to head nurse/supervisor and circulating nurse positions in the surgical and obstetrical suites. An operating-room technician may assist in circulating duties under the direct supervision of a qualified registered nurse.

STANDARD IV: Individualized, goal-directed nursing care shall be provided to patients through the use of the nursing process.

INTERPRETATION: The nursing process (assessment, planning, intervention, evaluation) shall be documented for each hospitalized patient from admission through discharge. Each patient's nursing needs shall be assessed by a registered nurse at the time of admission or within the period established by nursing department/service policy. These assessment data shall be consistent with the medical plan of care and shall be available to all nursing personnel involved in the care of the patient.

A registered nurse must plan each patient's nursing care and, whenever possible, nursing goals should be mutually set with the patient and/or family. Goals shall be based on the nursing assessment and shall be realistic, measurable, and consistent with the therapy prescribed by the responsible medical practitioner. Patient education and patient/family knowledge of self-care shall be given special consideration in the nursing plan. The instructions and counseling given to the patient must be consistent with that of the responsible medical practitioner. The plan of care must be documented and should reflect current standards of nursing practice. The plan shall include nursing measures that will facilitate the medical care prescribed and that will restore, maintain, or promote the patient's well-being. As appropriate, such measures should include physiological, psychosocial, and environmental factors; patient/family education; and patient discharge planning. The scope of the plan shall be determined by the anticipated needs of the patient and shall be revised as the needs of the patient change. Exceptions to the requirement for a care plan shall be defined in writing.

Documentation of nursing care shall be pertinent and concise, and shall reflect the patient's status. Nursing documentation should address the patient's needs, problems, capabilities, and limitations. Nursing intervention and patient response must be noted. When a patient is transferred within or discharged from the hospital, a nurse shall note the patient's status in the medical record. As appropriate, patients who are discharged from the hospital requiring nursing care should receive instructions and individualized counseling prior to discharge, and evidence of the instructions and the patient's or family's understanding of these instructions should be noted in the medical record. Such instructions and counseling must be consistent with the responsible medical practitioner's instructions.

The nursing department/service is encouraged to standardize documentation of routine elements of care and repeated monitoring of, for example, personal hygiene, administration of medication, and physiological parameters.

STANDARD V: Nursing department/service personnel shall be prepared through appropriate education and training programs for their responsibilities in the provision of nursing care.

INTERPRETATION: Education/training programs for nursing department/service personnel shall be ongoing and designed to augment their knowledge of pertinent new developments in patient care and to maintain current competence. The scope and complexity of the program shall be based on the documented educational needs of nursing staff personnel and the resources available to meet those needs. The needs shall be identified, at least in part, through the findings of the review and evaluation of nursing care and nursing department/service monitoring activities. The extent of participation of each nursing staff member shall be documented.

The individual responsible for developing and coordinating nursing educational/training programs should be knowledgeable in educational methods and current nursing practice. Registered nurses who provide direct patient care shall contribute to such programs. An evaluation of the educational activities should be performed periodically. The educational programs shall include instruction in the safety and infection control requirements described elsewhere in this *Manual*.

Cardiopulmonary resuscitation training shall be conducted as often as necessary, but not less than annually, except for nursing staff members who can otherwise document their competence.

Nursing department/service personnel, at least on the supervisory level, should also participate in outside meetings that are relevant to their patient care responsibilities, and such participation should be documented. Nursing staff members should be encouraged to participate in any available pertinent self-assessment programs.

New nursing department/service personnel shall receive an orientation of sufficient duration and content to prepare them for their specific duties and responsibilities in the hospital. The orientation shall be based on the educational needs identified by assessment of the individual's ability, knowledge, and skills. Any necessary instruction shall be provided nursing service personnel before they administer direct patient care. Prior to their performing nursing functions within a patient care area, nursing personnel who are not hospital employees must be provided any required orientation by the nursing department/service.

Pertinent professional books and current nursing periodicals should be made available to nursing personnel. Appropriate reference material should be made available to each patient care unit.

STANDARD VI: Written policies and procedures that reflect optimal standards of nursing practice shall guide the provision of nursing care.

INTERPRETATION: Written standards of nursing practice and related policies and procedures shall define and describe the scope and conduct of patient care provided by the nursing staff. These standards, policies, and procedures shall be reviewed at least annually, revised as necessary, dated to indicate the time of the last review, signed by the responsible reviewing authority, and implemented. Nursing department/service policies and procedures shall relate at least to:

- assignment of nursing care consistent with patient needs, as determined by the nursing process;
- acknowledgment, coordination, and implementation of the diagnostic and therapeutic orders of medical staff members;
- medication administration;
- confidentiality of information;
- the role of the nursing staff in discharge planning;
- the role of the nursing staff in patient and family education;
- maintenance of required records, reports, and statistical information;
- cardiopulmonary resuscitation;
- patient, employee, and visitor safety; and
- the scope of activity of volunteers or paid attendants.

Additional policies and procedures are usually required for units in which special care is provided. Current hospital and medical staff policies and procedures that affect the nursing staff's provision of care shall also be available in each patient care area.

STANDARD VII: The nursing department/service shall provide mechanisms for the regular review and evaluation of the quality and appropriateness of nursing department/service practice and functions. Such mechanisms shall be designed to attain optimal achievable standards of nursing care.

INTERPRETATION: The nurse administrator shall be responsible for assuring that a review and evaluation of the quality and appropriateness of nursing care is accomplished in a timely manner. The review and evaluation may be performed by the nursing department/service as a whole or by a designated representative committee, or by the professional nursing staff assigned to clinical departments, services, or units. When possible, nursing quality assurance efforts should be integrated with similar activities in the hospital. The review and evaluation shall be based upon written criteria, shall be performed at least quarterly, and should examine the provision of nursing care and its effect on patients. Methods of review and evaluation may include, but are not necessarily limited to, patient observation or interview, specific monitoring functions, or use of the patient medical record. Nursing staff personnel who provide patient care shall participate in the review. When possible, the medical record department should help the nursing department/service perform medical record functions related to the nursing department's/service's review of nursing care. The quality and appropriateness of nursing care provided by personnel who are not hospital employees, that is, those obtained through agencies, registries, or other outside sources, shall be included in the regular review of nursing care.

A mechanism shall be designed to assure that pertinent findings from the evaluation of nursing care are disseminated within the nursing department/service, and that appropriate action is taken.

Reference to other nursing department/service requirements is made in the following sections of this *Manual:* Anesthesia Services, Dietetic Services, Emergency Services, Functional Safety and Sanitation, Home Care Services, Hospital Sponsored Ambulatory Care Services, Infection Control, Medical Record Services, Nuclear Medicine Services, Pharmaceutical Services, Professional Library Services, Quality Assurance, Radiology Services, Rehabilitation Programs/Services, Respiratory Care Services, Social Work Services, and Special Care Units.

Source: Redman, R. (Ed.). Nursing Services. *Accreditation manual for hospitals* (1980 ed.). Chicago: Joint Commission on Accreditation of Hospitals, 1978. Reprinted with permission.

Exhibit B

Purposes

The purposes of the Joint Commission on Accreditation of Hospitals, as stated in its certificate of incorporation, are:

1. to establish standards for the operation of hospitals and other health-related facilities and services;
2. to conduct survey and accreditation programs that will encourage members of the health professions, hospitals, and other health-related facilities and services voluntarily:
   a. to promote high quality of care in all aspects in order to give patients the optimal benefits that medical science has to offer,
   b. to apply certain basic principles of physical plant safety and maintenance, and of organization and administration of function for efficient care of the patient, and
   c. to maintain the essential services in the facilities through coordinated effort of the organized staffs and the governing bodies of the facilities;
3. to recognize compliance with standards by issuance of certificates of accreditation;
4. to conduct programs of education and research, and publish the results thereof, which will further the other purposes of the corporation, and to accept grants, gifts, bequests, and devices in support of the purposes of the corporation; and
5. to assume such other responsibilities and to conduct such other activities as are compatible with the operation of such standard-setting, survey and accreditation programs.

Historical Review

The Joint Commission on Accreditation of Hospitals is an outgrowth of the Hospital Standardization Program established by the American College of Surgeons in 1918 to encourage the adoption of a uniform medical record format that would facilitate the accurate recording of the patient's clinical course. The American College of Surgeons recognized the need for a system of standardization that would provide a means of identifying those institutions devoted to the highest ideals of medicine.

Although the American College of Surgeons' standardization program was successful, it grew to be a financial burden on the College, and participation by other national professional organizations was solicited in order to continue the program. In 1951, an event occurred which was unique in the history of medicine: five major associations of North American medicine and hospitals jointly created an organization whose sole purpose was to encourage the voluntary attainment of uniformly high standards of institutional medical care. The founding members of the Joint Commission on Accreditation of Hospitals were the American College of Surgeons, the American College of Physicians, the American Hospital Association, the American Medical Association, and the Canadian Medical Association. The Canadian Medical Association continued its participation in the Joint Commission until 1959 when the Canadian Council on Hospital Accreditation activated its own program.

The standards developed over a period of 35 years by the American College of Surgeons were adopted by the Joint Commission, and the hospitals listed by the Hospital Standardization Program were accepted as accredited. On January 1, 1952, the Joint Commission officially began the task of reviewing hospital survey reports, of granting accreditation based upon these reports, and of carefully reviewing the standards. After the first year's experience, these standards were amended in a few details. The standards were revised six times between 1953 and 1965.

In 1965, Public Law 89-97 (Medicare) was enacted. Reference to the Joint Commission in this law represented the confidence of Congress in the ability of the health care sector to voluntarily assess the quality of care being provided. Written into the Medicare Act was the provision that the hospitals participating in that program were to maintain the level of patient care that had come to be recognized as the norm. The standards of the Joint Commission are specifically referred to in the law, and the *Conditions of Participation for Hospitals,* subsequently promulgated and published by the Social Security Administration, reflected the 1965 standards of the Joint Commission.

One result of the 1965 Medicare legislation was the provision that hospitals accredited by the Joint Commission were automatically "deemed" to be in compliance with the federal Medicare *Conditions of Participation* and, thus, deemed to be eligible for participation in Medicare. (The 1972 Amendments to the Social Security Act, Public Law 92-603, provide for "validation" surveys of JCAH-accredited hospitals. This means that, while JCAH-accredited hospitals continue to be deemed eligible for participation in Medicare, the Secretary of the Department of Health, Education, and Welfare is authorized to validate JCAH findings, either on a selective sample basis or on the basis of substantial complaint.)

Recognizing that most of the nation's hospitals are eager to achieve a level higher than a required minimum, the Board of Commissioners, in August 1966, voted "to review, reevaluate, and rewrite the hospital accreditation standards and their supplemental interpretations to attain the following two objectives:

1. To raise and strengthen the standards from their present level of minimum essential to the level of optimal achievable and to assure their suitability to the state of the art.
2. To simplify and clarify the language of standards and interpretations to remove all possible ambiguities and misunderstandings."

Consequently, the standards underwent extensive revision, resulting in the 1970 edition, called, for the first time, the *Accreditation Manual for Hospitals*. Since then, the *Accreditation Manual for Hospitals* has undergone continuous review and revision to keep abreast of the state of the art.

Development of Standards

All JCAH standards have certain characteristics: they are valid, that is, they relate to the quality of care or services provided; they are optimal, reflecting the highest state of the art; they are achievable, meaning that compliance with them has been demonstrated in an existing facility; and, compliance with them is measurable.

The development of standards is an ongoing process. A standard is established because there is an identifiable need to measure or enhance the quality of a particular aspect of care or service. Innovations in techniques, advancements in knowledge, changes in governmental regulations, or the demand by consumers for accountability can bring about the need to revise or develop standards. Cost consciousness is an integral part of the standards development process.

Input for each standard is solicited from specialty organizations and experts in the area applicable to the standards under development or revision. In addition, those governmental agencies concerned with promulgating related standards and regulations are sent draft copies of proposed or revised JCAH standards for comment. Another important source of input is the feedback surveyors receive while conducting surveys. Individual health care professionals and other health care groups are encouraged to provide input through their respective delegations to the JCAH Board of Commissioners or through direct communication with the staff of JCAH. The development, review, and revision of standards is the responsibility of the Board's Standards and Survey Procedures Committee, and the standards must be approved by the full Board of Commissioners.

The constant process of revising the hospital standards could not be realized without the contributions and participation of hundreds of professionals and countless hospital- and health-related organizations. The Joint Commission wishes to acknowledge and commend the efforts of all these individuals and groups.

Implementation of Standards

Although the standards are comprehensive and applicable to all hospitals that may properly seek accreditation, the JCAH recognizes that the methods used to meet these standards may vary with the type and size of the hospital. Hospitals may arrange to obtain or share some outside services on a contractual basis. In such circumstances, the providing agencies should either be accredited by the appropriate accrediting body of the Joint Commission or be required to maintain the level of performance detailed in applicable standards. Governmental requirements prevail when they make a greater demand than JCAH's standards.

To assist hospital personnel in understanding the standards and their application, interpretative material is provided. These interpretations are intended to make the conditions of compliance more easily recognizable. Although a hospital may fail to achieve total compliance, there must be substantial overall compliance. There is a judgmental factor in each accreditation decision, and it is recognized that complete compliance with every standard and interpretation is rarely possible. Every hospital, however, should strive to achieve the optimal goals that the standards represent. In this effort, alternative innovative procedures may be acceptable, provided the hospital can demonstrate that the desired results have been attained. Thus, these interpretations should serve as a guide for hospitals in organizing and providing efficient patient care. They are not intended to establish any type of restriction on the practice of medicine itself, but rather to allow for variations in the practices conducted by well-trained, qualified practitioners.

Although a crucial demand facing hospitals today is for effective organization and internal relationships, it is not within the province of the Joint Commission to decree the details of implementation in this area. It is a fact that hospital governing bodies are responsible for the overall conduct of the hospital in a manner consonant with the hospital's objective of delivering a high quality of patient care. A clear statement to this effect should serve to dispel any confusion and to establish a sound basis for a realistic and workable set of relationships among the governing body, the hospital administration, and the medical staff. While these internal relationships are in the process of development and adjustment, it is essential that the responsibility of the hospital's governing body be stated, that the essential role of the chief executive officer acting on behalf of the governing body be recognized, that the role of the medical staff be stated, and that conflicting lines of authority and communication be avoided.

Summary

The JCAH assumes the role of evaluator, consultant, and educator. Its function is to help hospitals identify both their strengths and weaknesses in regard to JCAH standards, and to provide guidelines for improvement through consultation and education. A request by a hospital for a survey signifies a professionally motivated, voluntary commitment to self-evaluation and self-improvement.

The voluntary approach will survive if health care providers support and comply with principles, standards, and procedures that are sufficiently detailed and comprehensive to assure all that a higher quality of care is being provided, and that deviations will be identified and addressed.

Of paramount importance to the voluntary approach, then, is the continuing examination, the appropriate revision, and the proper implementation of these standards. As a result of its responsiveness to the needs of hospitals and their patients, the JCAH remains in the forefront of those dedicated to the evaluation and improvement of the quality of health care in the United States.

Editor's Note

Throughout this *Accreditation Manual for Hospitals* reference is made to documents or standards published by other organizations. Each such reference is to a specific document at a given point in time. Subsequent editions of any materials used as a reference do not automatically become the authoritative reference of the Joint Commission until approved as such by the Board of Commissioners.

Pronouns throughout this document have been chosen to provide ease in reading and are not meant to exclude reference to the opposite sex.

Guidelines for Legal Responsibilities in Everyday Practice

Guidelines on Physician/Nurse Communications

- Question the physician who wrote the order.
- If there is still disagreement,
    1. ask the doctor to implement the order, *or*
    2. seek administrative assistance, starting with the nurse manager.
- Follow the hospital policy.

Guidelines for Charting (Kerr, 1975)*

- Chart on every line.
  Vital information squeezed between lines is an "attorney's delight."
- Record observations, *not* value judgments.
  Write what you see, hear, smell, feel, and the results of special assessments.
- Avoid basket terms.
  Always chart observations to back up your evaluation. The term "good day" has a different meaning for each nurse and is dependent on the patient. Make the reader "see" the patient and the care given in your charting.
- Make cautious but sensible judgments.
  Nurses should assume more responsibility for their statements. The word "apparently" can be relegated to history.
- Avoid biased findings
  Chart your own observations; avoid being biased by the "experts."

Source: Kerr, A. Nurses' notes "That's where the goodies are!" *Nursing 75*, February 1975, 5, 34–41.

- Be careful not to show emotions in your charting.
- Utilize common sense.
- Read the doctor's progress notes to assure continuity with your own thoughts.
- Write what you mean; punctuation can make a difference.
- Emergency Room charting
  Be brief but include all necessary information. Adequate space should be provided to chart observations, treatments, and medications. The date should include the day, month, and year.

Guidelines for Medical Records

- Know the state, federal, and JCAH requirements for medical records.
- Know your state's law in relation to patient's access to his/her record.
- Establish agency policies on how medical records are to be kept, patient's access to his/her chart, requests for information from outsiders, and confidentiality.
- Know whether nurses are protected by privileged communication in your state.
- Provide inservice to inform staff about these areas.

Guidelines for Medication

- Check the physician's orders.
- Follow the five rights—the right drug, the right dose, the right time, the right route, and the right patient.
- Know the medication you are giving.
- Provide patient teaching about the medications.
- Question doctors' orders as needed.
- Observe reactions and document in the patient's record.

Guidelines for Intensive Care and Emergency Room

- Establish clear policies and procedures for the functions of nurses, especially to cover those overlapping areas between nursing and medicine.
- Assign to work in these areas nurses who are competent and knowledgeable about intensive care and emergency room nursing.

Guidelines for Incident Reports

- Remember negligence can occur not only from actual injury but also from what the nurse did prior to and after the injury.

- Document the facts on the special incident report as well as in the patient/client record with appropriate follow-up charting.
- Review incident reports periodically for trends in the types of incidents, types of patients involved, nursing units where frequent incidents occur, or particular nurses who are always involved.
- Utilize nursing audit to identify staff needs and provide the necessary in-service.

Guidelines for the Suicidal or Homicidal Patient (Kelly, 1976)*

- Any indication that a patient or employee has suicidal tendencies should be taken seriously and reported to the appropriate person.
- Generally a patient with known suicidal inclinations should not be left alone, even for a second, unless he/she is completely protected from self-harm by restraints or confinement.
- Items that a depressed person might use for suicidal purposes should be kept away from him/her. Observations should be reported accurately on the patient's chart.
- It is important to cooperate with the police and hospital authorities guarding a patient who is accused of homicide.
- Avoid unethical discussions of a homicide case involving a patient or employee.
- Keep complete and accurate records of all facts that might have bearing on the legal aspects of the case.
- Seek immediate help for nurses who show suicidal tendencies, or for their families.

Guidelines for Nursing Research

- Establish policies to clarify the nurse's role in research.
- Utilize the ANA Guidelines on Ethical Values.
- Know the role of the hospital committee on research, usually called the Human Experimentation Committee.
- Inform participating nurses about the details of the research.
- Find out whether the research has been approved by the hospital committee.

---

*Source: Kelly, L. Y. Keeping up with your legal responsibilities. *Nursing 76*, June 1976, *6*, 81–93.

A Brief Summary on Legal Responsibilities

Guidelines for Legal Responsibility of the Staff Nurse

1. Know your own strengths and weaknesses; practice only in areas where you are competent and prepared.
2. Know the Nurse Practice Act in your state.
3. Keep current on nursing through continuing education workshops, conferences, etc.
4. THINK—about patient safety in all your actions.
5. Read and understand the policies of your hospital.
6. Be willing to work on policy and procedure committees.
7. Protect yourself with professional liability insurance.
8. Communicate effectively, both verbally and in writing.
9. Chart all pertinent observations and occurrences during your shift.
10. Explain any nursing action to the patient so that he/she understands.
11. Inform the patient of his/her rights.
12. Utilize the nursing process.

Guidelines for Legal Responsibility of the Nurse Manager

1. Establish good interpersonal communication with staff, and follow through.
2. Adequate staffing.
3. Assign competent staff. Be aware of staff members' strengths and weaknessess in order to assign them to appropriate floors and patients. Look at their past performance as well as to license and certification.
4. Have written nursing policies and procedures which are continually revised. Policies and procedures can be subpoenaed in court, and

without them the hospital administration can be found negligent (Perry, 1978).*

5. Staff development and continuing education must be encouraged on all aspects of practice. Professional obsolescence occurs in nursing at 2.5 to 5 years after graduation unless education is updated (Creighton, 1975).** Just attending workshops is not enough; the knowledge must be applied in nursing practice.

6. Personnel policies and performance descriptions are important as they serve as evidence that the nurse manager is taking reasonable precautions to provide a competent staff.

7. Nursing rounds to identify potential and real problems.

8. Learn to recognize the suit-prone patient; alert staff and discuss how to deal with such a patient.

9. Make sure the working environment is safe.

10. Have adequate equipment and supplies.

---

*Source: Perry, S. Managing to avoid malpractice, part II. *Journal of Nursing Administration*, September 1978, *8*, 16–22.

**Source: Creighton, H. *Law every nurse should know.* Philadelphia: W. B. Saunders Co., 1975.

Statement on a Patient's Bill of Rights

1. The patient has the right to considerate and respectful care.
2. The patient has the right to obtain from his physician complete current information concerning his diagnosis, treatment, and prognosis in terms the patient can be reasonably expected to understand.
3. The patient has the right to receive from his physician information necessary to give informed consent prior to the start of any procedure and/or treatment. ... Where medically significant alternatives for care or treatment exist, or when the patient requests information concerning medical alternatives, the patient has the right to such information (and) to know the name of the person responsible for the procedures and/or treatment.
4. The patient has the right to refuse treatment to the extent permitted by law, and to be informed of the medical consequences of his action.
5. The patient has the right to every consideration of his privacy concerning his own medical care program.
6. The patient has the right to expect that all communications and records pertaining to his care should be treated as confidential.
7. The patient has the right to expect that within its capacity a hospital must make reasonable response to the request of a patient for services.
8. The patient has the right to obtain information as to any relationship of his hospital to other health care and educational institutions insofar as his care is concerned ... (and) any professional relationships among individuals, by name, who are treating him.
9. The patient has the right to be advised if the hospital proposes to engage in or perform human experimentation affecting his care or treatment ... (and) has the right to refuse to participate...
10. The patient has the right to expect reasonable continuity of care.

11. The patient has the right to examine and receive an explanation of his bill regardless of source of payment.
12. The patient has the right to know what hospital rules and regulations apply to his conduct as a patient.

Source: Reproduced, with permission, from a *Statement on a Patient's Bill of Rights*, copyright 1975, American Hospital Association.

See also Rights and Responsibilities of Patients, *1980 Accreditation Manual for Hospitals*, JCAH, 1979, pp. xiii–xvi.

Glossary

Accountability: Being answerable for one's actions.

ACT-U-AR: A self-*actu*alizing semin*ar* (also act-as-you-are, your best self), designed to help nurse managers sharpen their leadership skills and organizational effectiveness.

Agency: A business or service acting for others; a hospital, nursing home, mental health center, public health department, or other healthcare organization.

Amortize: To liquidate (a debt) by installment payments or payment into a sinking fund; to write off (capital expenditures) by prorating over a certain period of time.

Annual Budgetary Planning (ABP): An organized approach to program planning for quality patient care with cost containment through decentralized nursing responsibility for budget preparation and control.

Apperceptive Mass: The associational area of your brain; what you have to react with.

Authority: The sanction to act within a prescribed area of responsibility.

Behavioral Sciences: The sciences which study the activities of man and the lower animals by means of naturalistic observation and experimentation. They include: psychology, sociology, and social anthropology.

Budget, Capital Expenditures: The estimates of the purchase and/or carrying costs for capital acquisition; including new—as well as replacement and improvement of—equipment and buildings.

Budget, Operating: An itemized summary of probable expenses and income for a given period, including estimates of salary and nonsalary expenses, and estimates of patient and other revenues; sometimes called the "revenue and expense budget."

Case Nursing: A nursing modality using a caseload of one or more patients assigned to one RN who is responsible for their care.

Clinical Track: Career development and promotion via specialized clinical positions as contrasted with nursing management, education, and research positions.

Concept: An idea, a general understanding, thought, or notion that grows out of specific instances or occurrences.

Conceptualize: To form ideas, concepts, or theories; to perceive the broad integrative relationships of diverse elements.

Contract (for employment): A written agreement of conditions of employment between two or more parties; as between dean/faculty, hospital administrator/nursing administrator, nursing administrator/professional nursing staff.

Contract, Labor: The formalized agreement reached through collective bargaining between representatives of labor and management.

Controlling: The evaluating, measuring, and feedback function; the link between doing and planning in the management process.

Diagram: A schematic or plan; a graphic representation of relationships between parts of a whole.

Doing: The directing and implementation phase of the management process; carrying out the plans.

Element: A fundamental, essential, or irreducible constituent of a composite entity.

Function: Assigned duty or activity; specific occupation or role; thus the *management functions* are planning, doing, and controlling—the three cyclical components of the management process.

Functional Nursing: A nursing modality with division of labor according to tasks and routines; selected functions are assigned to all personnel with no one person being responsible for each patient's direct nursing care.

Gestalt: Form, figure, configuration; an integrated whole which is greater than the sum of its parts.

Goal: A specific statement of purpose; aim.

Head Nurse: The nurse manager with 24-hour responsibility on a single patient care unit for clinical nursing care, patient teaching, staff development, and unit management.

Healthcare: The process of maintaining optimal functioning of an organism with freedom from disease and abnormality; as an adjective, descriptive of those persons or agencies devoted to assisting others in maintaining or returning to a normal, healthy condition.

Human Mode: Those aspects of management, nursing, and patient care that focus on the motivation and behavior of the patients and the nursing staff, emphasizing the interpersonal skills in nursing.

Identity Group: A small number of one's peers or co-workers sharing common goals. (See also **Knee Group**.)

Job Description: A specification of the duties, conditions, and requirements of a particular job; prepared through a job analysis, usually for wage classification purposes. Sometimes performance standards are included. (See also **Performance Description;** sometimes called a Job Performance Description.)

Job Enrichment: Structuring jobs so they are more satisfying to employees.

Job Evaluation: The management technique for determining the relative worth (value) of jobs in an organization as a basis for a wage and salary classification plan.

Job Performance Description: see **Performance Description.**

Knee Group: A discussion group of three to five persons seated in a circle of chairs pulled together so closely that the participants' knees touch. (See also **Identity Group.**)

Leader: One who has followers; one who guides or directs the activities of others.

Leadership: Using human mode skills in guiding and directing the activities of others.

Major Job Segments: The responsibilities and duties required of an employee to get the work done and meet objectives.

Management: The process of accomplishing results through the creative use of people's talents.

Management by Objectives (MBO): A results-oriented philosophy and system of managing, using mutually established objectives, target dates, and evaluation of performance. (See also **Nursing Objectives.**)

Management Functions: Planning (including organizing), doing (directing, implementing), and controlling. See also **Function.**

Management Track: Career development and promotion via administrative and nurse manager roles (including those in education) as contrasted with the clinically oriented promotional opportunities.

Matrix Organization: An organic, adaptive organization structure that provides for functional interdepartmental and interdisciplinary leadership to achieve common goals. Graphically this structure appears as a grid (matrix) with hierarchical (vertical) coordination through departmentalization and the formal chain of command, and simultaneous lateral (horizontal) coordination among departments at each level.

Model: A tentative ideational structure used as a testing device; the structural relationships among the elements of a concept or system; the framework within which an idea exists; a means of communicating a concept.

Modular Nursing: A compromise between **primary nursing** and **team nursing**: a nursing unit is divided into modules (bed group areas) with an RN assigned to each module and to the same patients every day, with responsibility for the nursing process and coordinating other nursing personnel.

Motive Force: That element in the working relationship between two or more persons which determines whose plan of action is dominant; characterized by an ability to see the broad picture, a desire to change things, and a willingness to be measured by results.

Nurse Manager: A nurse whose regular performance responsibilities include the management of personnel and patient care. (See Chapter 1.)

Nursing Audit: A method (as part of a quality assurance program) for assuring documentation of the quality of nursing care in keeping with the standards of the agency, the nursing department, and the professional, governmental, and accrediting groups.

Nursing by Objectives (NBO): A results-oriented philosophy and system of managing a department of nursing using mutually established objectives, target dates for completion, and evaluation of performance.

Nursing Care: Delivery of direct care to patients.

Nursing Modality: The persistence of a general pattern among the nursing staff for delivering nursing care.

Nursing Process: The four cyclical steps of sizing up the patient's needs and problems (*assessing*), deciding what to do (*planning*), securing action (*implementing*), and seeing if the action helped with the needs and problems (*evaluating*).

Nursing Services: Delivery of direct care to patients plus those elements of nursing done on behalf of the patients but not necessarily in their presence.

Objective: A specific task-oriented statement of results to be achieved to accomplish a goal.

Objectives, Jointly Developed: Objectives mutually prepared by the nursing employee with the nurse manager of that person.

Organizational Development (OD): A process of creating a climate for organizational change and growth through the development and effective utilization of nursing personnel and other resources.

Patient Care Coordinator: The nurse manager who provides 24-hour administrative leadership for two or more patient care units.

Patient Classification: A system for identifying the nursing care needs of patients by categories.

Performance Appraisal: See **Performance Evaluation.**

Performance Description: A statement of the *purpose* of a job, the major performance *responsibilities* (grouped by the persons *to whom* the responsibilities exist), and *measures* of satisfactory performance. (See also **Job Description.**)

Performance Evaluation: The regular review and appraisal of personnel performance. (See also **Results-Oriented Performance Evaluation Program— ROPEP.**)

Philosophy: Those beliefs, principles, and values that serve as a basis for action and behavior.

Planning: Thinking ahead, determining what shall be done; the phase of the management process that includes organizing, establishing objectives, defining problems and opportunities, setting goals, and developing strategy and tactics for actions.

Primary Care: That care provided to healthcare consumers as they enter the community healthcare system, via the physician, family nurse practitioner, clinic, emergency room, home health agency, etc. (Not to be confused with **Primary Nursing.**) See also **Secondary** and **Tertiary Care.**

Primary Nurse: The RN who is accountable for a small caseload of patients from admission through discharge in a hospital setting in which primary nursing is the basic modality of care.

Primary Nursing: A nursing modality with one RN assigned and accountable for a small caseload of individual patients from their admission to discharge, permitting a one-to-one patient-nurse relationship (with the focus on the nursing process) and a problem-solving approach based on the patient's needs and problems. (Not to be confused with **Primary Care.**)

Problem-Oriented Nursing System (PONS): A process for assessing, planning, implementing, and evaluating patient care based on identified principles of nursing practice; involving the systematic recording of each patient's data base and identified problems; with an initial plan of care, progress notes, and discharge planning keyed to the problem list; and supported by a quality assurance program with inservice and continuing education as relevant.

Professional: A person with the knowledge, skills, experience, confidence, flexibility, and performance results that lead to recognition for a line of work.

Program Performance Plan (PPP): A long-range schedule of the interrelated steps required to effect a desired result, objective, or goal.

Quality Assurance Program (QAP): A planned approach to aid each healthcare agency in meeting patient care goals through compliance with the standards established by the accrediting agencies and professional groups.

Responsibility: A duty or activity a person is expected to perform; that for which a person is held accountable.

Results-Oriented Performance Evaluation Program (ROPEP): A method of establishing and implementing a performance appraisal plan for nursing personnel based on performance descriptions with measurable standards of quality and quantity.

Schedule: A timetable or production plan; in nursing management, it usually refers to the time sheets (or cyclical schedule) showing planned work days for personnel.

Scheduling: To plan or appoint for a certain time or date; to make up and enter on a schedule (time sheet).

Scientific Management: A type of management based on measurement plus control; the term was selected by Frederick Winslow Taylor ("the father of scientific management") and his colleagues in the early years of the twentieth century.

Secondary Care: That more specialized medical care provided to healthcare consumers in an acute care general hospital or similar facility, usually following **Primary Care** services.

Skill: Proficiency in a way of doing something using one's hands, body, and brain.

Staffing: To provide with a staff of employees.

Standard: An acknowledged measure of comparison for quantitative or qualitative value; criterion, norm.

Standards of Care: Clearly defined measures of comfort, techniques, clinical observation, perception, interpretation, and judgments used in initiating nursing actions and evaluating therapeutic results.

Standards of Performance: Written statements that define and provide a measure of how well employees are expected to carry out their responsibilities and meet their objectives.

Standards of Service: Clearly defined measures for the planning and managing of nursing care, staffing the units, making work assignments, keeping records, implementing policies and procedures, and maintaining interpersonal relations.

System: A group of interrelated elements forming a collective entity.

Target Date: The date by which an objective is to be achieved.

Team Nursing: A nursing modality with an RN serving as team leader for a group of nursing personnel working together to provide care to assigned patients; focus is on involving all personnel in group process, seeking best individual and combined efforts.

Technical Mode: Those aspects of management, nursing, and patient care that are dependent largely on treatments, systems, and procedures of a technical nature.

Technique: A design for an action plan, procedure, or program to assist the nurse manager perform one or more management functions.

Theory: Systematically organized knowledge applicable in a relatively wide variety of circumstances; especially a system of assumptions, accepted principles, and rules of procedure devised to analyze, predict, or otherwise explain the nature or behavior of a specified set of phenomena.

Third-Party Intervention: Use of a specific technique by a non-involved, objective, skillful third person to facilitate problem resolution by the two persons who own the problem.

Tertiary Care: That care offered by highly specialized providers, as in intensive-type care units of regional medical centers. Sometimes used to denote longer-term skilled care facilities and nursing homes.

Time Sheet: The planned personnel work schedule, and/or the record of days and hours worked.

Total Nursing: A nursing modality in which an RN is responsible for delivering all aspects of patient care on a single shift; used widely in intensive care units (CCU, ICU, SICU, PICU, NNICU).

Transactional Analysis in Problem Solving (TAPS): A model for effective problem solving and decision making based upon the study of ego states exhibited by human beings.

Unit Cluster: The grouping of like units by type of service (or related characteristics) for purposes of optimum patient care, staffing, scheduling, and budgetary planning and control.

Wide-Track Careers in Nursing (WTC): A viable system for providing selective career options on the clinical, management, education, and research tracks, using agency-developed criteria for continuing education opportunities and the related qualifying procedures; a vital adjunct to ROPEP.

Index

457

About the Authors

WARREN AND JOAN GANONG are a husband and wife healthcare management counseling team. They are president and vice-president of Ganong Healthcare Management Consultants and The Nursing Management Institute. Their consulting, workshop, and facilitating work takes them into practically every area of the healthcare industry. Their clients include general hospitals and medical centers, state and county agencies, VA hospitals, mental health clinics, longterm nursing and skilled care facilities, university and hospital schools of nursing, and other educational centers.

Joan began her career as a psychiatric aide, then became interested in nursing and received her diploma from St. Luke's Hospital School of Nursing, New York City. She studied at Hunter College for her B.S. in Education, and at the University of Maryland for her M.S. in Nursing. Presently she is a doctoral candidate in psychological counseling, Fielding Institute, Santa Barbara, California. Joan has held positions at every job level in nursing service and nursing education in hospitals such as St. Luke's in New York City, Johns Hopkins and Union Memorial in Baltimore, Maryland, and Presbyterian-University in Pittsburgh, Pennsylvania. She is an adjunct assistant professor in continuing education at the University of North Carolina School of Nursing in Chapel Hill. She also serves on the faculty of the University of Minnesota Independent Study Program in Patient Care administration.

Warren's background is in management engineering, labor relations, and organizational development—with a quarter century of consulting experience for healthcare agencies. His B.S. in Industrial Engineering is from Northeastern University, with graduate work at M.I.T. He is a certified management consultant, president of the North Carolina Chapter of the Institute of Management Consultants, and a member of the board of directors of the parent certifying organization, IMC. He has served in the past as president of the Association of Management Consultants, the Pittsburgh Management Consultants Association, and the Pittsburgh Chapter of the Society for Advancement of Management (now part of the American Management Associations, Inc.).

Joan and Warren teach extensively in university, school, business, and on-the-job settings. In their consulting work, the Ganongs place emphasis on helping personnel of client organizations to help themselves staff development in newer concepts, methods, techniques, and skills. Known as "the people people," they have written extensively in their fields. They publish the *HELP Series of Management Guides* and are the authors of *Cases in Nursing Management* (Aspen, 1979) and Nursing Job Performance Evaluation (T) (Aspen, 1980, manuscript in preparation).